Peripheral Vascular Disease

Editors

PRAKASH KRISHNAN
TYRONE COLLINS

INTERVENTIONAL CARDIOLOGY CLINICS

www.interventional.theclinics.com

Consulting Editors
SAMIN K. SHARMA
IGOR F. PALACIOS

October 2014 • Volume 3 • Number 4

ELSEVIER

1600 John F. Kennedy Boulevard • Suite 1800 • Philadelphia, Pennsylvania, 19103-2899

http://www.theclinics.com

INTERVENTIONAL CARDIOLOGY CLINICS Volume 3, Number 4
October 2014 ISSN 2211-7458, ISBN-13: 978-0-323-32616-2

Editor: Adrianne Brigido
Developmental Editor: Barbara Cohen-Kligerman

Interventional Cardiology Clinics (ISSN 2211-7458) is published quarterly by Elsevier Inc., 360 Park Avenue South, New York, NY 10010-1710. Months of issue are January, April, July, and October. Subscription prices are USD 195 per year for US individuals, USD 305 for US institutions, USD 130 per year for US students, USD 230 per year for Canadian individuals, USD 375 for Canadian institutions, USD 150 per year for Canadian students, USD 295 per year for international individuals, USD 375 for international institutions, and USD 150 per year for international students. To receive student/resident rate, orders must be accompanied by name of affiliated institution, date of term, and the *signature* of program/residency coordinator on institution letterhead. Orders will be billed at individual rate until proof of status is received. Foreign air speed delivery is included in all *Clinics* subscription prices. All prices are subject to change without notice. **POSTMASTER:** Send address changes to *Interventional Cardiology Clinics*, Elsevier Health Sciences Division, Subscription Customer Service, 3251 Riverport Lane, Maryland Heights, MO 63043. **Customer Service: Telephone: 1-800-654-2452** (U.S. and Canada); **1-314-447-8871** (outside U.S. and Canada). **Fax: 1-314-447-8029. E-mail: journalscustomerservice-usa@elsevier.com** (for print support); **journalsonlinesupport-usa@elsevier.com** (for online support).

Reprints. For copies of 100 or more of articles in this publication, please contact the Commercial Reprints Department, Elsevier Inc., 360 Park Avenue South, New York, NY 10010-1710. Tel.: 212-633-3874; Fax: 212-633-3820; E-mail: reprints@elsevier.com.

Contributors

CONSULTING EDITORS

SAMIN K. SHARMA, MD, FSCAI, FACC
Director of Clinical Cardiology; Director of Cardiac Catheterization Laboratory, Mount Sinai Medical Center, New York, New York

IGOR F. PALACIOS, MD, FSCAI
Director of Interventional Cardiology, Cardiology Division, Heart Center, Massachusetts General Hospital; Associate Professor of Medicine, Harvard Medical School, Boston, Massachusetts

EDITORS

PRAKASH KRISHNAN, MD, FACC
Director of Endovascular Services, Cardiac Catheterization Laboratory; Assistant Director of Mount Sinai Heart Network, Mount Sinai Heart; Assistant Professor of Medicine, Mount Sinai School of Medicine, New York, New York

TYRONE COLLINS, MD, FACC
John Ochsner Heart and Vascular Institute, Ochsner Medical Center, New Orleans, Louisiana

AUTHORS

ANVAR BABAEV, MD, PhD
Division of Cardiology, New York University Langone Medical Center, New York, New York

JAMES F. BENENATI, MD
Medical Director, Noninvasive Vascular Laboratory, Miami Cardiac and Vascular Institute, Miami, Florida; Clinical Associate Professor of Radiology, University of South Florida College of Medicine, Tampa, Florida

MARCIN BUJAK, MD, PhD
Section of Cardiovascular Medicine, Department of Internal Medicine, Yale University School of Medicine, New Haven, Connecticut

IAN DEL CONDE, MD
Cardiology and Vascular Medicine, Miami Cardiac and Vascular Institute, Miami, Florida; Clinical Associate Professor of Radiology, University of South Florida College of Medicine, Tampa, Florida

LARRY J. DIAZ-SANDOVAL, MD
Department of Clinical Research, College of Osteopathic Medicine, Michigan State University; Department of Medicine, Metro Health Hospital, Wyoming, Michigan

PHILLIP A. ERWIN, MD, PhD
Interventional Cardiology Fellow, Department of Cardiovascular Medicine, Heart and Vascular Institute, Cleveland Clinic, Cleveland, Ohio

JACQUELINE GAMBERDELLA, MS
Section of Cardiovascular Medicine, Department of Internal Medicine, Yale University School of Medicine, New Haven, Connecticut

WILLIAM A. GRAY, MD, FACC
Associate Professor of Clinical Medicine; Director of Endovascular Services, Department of Medicine, Columbia University Medical Center, NY Presbyterian Hospital, New York, New York

KARTHIK GUJJA, MD, MPH
The Zena and Michael A. Wiener Cardiovascular Institute, The Mount Sinai School of Medicine, New York, New York

JULIAN J. JAVIER, MD, FACC, FSCAI, FCCP
Naples Vein Center, Naples, Florida

VISHAL KAPUR, MD, FACC
Assistant Professor of Clinical Medicine, Department of Medicine, Icahn School of Medicine, Mount Sinai Medical Center, New York, New York

PRAKASH KRISHNAN, MD, FACC
Director of Endovascular Services, Cardiac Catheterization Laboratory; Assistant Director of Mount Sinai Heart Network, Mount Sinai Heart; Assistant Professor of Medicine, Mount Sinai School of Medicine, New York, New York

DAVID W. LEE, MD
Division of Cardiology, New York University Langone Medical Center, New York, New York

JUN LI, MD
Clinical and Research Fellow, Department of Medicine, Case Western Reserve University School of Medicine; Division of Cardiovascular Medicine, Harrington Heart and Vascular Institute, University Hospitals Case Medical Center, Cleveland, Ohio

CARLOS MENA, MD
Section of Cardiovascular Medicine, Department of Internal Medicine, Yale University School of Medicine, New Haven, Connecticut

D. CHRISTOPHER METZGER, MD
Wellmont CVA Heart Institute, Kingsport, Tennessee

J.A. MUSTAPHA, MD
Department of Clinical Research, College of Osteopathic Medicine, Michigan State University; Department of Medicine, Metro Health Hospital, Wyoming, Michigan

SAHIL A. PARIKH, MD, FACC, FSCAI
Assistant Professor, Division of Cardiovascular Medicine, Harrington Heart and Vascular Institute, University Hospitals Case Medical Center; Director, Interventional Cardiology Fellowship Program; Director, Experimental Interventional Cardiology Laboratory; Assistant Professor, Department of Medicine, Case Western Reserve University School of Medicine, Cleveland, Ohio

BHASKAR PURUSHOTTAM, MD
The Zena and Michael A. Wiener Cardiovascular Institute, Mount Sinai School of Medicine, New York, New York

ANITHA RAJAMANICKAM, MD
Department of Interventional Cardiology, The Zena and Michael A. Wiener Cardiovascular Institute, Mount Sinai School of Medicine, New York, New York

LOUAI RAZZOUK, MD
Division of Cardiology, New York University Langone Medical Center, New York, New York

MEHDI H. SHISHEHBOR, DO, MPH, PhD
Director of Endovascular Services; Associate Program Director, Interventional Cardiology, Department of Cardiovascular Medicine, Heart and Vascular Institute, Cleveland Clinic, Cleveland, Ohio

JOSE WILEY, MD, FACC, FACP, FSCAI
Assistant Professor of Medicine-Cardiology and Radiology; Associate Director of Endovascular Interventions, The Zena and Michael A. Wiener Cardiovascular Institute, The Mount Sinai School of Medicine, New York, New York

ADRIAN ZALEWSKI, BSc
The Zena and Michael A. Wiener Cardiovascular Institute, Mount Sinai School of Medicine, New York, New York

Contents

INTERVENTIONAL CARDIOLOGY CLINICS

FORTHCOMING ISSUES

January 2015
Transcatheter Aortic Valve Replacement
Susheel Kodali, *Editor*

April 2015
Transradial Angiography and Intervention
Sunil Rao, *Editor*

July 2015
Optical Coherence Tomography
Matthew Price, *Editor*

RECENT ISSUES

July 2014
Renal Complications in the Catheterization Laboratory
Hitinder S. Gurm, Judith Kooiman, *Editors*

April 2014
Approaches to Left Atrial Appendage Exclusion
Randall Lee and Moussa C. Mansour, *Editors*

January 2014
Carotid and Cerebrovascular Disease
Christopher J. White and Kenneth Rosenfield, *Editors*

ISSUES OF RELATED INTEREST

Cardiology Clinics, November 2014 (Vol. 31, No. 4)
Cardiovascular Intensive Care
Umesh K. Gidwani, Samin K. Sharma, and Annapoorna Kini, *Editors*
Available at: http://www.cardiology.theclinics.com/

Preface
Peripheral Artery Disease

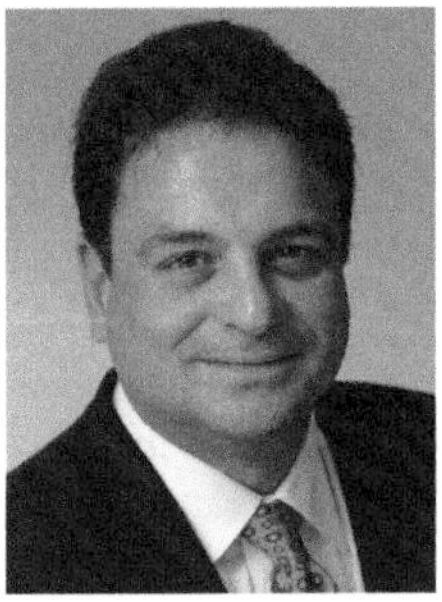
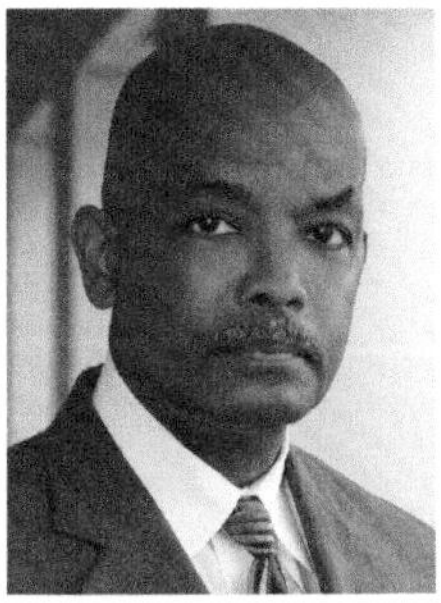

Prakash Krishnan, MD, FACC   Tyrone Collins, MD, FACC
Editors

Peripheral artery disease (PAD) is a very common condition affecting 12 to 20% of Americans age 65 and older. It occurs mostly in people older than 50 years and is a leading cause of disability among this population and in those with diabetes. PAD affects both men and women equally and the prevalence is higher among African Americans compared with non-Hispanic whites. Peripheral venous disease (PVD) is a significant public health problem with an estimated prevalence of varicose veins ranging from 7 to 60%, and the number of deep venous thrombosis/pulmonary embolisms is estimated at 300,000 to 600,000 each year in the adult population. The significant morbidity and mortality associated with PAD and PVD makes this disease state an important public health problem. The overlap of PAD and PVD with coronary artery disease has led interventional cardiologists to be more involved in the care of these patients.

The growth of endovascular techniques in the management of PAD has led to the increased nonsurgical treatment of the disease. The lack of formalized training and consensus among specialties has led to a wide variance on the approach to and treatment of PAD in various vascular beds. This issue of *Interventional Cardiology Clinics* provides the reader with evidence-based guidance as well as education about the fundamentals of treating patients with PAD and PVD.

The authors of the ensuing articles are experts and leaders in the field of vascular medicine and endovascular intervention. The text is written with an eye toward everyday PAD practice. The most up-to-date evidence-based approach and widely accepted interventional techniques are discussed to provide the reader a detailed overview of the screening, diagnosis, and treatment of PAD. The issue includes history and physical diagnosis as well as the use of noninvasive modalities to confirm the diagnosis and aid in the treatment of PAD. We have also focused articles on specific vascular beds, such as brachiocephalic, mesenteric, renal, and superficial femoral artery disease. Complex clinical presentations such as acute limb ischemia and critical limb ischemia as well as common venous conditions such as superficial venous insufficiency and deep venous disease have been included to make this issue of *Interventional Cardiology Clinics* a most comprehensive overview.

We would like to thank the authors for contributing their time, effort, and expertise to complete this issue of *Interventional Cardiology Clinics*.

We would also like to thank Dr Samin Sharma and Dr Igor Palacios for recognizing the adverse impact of PAD/PVD in cardiovascular patients and the importance of educating the interventional

Intervent Cardiol Clin 3 (2014) ix–x
http://dx.doi.org/10.1016/j.iccl.2014.07.006

cardiology community on its prevalence, diagnosis, and available treatment modalities.

Prakash Krishnan, MD, FACC
Department of Interventional Cardiology
The Zena and Michael A. Wiener Cardiovascular Institute
Mount Sinai Heart
Marie-Josée and Henry R. Kravis Center for Cardiovascular Health
Mount Sinai Medical Center
Mount Sinai School of Medicine
1 Gustave L. Levy Place, Box 1030
New York, NY 10029, USA

Tyrone Collins, MD, FACC
John Ochsner Heart and Vascular Institute
Ochsner Medical Center
1514 Jefferson Highway
New Orleans, LA 70121, USA

E-mail addresses:
prakash.krishnan@mountsinai.org (P. Krishnan)
tcollins@ochsner.org (T. Collins)

History and Physical Examination in Diagnosis of Peripheral Artery Disease

Anitha Rajamanickam, MD, Prakash Krishnan, MD*

KEYWORDS

• PAD • Physical exam • Diagnosis

KEY POINTS

- Peripheral artery disease (PAD), a disease of the arteries of the extremities caused by artery obstruction, may be silent or present with an assortment of symptoms and signs suggesting peripheral artery ischemia.
- Peripheral vascular disease includes PAD and disorders of the peripheral venous system and lymphatic system.
- Generally, PAD is synonymous with arteries of the limbs and pelvis, but it can be expanded to include the renal arteries, carotid arteries, mesenteric arteries, and the aorta.
- It is imperative to recognize and treat PAD early, as appropriate management of PAD can help avoid devastating complications such as limb amputation and death.

INTRODUCTION

Peripheral artery disease (PAD), defined as obstructive disease of the arteries of the extremities, may be silent or present with an assortment of signs and symptoms suggesting peripheral artery ischemia. In patients presenting with PAD in 1 vascular territory, 35% had disease in another territory, and 50% had cerebrovascular or coronary heart disease[1] and 3% had nonfatal myocardial infarction rate.[1] Both asymptomatic PAD and symptomatic PAD are independent risk factors for increased mortality.[2] The worldwide prevalence of PAD is between 3% and 12%. It is imperative to recognize and treat PAD early to avoid devastating complications like limb amputation and death. Peripheral vascular disease (PVD) includes PAD and disorders of the peripheral venous system (PeVD) and lymphatic system. Generally, PAD is synonymous with arteries of the limbs and pelvis but can be expanded to include the renal arteries, carotid arteries, mesenteric arteries, and the aorta (which are discussed in detail in elsewhere in this issue of *Interventional Cardiology Clinics*).

PATIENTS AT RISK FOR PAD

The most common etiology is atherosclerosis (collection of lipid fibrous material with or without calcification between the intima and media of large and medium-sized arteries causing focal or diffuse obstruction), although other disease processes like inflammatory, immune, and hypercoagulable disorders can cause signs and symptoms of arterial insufficiency. A multidisciplinary approach involving the primary care provider, podiatrist, vascular interventionalist, and/or vascular surgeon and plastic surgeon is ideal for the comprehensive care of the PAD patients. A thorough history and physical examination are important for identifying PAD, which is a very treatable condition. When

The authors have nothing to disclose.
Department of Interventional Cardiology, Zena and Michael A. Weiner Cardiovascular Institute, Mount Sinai School of Medicine, 1 Gustave L. Levy Place, Box 1030, New York, NY 10029, USA
* Corresponding author.
E-mail address: prakash.krishnan@mountsinai.org

Intervent Cardiol Clin 3 (2014) 461–467
http://dx.doi.org/10.1016/j.iccl.2014.06.007
2211-7458/14/$ – see front matter

recognized early and appropriately managed, complications that lead to limb loss can be minimized. All patients should have a comprehensive history taken and be examined for PAD, but patients with the risk factors shown in **Box 1** should be specifically examined for PAD.

SYMPTOMS

Symptoms of PAD depend upon the location and severity of stenosis and can be completely absent or range from mild extremity pain with moderate-to-severe exertion to limb- or life-threatening ischemia. Asymptomatic PAD usually is benign; however, the disease can progress rapidly, especially in smokers, hypertensive patients, diabetics, and patients with hyperlipidemia or chronic kidney disease.[4]

Claudication

The patient may complain of fatigue, aching, numbness, weakness, or heaviness in muscles, or pain of lower extremities with exertion. The primary and secondary sites of discomfort in the buttock, thigh, calf, or foot should be recorded, as well as the amount of exertion. Claudication strongly suggests PAD.

Box 1
Risk factors for peripheral artery disease

Age[3]

- Age ≥70 years
- Age 50–69 years with a history of smoking or diabetes
- Age 40–49 with diabetes and at least 1 other risk factor for atherosclerosis

Race: African Americans (men and women) and Hispanic American women[2,4]

Family history of a first-order relative with an abdominal aortic aneurysm or PAD

Smoking: most powerful risk predictor of PAD[5,6]

Coronary artery disease

Carotid artery disease

Renal artery disease

Diabetes and impaired glucose tolerance[5,6,8]

Hypertension[5,6]

Hyperlipidemia[5,6]

Hyperhomocysteinemia[6]

Metabolic syndrome

Chronic kidney disease, especially end-stage renal disease[5,7]

Elevated C-reactive protein

Leriche syndrome

Cardiac arrhythmias

Hypercoagulable states

Rest Pain

Any pain of the extremities at rest and its association with the upright or recumbent positions should be carefully evaluated. Ischemic rest pain is suspected if pain at rest occurs in the foot, toes, or instep and is aggravated by extremity elevation and improved by a dependent position. Almost always, ischemic rest pain worsens with leg exercise. Usually it does not present as nocturnal pain or cramps, but sometimes the pain is worse at night and relieved by sleeping in a chair with legs in a dependent position. Rest pain strongly suggests PAD.

Ulcers

Ulcers are any poorly healing or nonhealing wounds of the legs or feet. These can be caused by PAD or PVeD.

Complaints of Skin Changes

Thin, shiny, and brittle skin; thick opaque nails; hair loss on legs; and bluish/black discoloration of the extremities may be caused by PVeD or PAD.

Impotence

Severe symptomatic bilateral aortoiliac PAD almost always causes erectile dysfunction in men. Leriche syndrome is the triad of claudication, absent or diminished femoral pulses, and erectile dysfunction.

Other Symptoms

Edema of the symptomatic extremity may be caused by PAD, PVeD, or lymphatic disorders.

Complaints of paleness on leg elevation are suggestive of PAD.

Pain, tenderness, redness, and warmth in the extremities are suggestive of deep vein thrombosis (DVT) or thrombophlebitis.

Discoloration of the skin and ankles, swelling of the legs, and feelings of dull aching pain, heaviness, or cramping in the extremities may suggest venous insufficiency.

DIFFERENTIAL DIAGNOSIS OF CLAUDICATION

The Edinburgh Claudication Questionnaire has 91% specificity and 99% sensitivity for diagnosing PAD in symptomatic patients.[6] If the patient has pain when walking either in the calves (typical claudication) or in the thigh/buttock (defined as atypical claudication in the absence of calf pain) that increases with walking uphill or faster, the symptoms are 99.3% sensitive but only 13% specific for a diagnosis of PAD. If the patient also has relief with rest or standing (within 10 minutes), the specificity increases to 80%.[9] Multiple conditions mimic the symptoms of claudication (**Table 1**).

Buttock and Hip Claudication

This is seen in aortoiliac disease. The pain is aching in nature, presents immediately with or without weakness of the hip or thigh on walking, and subsides immediately with rest. Pulses in one or both groins are diminished, and males may present with impotence.

Thigh Claudication

PAD of the common femoral artery may cause claudication in the thigh, calf, or both. If the disease is isolated to the superficial femoral or popliteal arteries, the patients will have decreased distal pulses but normal femoral pulses.

Calf Claudication

This is the most common presentation. Claudication in the upper two-thirds of the calf is usually caused by superficial femoral PAD; in the lower third of the calf, it is usually caused by popliteal PAD. It presents as an increasingly aching pain that is consistently reproduced with exercise and quickly relieved with rest.

Foot Claudication

Isolated foot claudication is uncommon and represents PAD of the tibial and peroneal vessels.

CLASSIFICATION OF PAD BY SYMPTOMS

The Rutherford classification is the most commonly used classification and consists of 4 grades (**Box 2**).[11] The Fontaine classification is less commonly used (**Box 3**).[12–14]

PHYSICAL EXAMINATION

Ideally the patient should exposed from the waist down, but it is important to remove socks and shoes.

Skin

Inspect lower extremities and intertriginous areas for the following

- Color—may be black from hemostasis or brown from hemosiderin deposition. Acute limb ischemia presents as a white limb (extreme pallor) especially when compared with the other limb
- Trophic skin changes—thin, atrophic skin on the foot and lower extremity that shows pallor with elevation and rubor (redness) with dependency of the foot suggestive of ischemic PAD. Distal hair loss and hypertrophic nails are also seen with PAD
- Skin integrity and ulcers—these may be venous or arterial. Venous ulcers usually tend to be painless unless they have superimposed infection, whereas arterial ulcers are painful
- Scars or sites of prior ulcers
- Gangrene—wet or dry
- Varicose vein—presence of any varicose veins seen best with the patient standing upright

Palpation

Temperature

Starting distally, compare both extremities at similar levels with the back of the hand. A cool extremity suggests poor circulation and PAD.

Palpate varicose veins

If thrombophlebitis is present, veins will be hard and painful to touch.

Pitting edema

This should be tested for in dependent locations such as the dorsum of the foot and if present on the shins. If the patient has been in bed for a long period of time, the sacrum should be checked.

Pulse

Brachial, radial, ulnar, femoral, popliteal, dorsalis pedis, and posterior tibial sites should be checked. Also palpate the carotid and abdomen for aorta.

Pulse intensity should be assessed and recorded numerically as shown in **Box 4**.

For the carotid pulses, note the carotid upstroke and amplitude.

For the abdomen aorta, palpate just to the left of the midline in the epigastrium; make note of the presence of aortic pulsation, its maximal diameter, and whether it is expansile (suggests an aneurysm).

Examination for Arterial pulses

Dorsalis pedis artery pulse—on dorsal surface of the foot, running lateral to the extensor tendon of the first toe

Posterior tibial artery pulse—posterior and inferior to the medial malleolus of the tibia

Popliteal artery pulse—behind the knee in the posterior popliteal, typically done with both hands after flexing the knee of the patient to 45° while keeping the foot on the bed

Table 1
Differential diagnosis of PAD

Differential Diagnosis[10]	Main Location of Pain	Radiation of Pain	Characteristic of Pain	Exacerbating Factors	Relieving Factors
Arthritis of hip	Hip	Thigh Gluteal areas	Aching pain that is usually worse in the morning or upon waking up and depending on activity level or weather changes	Exercise (immediate)	Rest or sitting (slow relief)
Nerve compression	Hip	Down 1 leg Gluteal areas Lower Back	Sharp and stabbing Prior history of spine disorders	Exercise (immediate)	Rest or changing position (slow relief)
Spinal stenosis	Hip	Thigh Gluteal areas Lower Back	Sharp and may be accompanied by weakness Prior history of spine disorders	Exercise (after a period of time)	Rest or changing position (slow relief)
Venous claudication	Thigh	Entire leg Groin	Tight, throbbing aching pain Edema, visibly dilated veins, skin changes, lipodermatosclerosis and ulceration Numbness and tingling may be present	Standing or sitting with the feet in dependent position for prolonged periods	Walking and elevation of extremities (quick relief)
Arthritis of knee	Calf		Aching pain that is usually worse in the morning or upon waking up and depends on activity level or weather changes	Exercise (immediate)	Rest or sitting (slow relief)
Chronic compartment syndrome	Calf	Usually tenderness and pain is limited to anterior compartment	Pain is aching, squeezing, cramping or tight; seen in athletes, with bulky, well-developed calf muscles, with chronic exercise; presents commonly as bilateral pain	Exercise [gradually increasing pain often at a precise point during training]	Rest causes slow (10–20 min) but complete relief of pain, but elevation may provide quicker relief
Baker cyst	Thigh	Posterior knee pain	Pain is constant Swelling or a mass behind the knee	Exercise and prolonged standing and with hyperflexion of the knee	No relief with rest
Arthritis of foot	Foot and arch		Aching pain that is usually worse in the morning or upon waking up and depending on activity level or weather changes	Exercise	Improves with not bearing weight

Box 2
Rutherford classification of peripheral artery disease

Grade 0

- Category 0: Asymptomatic

Grade I

- Category 1: mild claudication
- Category 2: moderate claudication
- Category 3: severe claudication

Grade II

- Category 4: rest pain

Grade III

- Category 5: minor tissue loss not exceeding ulcer of the digits of the foot
- Category 6: major tissue loss; severe ischemic ulcers or frank gangrene

From Rutherford RB, Baker JD, Ernst C, et al. Recommended standards for reports dealing with lower extremity ischemia: revised version. J Vasc Surg 1997;26(3):517.

Femoral artery pulse—in the femoral triangle at the mid inguinal point which is located halfway between superior border of the symphisis in the mid line of the body and the anterior superior iliac crest.

Auscultation

Check both femoral arteries for the presence of bruits, especially if patient has had recent cannulation of the femoral artery or vein, as bruit suggests

Box 3
Fontaine classification of peripheral artery disease

1. Stage I: asymptomatic
2. Stage II: claudication
   i. Stage IIA: claudication at a distance greater than 200 m
   ii. Stage IIB: claudication at a distance less than 200 m
3. Stage III: rest pain
4. Stage IV: necrosis and/or gangrene of the limb

From Fontaine R, Kim M, Kieny R. Die chirugische Behandlung der peripheren Durchblutungsstörungen (Surgical treatment of peripheral circulation disorders). Helv Chir Acta 1954;21(5–6):499–533 [in German].

Box 4
Pulse intensity scoring

0 = Absent

1 = Diminished

2 = Normal

3 = Bounding

arteriovenous fistulas (AVFs) or pseudoaneurysms. AVFs present as a thrill or continuous bruit at the site of catheter insertion. A pseudoaneurysm is diagnosed by the presence of a pulsatile mass with a systolic bruit over the catheter insertion site. Pseudoaneurysms usually occur within 7 days after the sheath removal.

OTHER EXAMINATIONS

Capillary Refill

Compress the nail bed fully and release it. Normal refill time suggested by return of normal color to the nail bed should be less than 2 seconds.

Buerger Test

If capillary refill is abnormal, perform this test. First note the color of the patient feet and soles. Raise the patient's feet to 45° for at least 1 minute. If pallor or whiteness of the foot and sole rapidly develops, it suggests PAD. Then place the feet over the side of the bed, and the leg may turn cyanotic or blue in color. Next check for dependency. Sit the patient upright with feet in a dependent position. In normal patients, the feet return to normal color immediately. If they turn red, suspect PAD.

Blood Pressure

Check blood pressure in both arms and legs especially for asymmetry as it helps in identification of the level of obstruction.

Ankle–Brachial Pressure Index

This may be unreliable in patients with calcified arteries in the calf (often diabetic patients) or those with extensive edema, in which case the toe–brachial pressure index (TBPI) should be performed to aid in the diagnosis.

Allen Test/Barbeau Test

These should be used when knowledge of hand perfusion is needed.

Venous Refill with Dependency (Should Be < 30 s)

The vein should bulge outward within 30 seconds of elevation for 1 minute. Superficial veins of the leg empty into deep veins, but when venous valves are incompetent, retrograde filling occurs, causing varicose veins.

The Brodie–Trendelenburg Percussion Test

Place a finger over the distal part of the vein being examined and percuss the proximal part of the vein. Incompetence of valves in that vein is suggested if impulse is felt by the finger placed at the distal end.

Brodie–Trendelenburg Test

Start with the right leg and then the left. In a supine position, empty the superficial veins from a distal-to-proximal direction with the thumb or raise the hip to 90° to empty out the veins by gravity. Then press the thumb or tie a tourniquet just tight enough to compress the superficial veins but not the deep veins over the saphenofemoral junction (located about 4 cm below and 4 cm lateral to the pubic tubercle). Ask the patient to stand up. If the leg veins refill rapidly (normally the superficial saphenous vein will fill from below within 3–5 s), then the incompetence is located below the saphenofemoral junction in the deep or communicating vein. If there has been no rapid filling in 15 to 20 seconds, release the thumb or tourniquet; if there is now sudden filling, it indicates that the communicating veins are competent, but the superficial veins are incompetent. This test can be repeated using pressure at any point along the leg to figure out the level at which the veins are incompetent. It can be done above the knee to assess the midthigh perforators and below the knee to assess the short saphenous vein and the popliteal vein.[15]

Homans Sign

Homans sign is considered positive for DVT. A quick and forceful dorsiflexion of the patient's foot at the ankle while the knee is extended causes pain in the patient's calf. This is a safe test, although a single case repot of pulmonary embolism following calf pressure during a Doppler examination raised concerns. However, as it is neither sensitive nor specific test for DVT, it has fallen out of favor.[16]

REFERENCES

1. Fowkes FG, Low LP, Tuta S, et al, AGATHA Investigators. Ankle–brachial index and extent of atherothrombosis in 8891 patients with or at risk of vascular disease: results of the international AGATHA study. Eur Heart J 2006;27(15):1861–7.
2. Diehm C, Allenberg JR, Pittrow D, et al, German Epidemiological Trial on Ankle Brachial Index Study Group. Mortality and vascular morbidity in older adults with asymptomatic versus symptomatic peripheral artery disease. Circulation 2009;120(21):2053–61. http://dx.doi.org/10.1161/CIRCULATIONAHA. 109.8656003.
3. Writing Group Members, 2005 Writing Committee Members, ACCF/AHA Task Force Members. 2011 ACCF/AHA focused update of the guideline for the management of patients with peripheral artery disease (updating the 2005 guideline): a report of the American College of Cardiology Foundation/American Heart Association Task Force on practice guidelines. Circulation 2011;124:2020–45. http://dx.doi.org/10.1161/CIR.0b013e31822e80c3.
4. Murabito JM, D'Agostino RB, Silbershatz H, et al. Intermittent claudication. A risk profile from The Framingham Heart Study. Circulation 1997;96(1):44–9.
5. Selvin E, Erlinger TP. Prevalence of and risk factors for peripheral arterial disease in the United States: results from the National Health and Nutrition Examination Survey, 1999-2000. Circulation 2004;110(6):738–43.
6. Allison MA, Cushman M, Solomon C, et al. Ethnicity and risk factors for change in the ankle–brachial index: the multi-ethnic study of atherosclerosis. J Vasc Surg 2009;50(5):1049–56. http://dx.doi.org/10.1016/j.jvs.2009.05.061.
7. Rajagopalan S, Dellegrottaglie S, Furniss AL, et al. Peripheral arterial disease in patients with end-stage renal disease: observations from the Dialysis Outcomes and Practice Patterns Study (DOPPS). Circulation 2006;114(18):1914–22.
8. Belch J, MacCuish A, Campbell I, et al, Prevention of Progression of Arterial Disease and Diabetes Study Group, Diabetes Registry Group, Royal College of Physicians Edinburgh. The Prevention Of Progression of Arterial Disease And Diabetes (POPADAD) trial: factorial randomised placebo controlled trial of aspirin and antioxidants in patients with diabetes and asymptomatic peripheral arterial disease. BMJ 2008;337: a1840. http://dx.doi.org/10.1136/bmj.a1840.
9. Leng GC, Fowkes FG. The Edinburgh claudication questionnaire: an improved version of the WHO/Rose Questionnaire for use in epidemiological surveys. J Clin Epidemiol 1992;45:1104.
10. Dormandy JA, Rutherford RB. Management of peripheral arterial disease (PAD). TASC Working Group. TransAtlantic Inter-Society Consensus (TASC). J Vasc Surg 2000;31(1 Pt 2):S1–296.
11. Fontaine R, Kim M, Kieny R. Surgical treatment of peripheral circulation disorders. Helv Chir Acta 1954;21(5–6):499–533 [in German].
12. Norgren L, Hiatt WR, Dormandy JA. Inter-Society Consensus for the Management of Peripheral

Arterial Disease (TASC II). Eur J Vasc Endovasc Surg 2007;33(Suppl 1):S1–75. http://dx.doi.org/10.1016/j.ejvs.2006.09.024.
13. Norgren L, Hiatt WR, Dormandy JA, et al, TASC II Working Group. Inter-Society Consensus for the Management of Peripheral Arterial Disease (TASC II). J Vasc Surg 2007;45(Suppl S):S5–67. http://dx.doi.org/10.1016/j.jvs.2006.12.037.
14. Norgren L, Hiatt WR, Dormandy JA. Inter-Society Consensus for the Management of Peripheral Arterial Disease. Int Angiol 2007;26(2):81–157.
15. Trendelenburg F. Über die Unterbindung der Vena saphena magna bei Unterschenkelvaricen. Burns Beitr Klin Chir 1891;7:195–210.
16. Ebell MH. Evaluation of the patient with suspected deep vein thrombosis. J Fam Pract 2001;50(2):167–71.

Noninvasive Testing in Peripheral Arterial Disease

Ian Del Conde, MD[a,b,*], James F. Benenati, MD[b,c]

KEYWORDS

• Vascular test • Peripheral arterial disease • Vascular ultrasound • Ankle-brachial index
• Pulse volume recording • CT angiography • Magnetic resonance angiography

KEY POINTS

- The first test to perform in patients suspected of having peripheral artery disease is the ankle-brachial index (ABI).
- Patients undergoing evaluation for exertional leg discomfort, and who have normal or minimally decreased ABIs at rest, should undergo exercise ABIs.
- The level of disease in the lower extremities can be inferred by segmental limb pressures and pulse volume recordings.
- CT and MR angiography are very useful imaging studies (and in many instances, are largely interchangeable) for procedure planning in symptomatic patients with peripheral arterial disease.

In addition to a thorough clinical evaluation, most patients with suspected or established peripheral arterial disease (PAD) should undergo noninvasive vascular testing for objective assessment of the disease. The information gathered from these studies not only helps confirm the diagnosis and stratify patients, but is also useful for procedure planning, the assessment of outcomes, and for patient follow-up.

Noninvasive vascular testing can be broadly classified as functional (or physiologic) studies that provide information on the hemodynamic effects of PAD, and anatomic studies that provide detailed information about the location and other physical characteristics related to PAD. The presence and extent of limb ischemia can be gauged through physiologic studies, which include the ankle-brachial index (ABI), segmental limb pressures, pulse volume recordings (PVRs), and photoplethysmography (PPG). Computed tomography angiography (CTA) and magnetic resonance angiography (MRA) provide anatomic data. Duplex ultrasonography provides anatomic information and hemodynamic information.

ANKLE-BRACHIAL INDEX

Ankle-brachial index is the ratio of the systolic blood pressure measured at the ankle to the pressure measured at the brachial artery. An ABI is reported for each leg. The ABI informs on the presence of hemodynamically significant disease from the brachial arteries (as a surrogate of the thoracic aorta) down to the tibioperoneal arteries, without providing specific information on the level of obstruction. The ABI is usually the first diagnostic test to be performed in the evaluation of patients with PAD. The test is noninvasive, quick and easy to perform, and has good reproducibility. The blood pressure is measured by assessing

The authors have nothing to disclose.
[a] Cardiology and Vascular Medicine, Miami Cardiac and Vascular Institute, 8900 North Kendall Drive, Miami, FL 33176, USA; [b] University of South Florida College of Medicine, Tampa, FL 33612, USA; [c] Miami Cardiac and Vascular Institute, 8900 North Kendall Drive, Miami, FL 33176, USA
* Corresponding author. Cardiology and Vascular Medicine, Miami Cardiac and Vascular Institute, 8900 North Kendall Drive, Miami, FL 33176.
E-mail address: land@baptisthealth.net

Intervent Cardiol Clin 3 (2014) 469–478
http://dx.doi.org/10.1016/j.iccl.2014.06.006
2211-7458/14/$ – see front matter

blood flow distal to an inflated cuff (the width of the cuff should be at least 40% of the limb circumference). The two most common methods for measuring blood pressure are using a handheld Doppler ultrasound probe to assess arterial blood flow distal to the cuff, and by oscillometry. Other methods, including pulse palpation and auscultation, or PPG, tend to be less accurate and reproducible.[1]

The bilateral brachial systolic blood pressures should be comparable; a pressure gradient between both arms greater than 15 mm Hg should alert about the possibility of innominate, subclavian, or axillary artery stenosis. The ABI of each leg should be calculated by dividing the higher of the posterior tibialis (PT) or dorsalis pedis (DP) pressure by the higher of the two brachial systolic blood pressures (**Fig. 1**). The sensitivity and specificity of the ABI for the diagnosis of PAD is approximately 72% and 96%, respectively.[1,2] ABI calculations using the lower, rather than the higher, of the DP or PT pressures results in a lower sensitivity but greater specificity for the detection of PAD. A normal ABI exists when the ratio between the ankle and brachial systolic pressures equals 1.0. Although the general consensus is that an ABI of 0.9 or less is required for the diagnosis of PAD, an ABI between 0.91 and 0.99 should be considered borderline and indicates increased cardiovascular risk (see later). An ABI of 0.4 to 0.9 reflects mild to moderate disease, whereas an ABI below 0.4 is consistent with severe PVD. The absolute ABI does not always correlate with the clinical status of the patient, and rather provides a rough index of the severity of PAD.

In addition to its value for the diagnosis of PAD, the ABI is also an independent indicator of the risk of cardiovascular events, including cardiovascular death, major coronary events, and stroke. The relationship between ABI in the *x* axis, and cardiovascular events in the *y* axis, is represented in a reverse J-shaped curve, where the lowest level of risk (normal) is from ABI 1.11 to 1.40, with increasing cardiovascular risk for ABI less than 1.10 and ABI greater than 1.40.[3]

An important pitfall of the ABI in detecting PAD is that by definition, the ABI ratio is calculated using the higher systolic pressure of the DP or PT pulses. Therefore, the more diseased artery supplying the region (or angiosome[4]) where an ischemic ulcer may be located could be missed in the ABI interpretation. For example, a patient with a nonhealing ulcer in the heel, with a brachial systolic blood pressure of 120 mm Hg, a DP systolic blood pressure of 100 mm Hg, and a PT

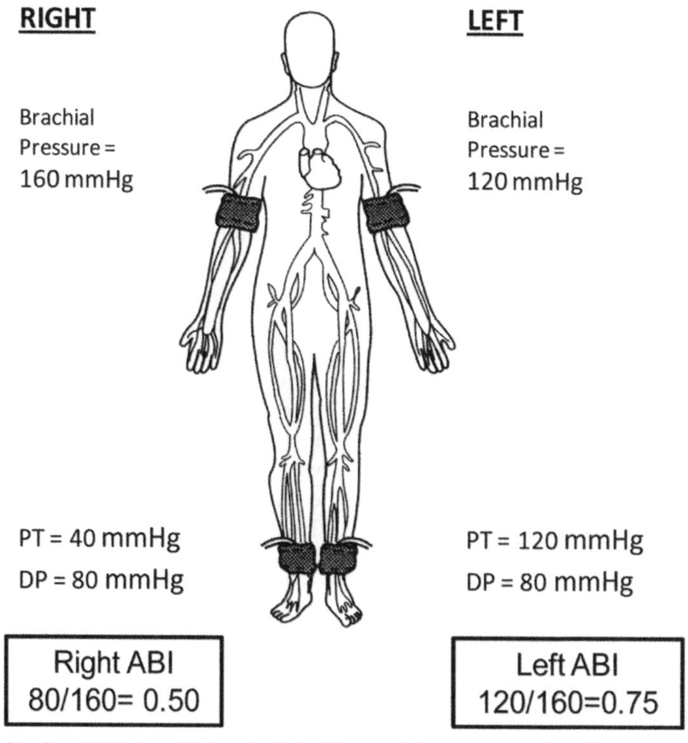

Fig. 1. Ankle-brachial index (ABI). An ABI is calculated for each lower extremity. The numerator is the ipsilateral DP or PT systolic pressure, whichever is higher. The denominator for the bilateral ABIs is the higher of the two brachial pressures.

systolic blood pressure of 40 mm Hg may be reported as having a mildly decreased ABI of 0.83, when in reality, the ABI of the artery that supplies the heel (where the ulcer is) is only 0.33. It would be an error to assume that the patient has mild PAD given the ABI of 0.83.

In the interpretation of an ABI, not only should the ratio of the two blood pressures be considered, but also the absolute ankle pressure in millimeters of mercury. This is especially important in patients presenting with limb ulceration, in which an ischemic cause is considered. Ankle pressures less than 50 mm Hg indicate severe PAD (usually multilevel disease) and suggest that an ischemic wound may not have sufficient perfusion to heal.

Abnormally High ABI

When the DP and PT arteries become heavily calcified, they may not compress normally during blood pressure cuff inflation, thereby giving an abnormally high ABI that is not reflective of the true systolic pressure at the ankle. The true ABI can therefore not be determined. Occasionally, these arteries may be noncompressible despite cuff pressures greater than 250 mm Hg, in which case the ABI cannot be calculated. Such calcification is often seen in patients with severe renal insufficiency (especially dialysis patients), medial calcinosis, or with long-standing diabetes mellitus. If such a situation is suspected or encountered, the distal limb blood pressure can be taken at the great toe using PPG, because the toe vessels rarely calcify. The ratio between the great toe and brachial systolic pressures is called the toe-brachial index. A normal toe-brachial index is considered as 0.75 or higher.

Exercise ABI

When a patient is being evaluated for leg discomfort when walking, and the ABI at rest is normal or only mildly reduced in a way that does not fully explain the patient's symptoms, the ABI should be measured after exercise. This strategy is useful in excluding disease in patients with lower extremity discomfort and "pseudoclaudication" secondary to other conditions, such as spinal stenosis. Ideally, the patient should exercise to the point of reproducing the exertional leg symptoms. Generally, most noninvasive vascular laboratories use the Gardner protocol, which is a standardized, constant-speed, constant-grade, exercise protocol used in the investigation of PAD. Patients walk on a treadmill at a 12-degree incline, a speed of 2 mph, and for at least 5 minutes or symptom-limited.[5] Other graded exercise protocols, such as the Bruce protocol, are not used because the rapid increase in speed and incline limits the assessment of exercise tolerance in claudicants. Patients who are unable to walk can be exercised with repeated pedal-plantar flexion. A decrease of at least 20 mm Hg and the ankle pressures suggest hemodynamically significant PAD. A normal postexercise ABI, or stable ankle pressures, virtually excludes PAD as the cause of the patient's claudication.

SEGMENTAL LIMB PRESSURES

Measurement of segmental blood pressures can help localize the level of occlusive disease in PAD. Blood pressure is measured at different levels of the lower extremities using adequately sized cuffs. The cuffs are placed on the thigh (either one in the upper thigh and one in the lower thigh; or just one lower thigh cuff), calf, ankle, and metatarsal region of the foot (**Fig. 2**). The blood pressure is assessed at the artery distal to the cuff using a handheld Doppler ultrasound. Oscillometric blood pressure determinations can also be used. The thigh pressure should be greater than or equal to 30 mm Hg greater than the reference arm pressure. A pressure gradient between any two adjacent levels in the lower extremities is considered normal if it is less than 20 mm Hg. A gradient greater than or equal to 30 mm Hg indicates a hemodynamically significant lesion in the segment proximal to the pressure decrease (**Table 1**). A "horizontal" pressure difference of greater than or equal to 30 mm Hg between the right and left limbs at the same level may indicate the presence of disease at or above the segment of the limb with the pressure decreased. Pressure gradients alone should not be the sole determinants for the diagnosis of significant PAD; PVRs at the same segments should also be considered (see next).

An important pitfall of segmental limb pressure assessment relates to vessel calcification and decreased compressibility, which can obscure a significant pressure gradient and result in a false negative result.

PULSE VOLUME RECORDINGS

Pulse volume recordings tracings depict changes in the volume of the limb during arterial pulsations. The cuffs are located at the same levels as for segmental limb pressures (see **Fig. 2**). Most modern systems used in segmental limb pressures also allow PVRs. The cuffs are inflated to approximately 60 to 65 mm Hg. A normal PVR waveform is similar to the waveform seen with intra-arterial blood pressure tracings, and consists of a rapid systolic upstroke, a rapid initial downstroke, a

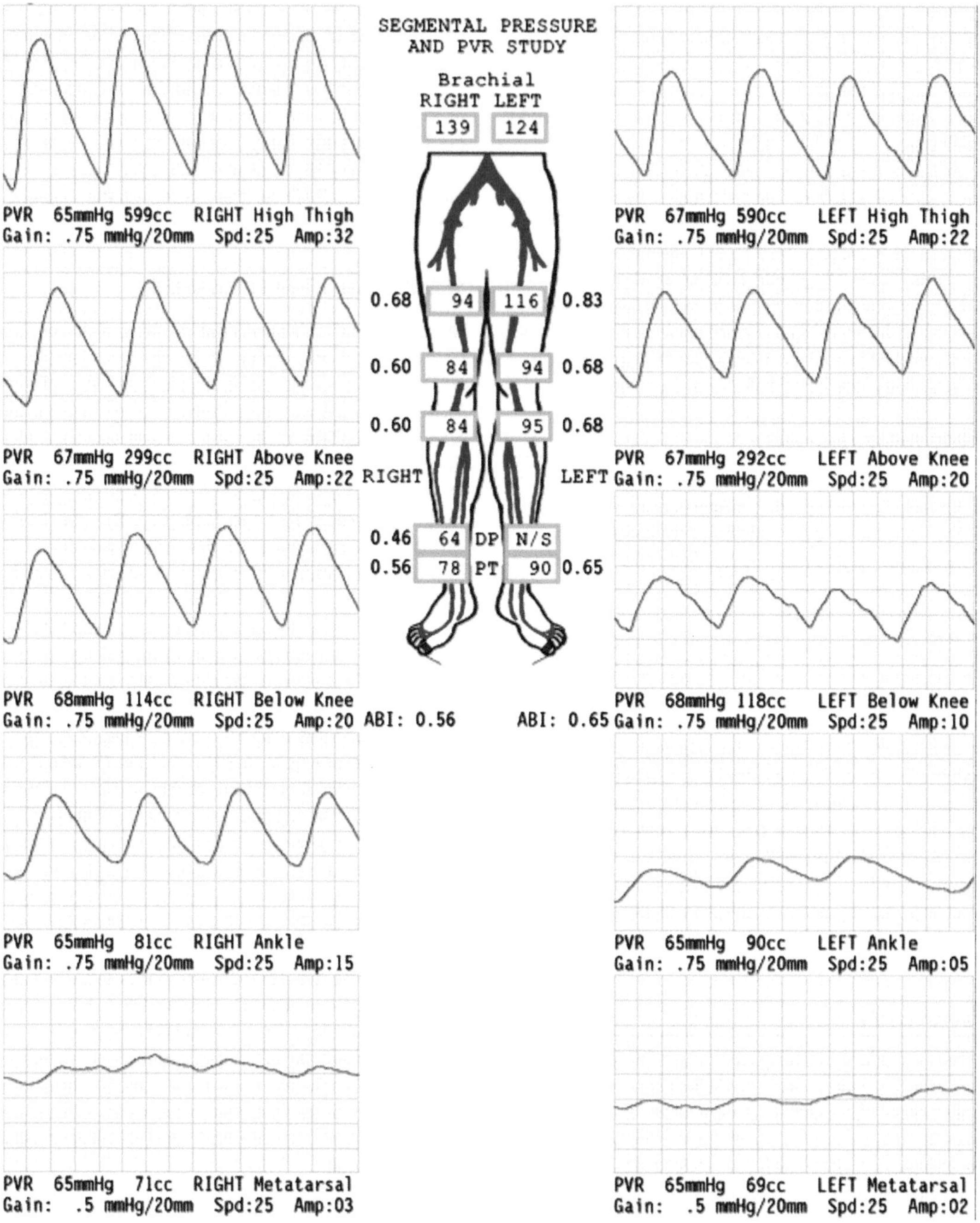

Fig. 2. Noninvasive, physiologic arterial study of the bilateral lower extremities. The ABIs, segmental limb pressures, and PVRs are shown. The right ABI is 78/139 = 0.56; the left ABI is 90/139 = 0.65. There was no signal in the left DP. Segmental limb pressures were obtained using the four-cuff method. The numbers inside the blue boxes represent the systolic pressures at each of the four levels: high thigh, low thigh, calf, and ankle (the DP and PT pressures are reported separately, but both are obtained at the ankle level). The PVR waveforms are obtained at the sites indicated in the lower right corner of each tracing box. Under normal conditions, the calf PVR waveforms should augment, and have an amplitude (Amp) at least 50% greater than the thigh waveforms. There is a significant deterioration of the left calf PVR waveforms; this indicates superficial femoral artery occlusive disease. The left ankle and metatarsal PVRs are markedly blunted, consistent with significant occlusive disease.

Table 1
Segmental limb pressures and PVR interpretation, four-cuff method

Location of Gradient	Interpretation
Brachial to brachial	Subclavian (or innominate), or axillary stenosis
Arm to unilateral high-thigh	Stenosis in either the common iliac, external iliac, common femoral, or the proximal superficial femoral arteries
Arm to bilateral high-thigh	Bilateral aortoiliac or iliofemoral stenoses, or aortic disease
High-thigh to low-thigh	Superficial femoral artery stenosis
Low-thigh to calf	Distal superficial femoral artery and/or popliteal artery stenosis
Calf to ankle	Tibioperoneal (or infrapopliteal) disease
Ankle to transmetatarsal or toe	Small vessel disease or vasospasm

The thigh pressure should be ≥30 mm Hg greater than the reference arm pressure. A pressure gradient greater than 20 mm Hg between adjacent levels in the lower extremities is abnormal.

prominent dichrotic notch, and smooth late equalization in the remainder of diastole. Waveforms obtained distal to a hemodynamically significant stenotic lesion usually have a delayed upstroke, decreased amplitude, and disappearance of the dichrotic notch. With severe disease, the waveforms ultimately become flat or nonpulsatile. The level of a stenosis therefore can be inferred based on the PVR waveforms.

PVR waveforms obtained at the level of the calf should have at least a 50% greater amplitude (termed augmentation) compared with the thigh PVR waveforms. A decrease in the amplitude (or failure to augment) of the calf PVR relative to that in the thigh suggests hemodynamically significant stenosis at the level of the superficial femoral or popliteal arteries. Blunted waveforms at the level of the thigh suggest disease above the level of the cuff, involving either the common iliac, external iliac, common femoral, or the proximal superficial femoral arteries. If blunted waveforms are noted in the thigh cuffs bilaterally, the possibility of bilateral aortoiliac or aortic disease (eg, mid aortic syndrome) should be considered. When faced with a blunted thigh PVR waveform, it is important that clinicians determine whether there is inflow disease (aortoiliac) or superficial femoral artery disease, because the management may be different. Continuous-wave Doppler interrogation at the common femoral artery can help distinguish these two possibilities.

Continuous Wave Doppler

A complete PVR study should include Doppler interrogation of the common femoral arteries, using either pulse-wave Doppler in a duplex ultrasound machine, or continuous-wave Doppler using a hand-held device. Both provide essentially the same information. A normal lower extremity arterial Doppler waveform is triphasic with a sharp systolic upstroke, a short reverse flow component, and a smaller forward flow component later in diastole. In cases of proximal stenosis, these waveforms become abnormal. Initially, the diastolic forward flow component disappears, giving rise to biphasic waveforms. With increasing severity of obstruction, the waveforms become monophasic with loss of diastolic reversal; there is a delayed upstroke, a rounded (instead of sharp) peak, and there may be increased diastolic forward flow (**Fig. 3**). A monophasic Doppler signal at the common femoral artery suggests aortoiliac disease.

TOE PHOTOPLETHYSMOGRAPHY

Ten-toe PPG should be part of a complete lower extremity noninvasive arterial evaluation. PPG is performed by placing a strapped sensor in the distal end of each toe to measure changes and cutaneous blood flow. Toe PPG tracings showed be obtained with the patient as warm as possible. Blood attenuates light of proportion to its content and tissue. Increased blood flow results in decreased reflection. A normal toe PPG tracing consists of a rapid upstroke, sharp systolic peak

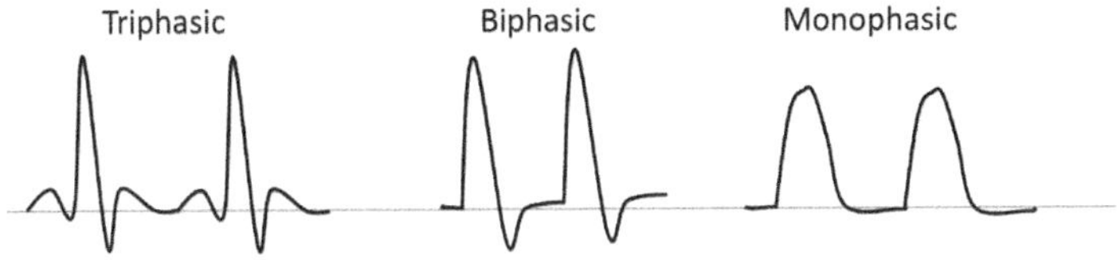

Fig. 3. Schematic representation of arterial Doppler signals in the lower extremities. See text for details.

with reflected wave. With decreased blood flow (eg, as seen with a proximal severe stenosis or vasospasm), the waveforms become dampened and with low amplitude.

ARTERIAL DUPLEX ULTRASOUND

A basic understanding of the principles of ultrasonography is essential for a complete understanding of vascular ultrasound studies. Vascular ultrasound is based on the principle described by Christian Doppler, consisting of a shift or difference between the frequency of an emitted sound beam, and the frequency of the reflected sound beam.[6] The frequency of sound waves used in diagnostic vascular ultrasound is measured in megahertz, which is inaudible to the human ear.

Vascular ultrasound studies consist of B-mode (also called grayscale imaging) and pulse-wave Doppler ultrasound, which includes color Doppler and spectral waveform analysis and flow velocity determinations.[7] The sensitivity of Doppler ultrasound to detect significant PAD is in the range of 92% to 95%, with specificity greater than 97%.[6,8] Whereas the B-mode and color Doppler assessment provides useful anatomic information related to the location and morphology of vascular lesions, including stenosis, occlusions, and aneurysms, spectral waveform analyses and velocity determinations provide quantitative and qualitative hemodynamic information related to stenosis.

Lower extremity arterial duplex ultrasonography is usually performed with a 5- or 7-MHz linear array transducer. The lower extremity arterial system is systematically examined by segments, typically going from proximal to distal: distal aorta, common iliac artery, external iliac artery, common femoral artery, common femoral artery bifurcation into the superficial femoral artery and profunda femoris, superficial femoral artery from proximal to distal, popliteal artery, trifurcation, anterior tibial artery, posterior tibial artery, and peroneal artery. Each segment is carefully examined using B-mode in the short axis view to assess the vessel wall and determine the presence of atherosclerotic plaque. Suspected stenotic lesions and atherosclerotic plaque should be assessed in long axis and in cross-section. Color Doppler is used to assess flow characteristics and areas of turbulence; pulse-wave Doppler examination is used for spectral waveform analysis, and determinations of peak- and end-systolic velocities (**Figs. 4** and **5**).[6]

Waveform Analysis

Normal Doppler signals should be triphasic. A change from triphasic to biphasic may carry significance; however, in some patients biphasic

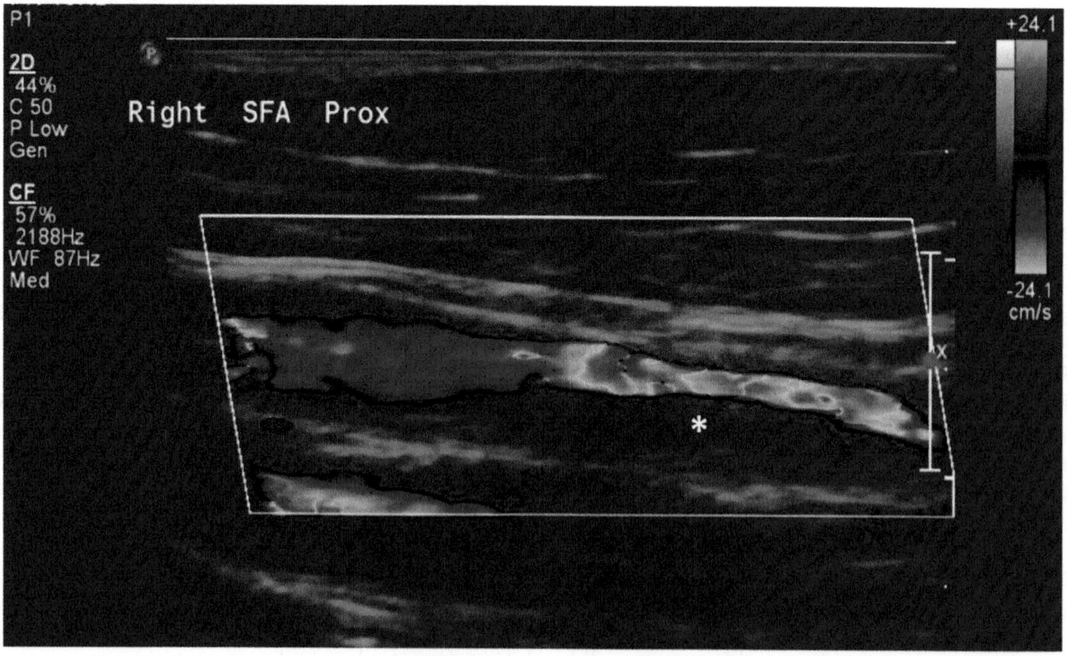

Fig. 4. Duplex ultrasound examination. A smooth, long-segment stenosis is seen in the right proximal superficial femoral artery. Significant atherosclerotic plaque is seen on grayscale (*asterisk*). Color Doppler highlights the degree of luminal narrowing, and demonstrates increased flow velocities with eventual aliasing and turbulence.

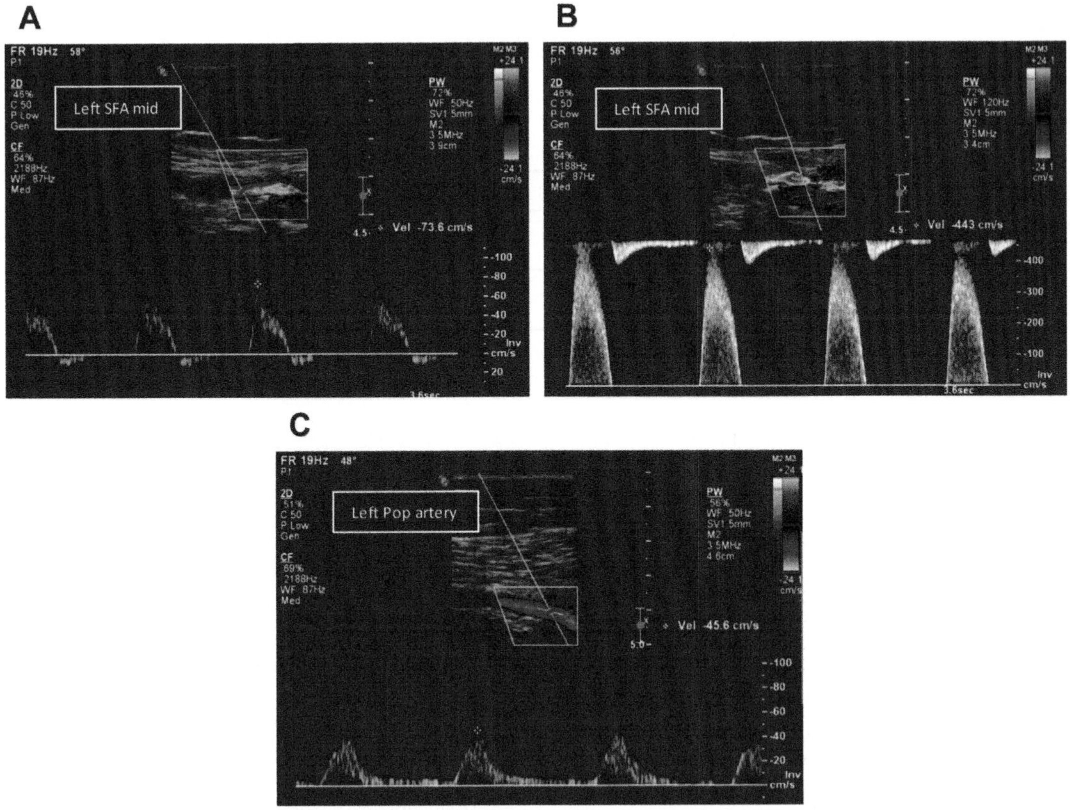

Fig. 5. Spectral waveforms. A stenosis in the left mid-superficial femoral artery is seen on color Doppler in the inserted box. (*A*) The spectral Doppler waveforms prestenosis are biphasic, with a normal upstroke and a peak systolic velocity of 73.6 cm/s. (*B*) Velocities at the site of stenosis are markedly elevated, with a PSV of 443 cm/s, consistent with a greater than 75% stenosis (velocity ratio = 443/73.6 = 6.0). (*C*) Waveforms obtained distal to the stenosis are monophasic, tardus et parvus, and with persistent diastolic flow.

flow patterns may be normal. Monophasic waveforms with prominent diastolic flow are always abnormal and are usually seen distal to severe stenosis or occlusion. Waveforms in areas of severe stenosis often demonstrate high velocities and spectral broadening, reflecting turbulent blood flow (see **Fig. 5**). It should be noted, however, that technical errors, such as increased gain, can also give an appearance of spectral broadening, even in the absence of disease. Poststenotic waveforms are characterized by slow and blunted upstrokes in what is termed "parvus et tardus" morphology, reflecting the same hemodynamic derangements seen, for example, in severe aortic stenosis.

Velocity Criteria

In contrast to echocardiography, flow velocities in vascular ultrasonography can easily be overestimated (thereby overestimating severity of the lesion) if the measurements are taken at an incorrect Doppler angle. The ideal Doppler angle for vascular examinations is 60 degrees, obtained at the center stream and parallel to the walls. Generally, peak systolic velocities (PSVs) in the lower extremity arterial system range from around 120 ± 20 cm/s in the iliac arteries, to 70 ± 10 cm/s in the popliteal or tibioperoneal arteries. As described in the Bernoulli principle, flow velocities increase at sites of stenosis (see **Fig. 5**). A direct correlation exists between the degree of stenosis and the PSVs. However, absolute PSVs should never be taken alone for the estimation of stenosis. Rather, it is the ratio between the PSV at the area of most severe stenosis to the PSV proximal to stenosis that correlates best with the degree of stenosis by angiography. Although numerous ultrasound criteria have been promulgated for the estimation of stenosis, the criterion we use in our laboratory is shown in **Table 2**. Accuracy of duplex depends on the quality of the examinations, which should ideally be performed by dedicated vascular ultrasonographers. Additionally, results obtained by duplex should be correlated with digital subtraction angiography or CTA as gold standards

Table 2
Duplex ultrasound velocity criteria for the estimation of the degree of stenosis in the arteries of the lower extremities

Degree of Stenosis by Angiography	Stenotic:Prestenotic PSV Ratio	Waveform and B-mode Analysis
<50%	<2:1 ratio	Triphasic waveform, no plaque
50%–74%	2:1 ratio	Monophasic waveform (biphasic possible) Significant plaque present
≥75%	4:1 ratio	Monophasic waveforms, PSV often >400 cm/s Significant plaque present
Occluded segment	—	Preocclusive thump, no flow seen Plaque or hypoechoic material (thrombus) present

to provide reassurance of the accuracy of the vascular laboratory.

Surveillance After Endovascular Intervention

There are data that suggest that surveillance with duplex ultrasound following endovascular and surgical revascularization translate into improved patency rates.[9–12] The velocity criteria used to assess degree of stenosis in native arteries should not be applied to stented arteries. Endovascular stents decrease arterial wall compliance, which in turn results in increased flow velocities within the stented segment, even in the absence of restenosis. The velocity criteria used to detect stenosis in unstented arteries is therefore unreliable. The presence of in-stent restenosis is generally determined based on the visualization on B-mode of intimal thickening within the stent, turbulent flow on dolor Doppler, and increased flow velocities compared with those proximal to the stent. According to the American College of Cardiology 2012 Appropriate Use Criteria for Peripheral Vascular Ultrasound Guidelines (endorsed by numerous other organizations), it is appropriate for asymptomatic patients to have a baseline examination within 1 month of intervention, and yearly thereafter.[13]

Surveillance After Surgical Bypass Grafting

Surgical bypass grafts are at risk of developing stenosis and occlusion. Once the graft becomes thrombosed, secondary patency rates are dismal. If a stenosis is detected and intervened on before graft thrombosis, up to 80% of the grafts can be salvaged (primary assisted patency).[11,12] Therefore, it is critical that patients who have undergone surgical bypass graft revascularization enter into a well-organized surveillance program using vascular ultrasound and ABIs for the early detection of a failing graft. The 2012 American College of Cardiology Appropriate Use Criteria endorse a baseline examination within 1 month of revascularization, at 6 to 8 months within the first year following the procedure, and yearly thereafter, even in asymptomatic patients or those with stable symptoms.[13]

The duplex ultrasound protocol for graft surveillance is similar to the one used in native vessels. The inflow artery to the bypass graft should be thoroughly assessed, measuring the PSV at a Doppler angle of 60 degrees. The proximal anastomosis, proximal, mid, and distal graft, distal anastomosis, and outflow artery should also be carefully interrogated. Peak systolic and end-diastolic velocities are obtained at each segment and compared with the proximal segment. If the ratio of the PSV within a stenotic segment to the proximal segment is greater than 2, this suggests a 50% to 75% stenosis. Additionally, low-flow velocities (eg, below 20 cm/s) should alert of impending graft failure.

CT ANGIOGRAPHY

CT angiography (CTA) has become one of the most valuable noninvasive imaging modalities for the assessment of vascular diseases.[14] The main indication for CTA is procedure planning in symptomatic patients with PAD. CTA findings can assist the decision of whether to revascularize a patient surgically or through an endovascular approach. With current 64- and 256-slice CT technology, the peripheral vascular system can be evaluated with high spatial resolution during a single acquisition and a single intravenous injection of contrast dye. Actual scanning times generally occur in the range of 20 seconds, minimizing motion artifact. Although a detailed description of the different CTA protocols used in the assessment of arterial diseases is beyond the scope of this article, readers are referred to comprehensive reviews on the topic.[14,15] Modern reconstruction packages allow the three-dimensional presentation of volumetric information, which can be of significant value in vascular interpretation (**Fig. 6**). An additional feature available in CTA, but not MRA, is curved multiplanar reconstructions, which allow the detailed inspection of the vessel in its long axis to always stay in plane while the image is scrolled.

An important limitation of CTA is that the presence of heavy calcification of the vessel wall, and even the presence of endovascular stents, limit visualization of the arterial lumen and therefore limit the assessment of the degree of stenosis. This is especially true in the tibioperoneal arteries. The sensitivity and specificity of CTA (four-slice system) for the diagnosis of stenosis greater than 50% in the peripheral arteries is 92% and 93%,[15,16] respectively, and is even higher in more modern systems. Common contraindications to the use of CTA are renal dysfunction, contrast dye allergy, and ionizing radiation. A typical CTA of the aorta with bilateral runoffs requires 100 to 140 mL of intravenous contrast dye for adequate vessel opacification and visualization.

MAGNETIC RESONANCE ANGIOGRAPHY

Magnetic resonance angiography (MRA) is an excellent noninvasive vascular imaging modality. In a recent pooled analysis, MRA had a sensitivity and specificity for the detection of significant stenotic lesions of approximately 95% and 96%, respectively.[17] Similar to CTA, the main indication of MRA in patients with PAD is in the preinterventional evaluation. In addition, MRA is particularly useful in the characterization of arterial wall diseases, such atherosclerosis, vasculitis or vessel wall inflammation, intramural hematoma, aneurysms, and dissections. A detailed description of all of the sequences and protocols used in MRA imaging is beyond the scope of this review; readers are referred to excellent reviews on this topic.[18,19] Compared with CTA, current MRA techniques have more limited spatial resolution, which decreases the sensitivity to detect subtle lesions. Another limitation of MRA relates to motion artifact. Relatively longer acquisition times compared with CTA often result in blurring and image degradation that may lead to overestimation or underestimation of the severity of a stenotic lesion. Important advantages of MRA over CTA are avoidance of ionizing radiation, and use of nonnephrotoxic contrast agents, although nephrogenic systemic fibrosis can occur in patients with significant renal dysfunction (estimated glomerular filtration rate <30 mL/min/1.73 m^2) who receive gadolinium. An important disadvantage of MRA is that it cannot be performed in many patients with metallic implants, such as pacemakers

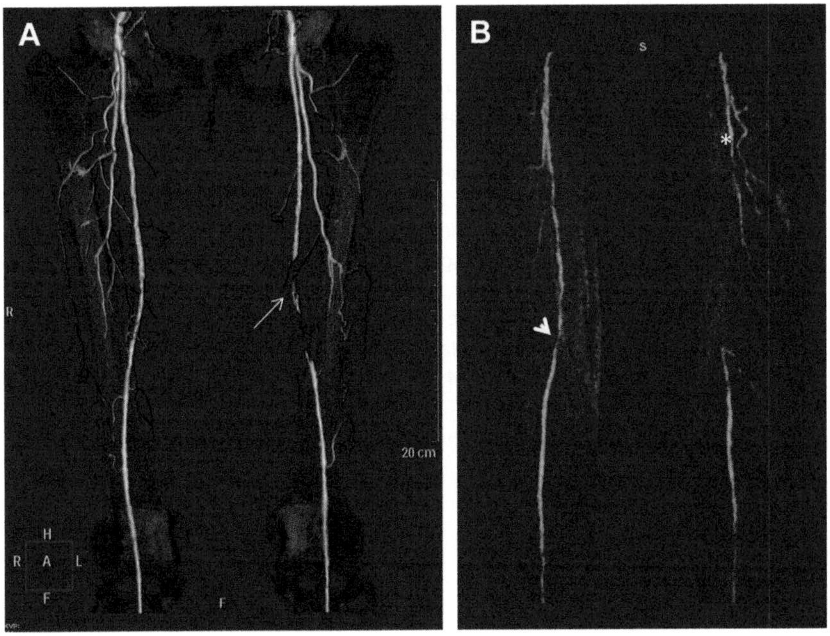

Fig. 6. (*A*) CTA with three-dimensional reconstruction. A short-segment occlusion of the mid left superficial femoral artery is seen (*arrow*), with distal reconstitution via collaterals. (*B*) MRA with maximum intensity projections of the bilateral superficial femoral arteries. There is a long-segment occlusion of the left superficial femoral artery at its origin (*asterisk*). On the right, there is diffuse disease in the superficial femoral artery, with evidence of significant stenosis (*arrowhead*). Note: the images in *A* and *B* are from different patients.

(although MRI-safe permanent pacemaker are now available and approved by the Food and Drug Administration), epicardial pacer wires, aneurysm clips, and some metallic implants; most contemporary inferior vena cava filters are MRA-safe.

SUMMARY

The vascular laboratory, CTA, and MRA techniques allow accurate and noninvasive assessment of the presence and severity of PAD. The functional tests, such as ABIs and PVRs, often provide the most important objective information on the presence of limb ischemia. Duplex ultrasound, CTA, and MRA provide more anatomic information related to the disease, which is important in procedure planning. A solid understanding of the principles, indications, and limitations of each of these modalities is critical for the correct interpretation and clinical use of these tests.

REFERENCES

1. Aboyans V, Criqui MH, Abraham P, et al. Measurement and interpretation of the ankle-brachial index: a scientific statement from the American Heart Association. Circulation 2012;126:2890–909.
2. Wikstrom J, Hansen T, Johansson L, et al. Ankle brachial index <0.9 underestimates the prevalence of peripheral artery occlusive disease assessed with whole-body magnetic resonance angiography in the elderly. Acta Radiol 2008;49:143–9.
3. Ankle Brachial Index Collaboration, Fowkes FG, Murray GD, Butcher I, et al. Ankle brachial index combined with Framingham Risk Score to predict cardiovascular events and mortality: a meta-analysis. JAMA 2008;300:197–208.
4. Taylor GI, Pan WR. Angiosomes of the leg: anatomic study and clinical implications. Plast Reconstr Surg 1998;102:599–616 [discussion: 617–8].
5. Gardner AW, Skinner JS, Cantwell BW, et al. Prediction of claudication pain from clinical measurements obtained at rest. Med Sci Sports Exerc 1992;24: 163–70.
6. Zierler RE. Strandness's duplex scanning in vascular disorders. Philadelphia: Wolters Kluwer; 2002.
7. Stewart JH, Grubb M. Understanding vascular ultrasonography. Mayo Clin Proc 1992;67:1186–96.
8. Moneta GL, Yeager RA, Antonovic R, et al. Accuracy of lower extremity arterial duplex mapping. J Vasc Surg 1992;15:275–83 [discussion: 283–4].
9. Idu MM, Blankenstein JD, de Gier P, et al. Impact of a color-flow duplex surveillance program on infrainguinal vein graft patency: a five-year experience. J Vasc Surg 1993;17:42–52 [discussion: 52–3].
10. Lundell A, Lindblad B, Bergqvist D, et al. Femoropopliteal-crural graft patency is improved by an intensive surveillance program: a prospective randomized study. J Vasc Surg 1995;21:26–33 [discussion: 33–4].
11. Bandyk DF. Vascular laboratory surveillance after intervention. Guest editorial. Perspect Vasc Surg Endovasc Ther 2007;19:353.
12. Bandyk DF, Chauvapun JP. Duplex ultrasound surveillance can be worthwhile after arterial intervention. Perspect Vasc Surg Endovasc Ther 2007;19: 354–9 [discussion: 360–1].
13. 2012 appropriate use criteria for peripheral vascular ultrasound and physiological testing part I: arterial ultrasound and physiological testing: a report of the American College of Cardiology Foundation appropriate use criteria task force. J Am Coll Cardiol 2012;60:242–76.
14. Ligon BL. Biography: history of developments in imaging techniques: Egas Moniz and angiography. Semin Pediatr Infect Dis 2003;14:173–81.
15. Met R, Bipat S, Legemate DA, et al. Diagnostic performance of computed tomography angiography in peripheral arterial disease: a systematic review and meta-analysis. JAMA 2009;301:415–24.
16. Schernthaner R, Stadler A, Lomoschitz F, et al. Multidetector CT angiography in the assessment of peripheral arterial occlusive disease: accuracy in detecting the severity, number, and length of stenoses. Eur Radiol 2008;18:665–71.
17. Menke J, Larsen J. Meta-analysis: accuracy of contrast-enhanced magnetic resonance angiography for assessing steno-occlusions in peripheral arterial disease. Ann Intern Med 2010;153:325–34.
18. Ersoy H, Rybicki FJ. MR angiography of the lower extremities. AJR Am J Roentgenol 2008;190:1675–84.
19. Ho VB, Corse WR. MR angiography of the abdominal aorta and peripheral vessels. Radiol Clin North Am 2003;41:115–44.

Endovascular Management of Brachiocephalic Disease

D. Christopher Metzger, MD

KEYWORDS

• Subclavian • Stent • Balloon • Subclavian steal • LIMA steal

KEY POINTS

- Brachiocephalic lesions are amenable to endovascular treatment; however, these treatments have significant risks associated with them and require modified procedural techniques.
- All interventions require careful preprocedural evaluation and consultation, with careful weighing of the risks and benefits of endovascular intervention versus the natural history of the disease with medical therapy or surgical intervention.
- Brachiocephalic endovascular interventions should be performed only by experienced operators with extensive previous carotid and endovascular experience in appropriate adequately equipped venues.
- Most brachiocephalic disease also has surgical options for treatment, which should be carefully considered in a vascular team approach.

INTRODUCTION

Atherosclerotic obstructive disease in the brachiocephalic vessels can lead to significant morbidity and mortality.[1] Either via obstructive or embolic consequences, lesions in these vessels can cause strokes in the cerebral regions or posterior circulation, or can lead to significant symptoms of vertebrobasilar insufficiency, arm claudication, or coronary insufficiency, among other manifestations. Endovascular treatment has emerged as a frontline therapy for treatment of many obstructive brachiocephalic lesions, with improving results in multiple studies, even in the highest risk patients.[2–14]

This article provides a practical guideline for endovascular treatment of brachiocephalic lesions, offering guidance based on personal experience at a high-volume center; lessons learned; and experiences gleaned from other high-volume operators, meetings, and text books. Detailed instructions for cervical carotid interventions have been described previously.[15] This article reviews techniques for treating innominate, ostial common carotid, subclavian artery, and ostial vertebral lesions, as well as several unique situations encountered during brachiocephalic interventions. It is hoped that this article can serve as an illustrated reference for operators to refer to as they appropriately apply endovascular treatment of brachiocephalic lesions in their own practices.

BACKGROUND CONSIDERATIONS FOR BRACHIOCEPHALIC OPERATORS

All brachiocephalic interventions have potential for severe cerebrovascular complications, including stroke and the locked-in syndrome. All operators who treat these lesions should therefore have appropriate endovascular training and experience before they undertake performance of these interventions independently. Even for routine subclavian interventions, and for all other interventions discussed in this article, operators should have met all of their specific society's position paper minimum requirements (eg, interventional radiology, interventional cardiology, vascular surgery)

The author has nothing to disclose.
Wellmont CVA Heart Institute, 2050 Meadowview Parkway, Kingsport, TN 37660, USA
E-mail address: cmetzger@mycva.com

Intervent Cardiol Clin 3 (2014) 479–491
http://dx.doi.org/10.1016/j.iccl.2014.07.005
2211-7458/14/$ – see front matter

before treating brachiocephalic lesions. Furthermore, for treatment of any innominate, carotid, or vertebral lesion, operators should be trained and credentialed for performance of carotid stenting and potentially neurologic rescue procedures before treating these lesions. In addition, because these interventions carry a significant risk and there are other treatment options, it is imperative to perform formal consultation with the patient and family before any brachiocephalic intervention. These interventions should never be performed as an ad hoc or drive-by procedure without proper discussions and documentation. The same principles for pretreatment with antiplatelet therapy and patient preparation that apply to carotid interventions should apply to brachiocephalic interventions.

BRACHIOCEPHALIC ANGIOGRAPHIC GUIDELINES

Brachiocephalic interventions require precise stent placement, as discussed later. It is important that the angiography suite has excellent imaging capabilities and experienced personnel. Digital subtracted angiography, a wide range of magnifications, and a wide arc of camera angulations immediately available are essential. The ability to perform preintervention and postintervention cerebral angiography and potential intervention is also important, as is the immediate availability of all potentially needed equipment for the intervention and/or bailout interventions.

The standard arch aortogram is performed first in a left anterior oblique (LAO) (40°) projection with digital subtraction (see **Figs. 1** and **20**). This aortogram is performed with the catheter just proximal to the brachiocephalic vessel and with the largest field possible, the catheter and brachiocephalic vessel origins placed at the bottom of the field, and imaging as much as possible above this (**Fig. 1**). Imaging should be performed for long enough to ensure that any retrograde filling is captured during the aortography (**Fig. 2**). A second arch aortogram may be performed as needed for further delineation of the innominate artery (usually a 20° right anterior oblique [RAO], 20° caudal view; see **Fig. 21**). Precise angiography and stenting of the ostium of the innominate, left common carotid, and left subclavian arteries is best accomplished in the 40° LAO projection. The origin of the left vertebral artery and its relationship to the left subclavian artery are best delineated in an RAO cranial projection (eg, 40° RAO, 15° cranial; **Fig. 3**; see **Figs. 5** and **6**), and imaging of the ostium of the right vertebral artery and its relation to the right subclavian artery are also best in a contralateral cranial projection (~40° LAO, 15° cranial). The distal innominate bifurcation and ostia of both the right subclavian and right common carotid arteries are best imaged in a 20° caudal, 20° RAO projection.

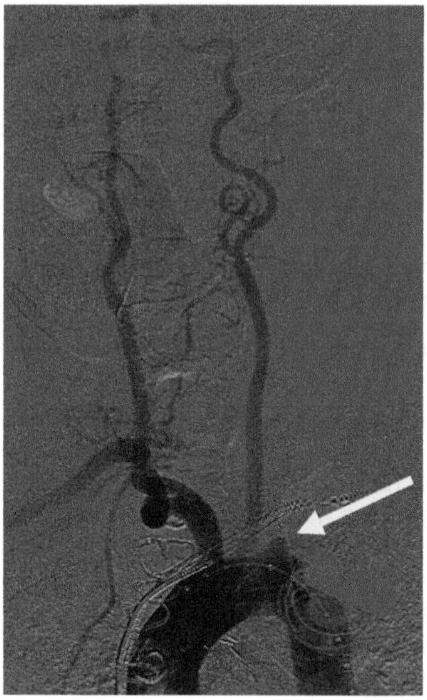

Fig. 1. Left anterior oblique arch aortogram showing left subclavian occlusion (*arrow*).

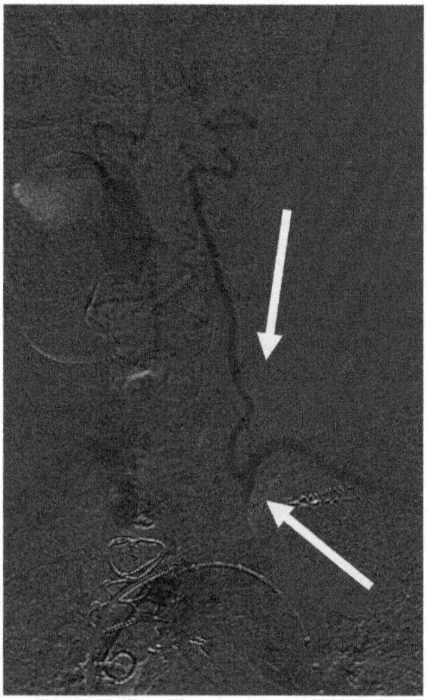

Fig. 2. Delayed arch aortogram showing retrograde filling of the left vertebral and subclavian arteries (*arrows*).

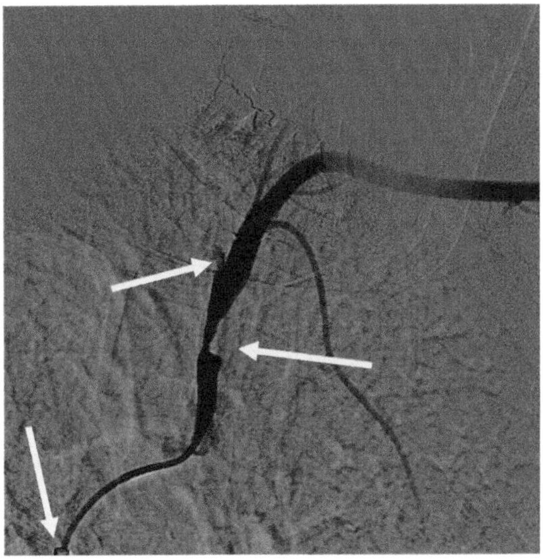

Fig. 3. RAO cranial angiogram showing subclavian stenosis and relationship to left vertebral origin. *Arrows* show guiding catheter, subclavian stenosis, and origin of left vertebral artery.

Each type of brachiocephalic intervention is reviewed individually here, including special situations, using case examples. In addition to previous consultation with all patients, dual antiplatelet therapy, and appropriate patient preparation, it is important to manage anticoagulation accurately throughout these procedures. This management can be accomplished either with bivalirudin or heparin, carefully documenting therapeutic activated coagulation times, with consideration of an intraprocedural heparin drip for potentially longer cases when heparin is selected.

Left Subclavian Interventions

Most left subclavian lesions are ostial or proximal. In general, the natural history is benign, and accordingly these should only be treated (and are only reimbursed) for appropriate indications, which include lifestyle-limiting arm claudication, vertebrobasilar insufficiency symptoms, or cardiac ischemia caused by decreased flow to a left internal mammary bypass graft. At our institution, we think that most proximal left subclavian artery non–chronic total occlusion (non-CTO) lesions are best treated from femoral artery access (even if treated from brachial or radial access, femoral access is usually needed for angiographic guidance for precisely positioning the ostial component of the stent). For most nonoccluded proximal lesions, we place a 7-French (Fr) shuttle sheath in the descending aorta after arch aortography and anticoagulation. In most cases, we use a 4-Fr or 5-Fr, 125-cm neurodiagnostic catheter through the shuttle sheath (see **Fig. 3**), and wire with an exchange length 0.035 inch angled Glidewire. For extremely complex lesions, exchange length 0.014 inch or 0.018 inch wires may be needed. We then use the catheter to exchange for a 0.035 inch supportive wire. We predilate almost all lesions. This predilatation is performed conservatively (usually balloons of 4–6 mm), and we perform angiography with the uninflated balloon in position in 2 views to help select the stent length after predilatation (**Figs. 4** and **5**). We use an LAO 40° angiogram to position the balloon in the ostium (see **Fig. 4**), and a contralateral cranial view to determine the proximity of the distal end of the balloon to the vertebral artery origin (see **Fig. 5**). Often we use a 40-mm balloon, position the distal end, estimate the stent length that will be needed, and allow the proximal end of the balloon to be in the aorta during predilatation. We usually use a 5-mm or 6-mm diameter balloon. After predilatation and careful sheath aspiration, subtracted angiography is repeated, and the stent is selected. A 7-mm or 8-mm balloon-expandable stent is used in most cases (balloon-expandable stents have better radial strength and precise positioning for these lesions). We again carefully position the stent in 2 views (**Figs. 6** and **7**), and carefully withdraw the shuttle sheath (ensuring that the shoulder of the balloon does not engage the sheath during stent deployment). After stent deployment, the stent balloon is used to reengage the sheath within the proximal stent, and then removed. Aspiration is carefully performed, and subtracted angiograms obtained in 2 views. The stent result is carefully assessed,

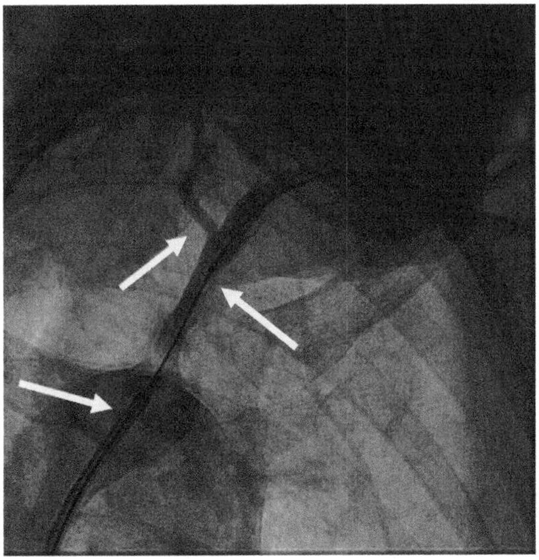

Fig. 4. RAO cranial angiogram with balloon to estimate the stent length needed. *Arrows* show guiding catheter position, balloon length, and origin of the left vertebral artery.

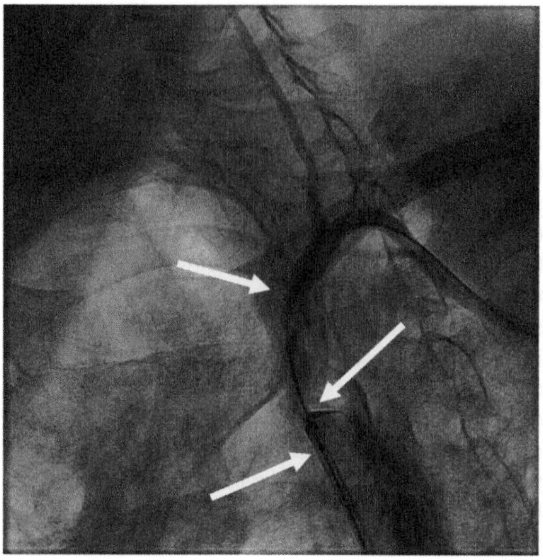

Fig. 5. Left anterior oblique 40° angiogram to assess the ostium for stent length decisions. *Arrows* show guiding catheter and both ends of the balloon.

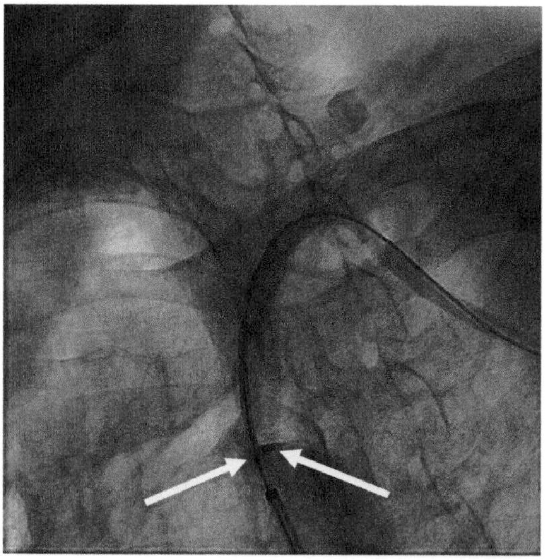

Fig. 7. Left anterior oblique angiogram to position proximal end of stent. *Arrows* show proximal end of the stent relative to the aortic arch.

and we also ensure that there is excellent flow into the vertebral and internal mammary arteries (**Fig. 8**). Postdilatation is performed only if necessary. If angiograms are satisfactory and the patient's neurologic examination is unchanged, we remove the wire and close the arteriotomy with a closure device in appropriate patients.

In most cases, we do not use distal embolic protection during subclavian artery intervention. In general, distal embolic protection has little benefit and adds significantly to the risk and complexity of the procedure. As with all interventions, there are occasional appropriate indications for the use of embolic protection devices. The use of covered stents (discussed later) can afford a degree of embolic protection for some higher risk lesions.

Covered balloon-expandable stents may have advantages for some cases. Examples potentially include ulcerated or ectatic lesions, high embolic risk lesions, heavily calcified lesions, or in-stent restenosis (**Figs. 9** and **10**). Great care should be taken to make sure the vertebral artery origin is not covered by the stent graft. If we think that an 8-mm covered stent will be used, we use an 8-Fr

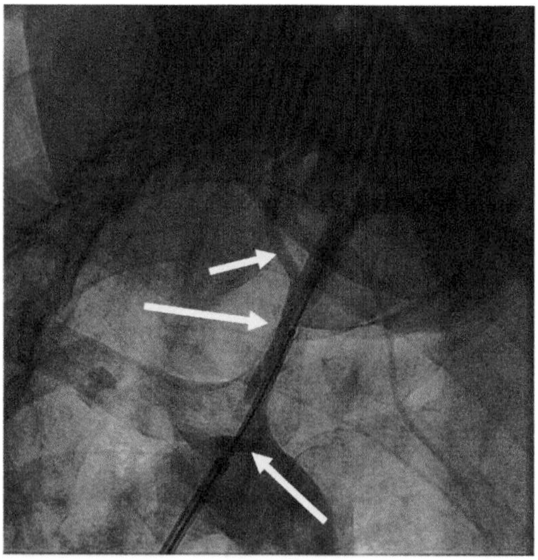

Fig. 6. RAO cranial angiogram to determine distal stent position relative to left vertebral artery. *Arrows* show proximal and distal ends of the stent and the origin of the left vertebral artery.

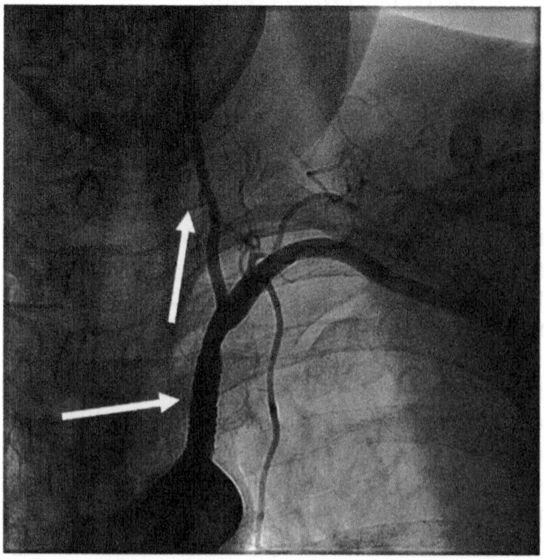

Fig. 8. Final angiogram after subclavian stent. *Arrows* show the widely patent stent and antegrade flow in the left vertebral artery.

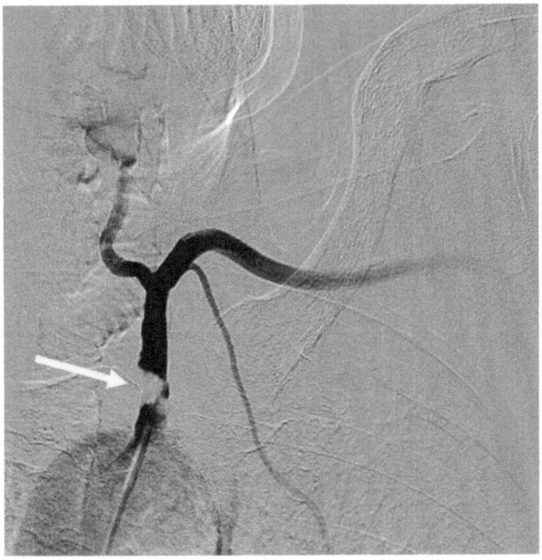

Fig. 9. Heavily calcified, eccentric left subclavian lesion (*arrow*).

shuttle sheath to provide additional room for angiography.

Left subclavian intervention with vertebral artery involvement

Subclavian lesions that involve the origin of the vertebral artery require special treatment (**Fig. 11**). We often use dual access with brachial or radial access in addition to femoral access. Important vertebral arteries can be wired with a 0.014 inch wire from arm access. After predilatation, the subclavian lesion and vertebral artery are reassessed. If the subclavian lesion and stent location spans the origin of the vertebral artery, we strongly consider use of a nitinol stent. After predilatation, we place the nitinol stent across the origin of the vertebral artery, avoiding the origin of the internal mammary if possible (**Fig. 12**). Before postdilating the nitinol stent, it is important that the 0.014 inch guidewire is placed through the nitinol stent tines into the vertebral artery. Postdilatations are then performed within the nitinol stent (**Fig. 13**). If there is significant narrowing of the vertebral artery, it is then easy to dilate this with

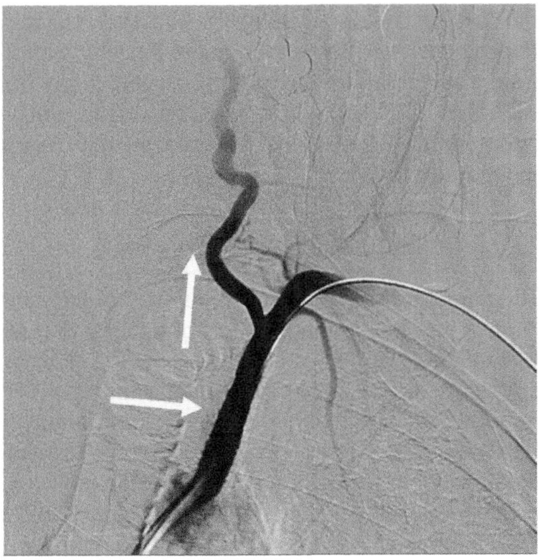

Fig. 10. Final angiogram after covered stent. *Arrows* show widely patent stent and antegrade flow into left vertebral artery.

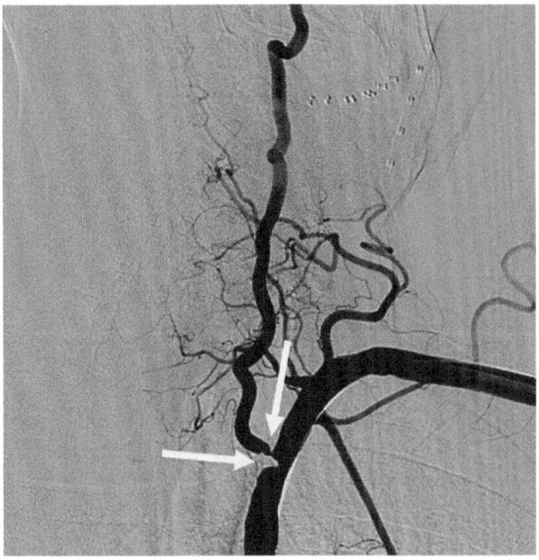

Fig. 11. Dual access to treat left subclavian and vertebral lesions. *Arrows* show left subclavian artery stenosis and ostial stenosis in the left vertebral artery.

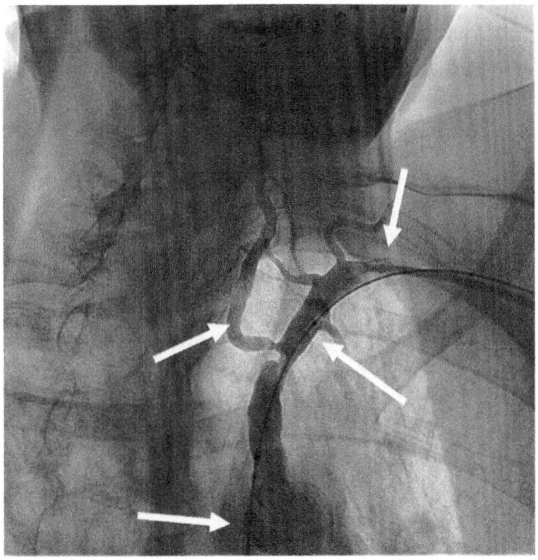

Fig. 12. Positioning nitinol stent after predilatation of left subclavian and vertebral arteries. *Arrows* show the guiding catheter, positions from the femoral artery and the left brachial artery access sites, and the distal end of the stent relative to the vertebral artery and the left internal mammary artery.

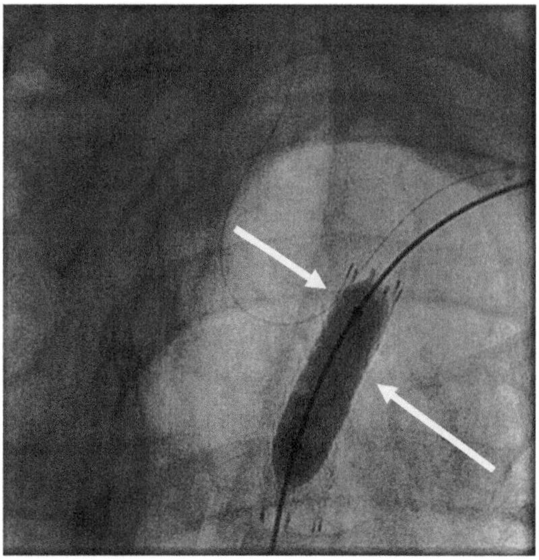

Fig. 13. Post-dilatation of a nitinol stent after rewiring through the stent into the vertebral artery. *Arrows* show wire in the left vertebral artery and the post-dilatation inflation.

a low-profile 0.014 inch balloon, and provisional stents can be placed as indicated (**Fig. 14**). This procedure can be performed either via femoral or arm access. Kissing balloon angioplasty is not needed in this location even if a stent is placed in the vertebral artery (**Fig. 15**). Careful technique and good judgment are needed for vertebral intervention in the setting of subclavian intervention (discussed later).

Left subclavian artery CTOs

Subclavian CTOs require careful consideration because the interventions are more challenging

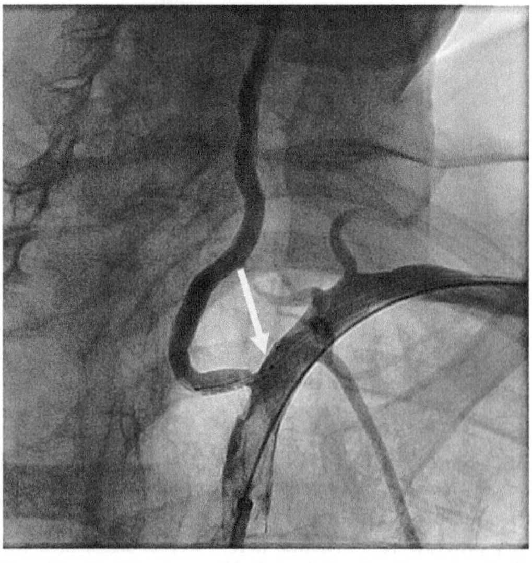

Fig. 14. Positioning of left vertebral artery stent via brachial access (*arrow*).

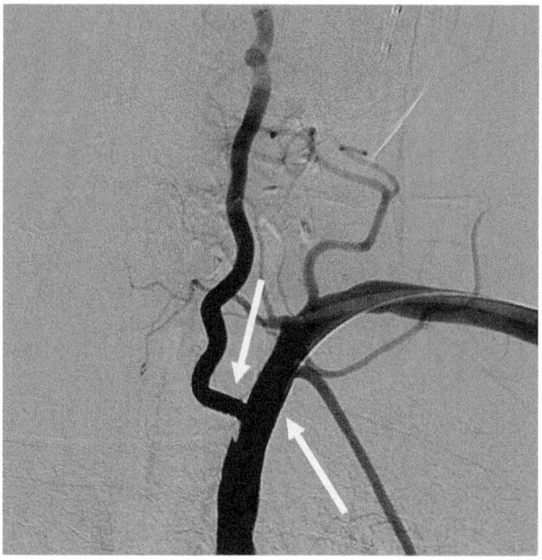

Fig. 15. Final angiogram after left subclavian and vertebral stents. *Arrows* show widely patent stents in the left subclavian and left vertebral arteries.

and the lesions are generally low risk. They should only be treated by experienced operators with significant symptoms and documented indications. Most lesions require dual access. Arm access is more challenging because of diminished pulses in the radial or brachial regions, and ultrasonography guidance or road mapping is frequently used to assist with access. It is important to ascertain with aortography and angiography the location of the distal end of the occlusion and its proximity to the vertebral artery. For ostial subclavian occlusions, there is usually insufficient support to cross them from femoral access, and a pigtail catheter in the aorta and a long sheath in the arm can be used to perform road mapping to guide the intervention from the radial or brachial approach (**Fig. 16**). Standard CTO techniques are then used, and it is imperative to avoid dissections that would extend into the vertebral artery.

Right Subclavian Artery Interventions

The same principles discussed earlier for left subclavian interventions apply to right subclavian interventions. However, there are some special considerations for the right subclavian artery. In general, lesions in the proximal right subclavian artery have a disproportionately high degree of calcification, increasing the technical difficulties and procedural risks. In addition, they are usually ostial in location, and in close proximity to the right common carotid artery. Precise positioning is imperative, because there is usually a short distance between the right common carotid artery for the

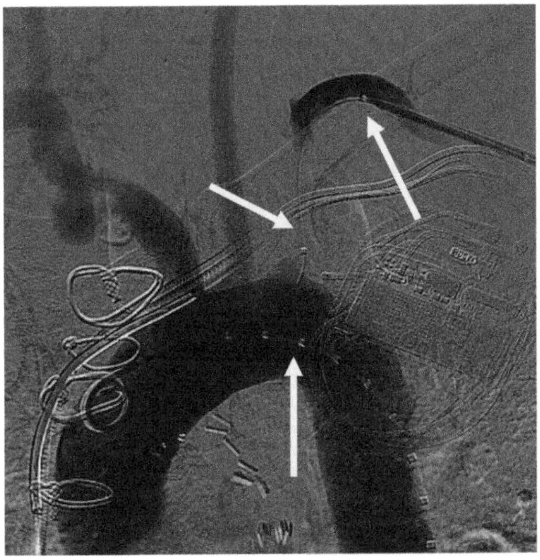

Fig. 16. Dual access with pigtail from femoral access and sheath via left brachial access to cross the CTO. *Arrows* show pigtail catheter in the aorta, guidewire, and left brachial sheath.

proximal end of the stent and the right vertebral artery for the distal end of the stent. There is also more angulation involving the innominate artery to access these lesions compared with the left subclavian artery. As such, interventions for the right subclavian artery require a careful risk/benefit ratio assessment.

For right subclavian interventions, the proximal vessel is usually best imaged in a 20° RAO, 20° caudal projection (**Figs. 17** and **18**), and the distal

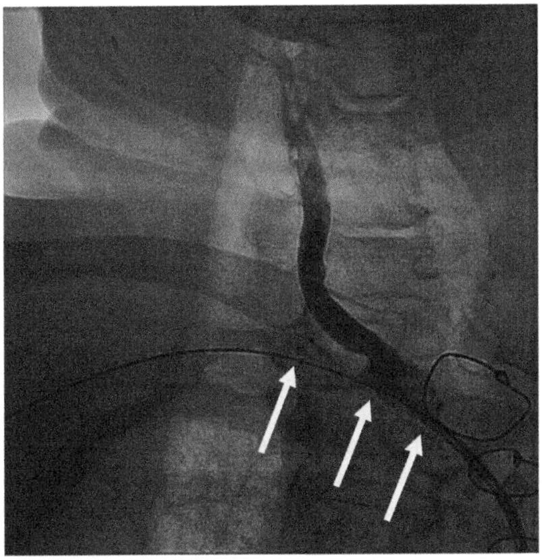

Fig. 17. Positioning right subclavian PTA balloon in RAO caudal image through 7-F shuttle sheath. *Arrows* show both ends of balloon and the tip of the guiding sheath.

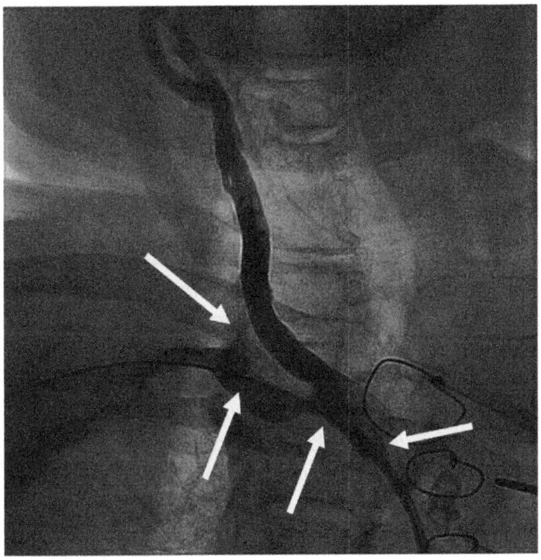

Fig. 18. Positioning stent in RAO caudal view. *Arrows* show both ends of the stent, guiding catheter tip, and origin of the right vertebral artery.

end imaged in a contralateral cranial projection with attention to the origin of the right vertebral artery. Shorter stents with precise positioning are usually required (see **Fig. 18**; **Fig. 19**), and balloon-expandable stents are almost always best.

Surgical alternatives for treating subclavian artery disease

It is important for all endovascular operators to remember that there are excellent surgical revascularization options for treatment of subclavian artery occlusive disease. A common carotid artery to subclavian bypass operation is a predictable and

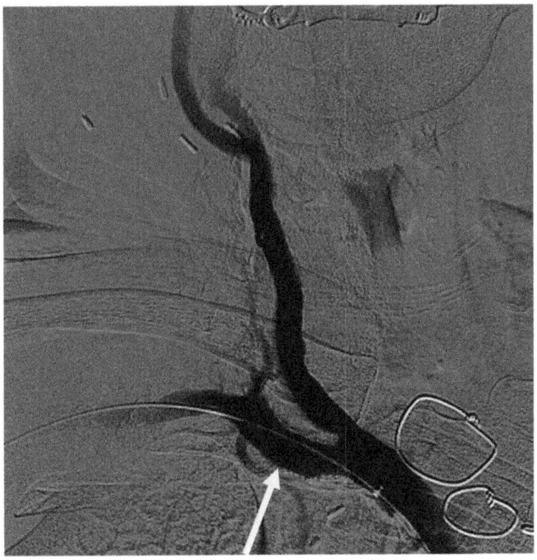

Fig. 19. Final angiogram after stenting.

durable procedure when performed by an experienced surgeon. Consultation with vascular surgical colleagues is recommended, especially for complex subclavian lesions and/or lower-volume endovascular operators.

Ostial Left Common Carotid Artery Interventions

We use femoral access for most ostial left common carotid artery interventions (the exception is an ostial left common carotid lesion with a bovine arch, which we may approach from right brachial access). After arch aortography and initiation of anticoagulation (usually bivalirudin for us), we place a 7-Fr shuttle sheath in the descending thoracic aorta. We think that distal embolic protection should be used for most of these procedures with the following modified technique. A 125-cm neurodiagnostic catheter (selected after reviewing the arch aortogram) is directed toward the ostium of the left common carotid artery using a no-touch technique. We use an exchange length Workhorse BareWire to wire the left internal carotid artery carefully. We then use an exchange length steerable 0.018 inch wire (we like the V-18 wire) to wire the external carotid artery (if patent and able to be wired). It is important to use exchange length wires, because the balloon-expandable stents are over-the-wire devices, and this leaves more options for retrieval devices and avoids wire trapping with the stents. The shuttle sheath is then advanced over the neurodiagnostic catheter to the common carotid artery origin. The neurodiagnostic catheter is then withdrawn, leaving the wires in place and the shuttle sheath adjacent to the common carotid artery origin (another reason exchange length wires are required). A roadmap or subtracted angiogram is then performed with a large imaging field to visualize the ostium of the common carotid artery and the landing zone for the distal embolic protection system. Using this image, the distal embolic protection system (we use a Nav6 device; Abbott Vascular, Santa Clara, CA, because it has an independent exchange length wire and is less likely to move during the intervention) is advanced and deployed in the distal internal carotid artery (see **Fig. 22**). Over the embolic protection wire, we then perform predilatation with a 6-mm 0.014 inch compatible balloon. We consider a rapid exchange scoring balloon such as the VascuTrak (Bard Peripheral Vascular, Tempe, AZ) balloon to avoid device slippage and because of its very short rapid exchange system, minimizing wire movement of the second external carotid artery wire during balloon removal. Angiography or road mapping are used with the balloon in place to help with stent size selection. After careful aspiration of the sheath and repeat angiography, a balloon-expandable stent is selected. In most cases this is an 8 × 17–19, or 8 × 27–29 balloon-expandable stent. It is very important that the over-the-wire stent is placed over both exchange length wires to provide additional support (in effect, a 0.032 wire is created), and also to avoid trapping of one of the wires. The stent is advanced and carefully positioned with angiography, ensuring that there is complete coverage of the ostial lesion. The more angulation in the arch, the more the stent may need to protrude into the arch, because the distal inferior aspect of the stent needs to cover the origin of the common carotid artery. The sheath is then carefully withdrawn, position of the stent is reconfirmed, and the stent balloon is inflated, avoiding contact with the balloon shoulder and the shuttle sheath during inflation (see **Figs. 23** and **24**). If needed because of ostial underexpansion, the stent balloon can be withdrawn partially into the arch and a higher inflation performed. As with all carotid artery interventions, repeated and aggressive angioplasty should be minimized to avoid embolic complications. After stent deployment, the stent balloon is used to help reengage the sheath within the stent. An assistant carefully holds the sheath in place and operates the fluoroscopy pedal while the operator carefully withdraws the stent balloon over both exchange length wires. After aspiration, subtracted angiography is repeated. If there is a satisfactory angiographic result, cerebral angiograms are obtained. Following neurologic evaluation, the distal embolic protection system is then removed. Because the stent often protrudes into the aortic arch, this may be more difficult. We sometimes use a bent-tip retrieval device. If this device does not work, a vertebral catheter can be advanced and used as a modified retrieval device (over the exchange length wire).

Innominate Artery Interventions

The techniques described for treatment of ostial left common carotid artery lesions apply in general to innominate artery interventions with the following modifications (**Figs. 20–24**). We often consider an 8-Fr shuttle sheath to easily accommodate a 10-mm balloon-expandable stent and also provide the ability for angiography around this device and easier stent balloon withdrawal following stenting. Balloon inflation times should be minimized as both the right cerebral and right posterior circulations are hypoperfused during each inflation. We also think that distal embolic protection should be used for most innominate

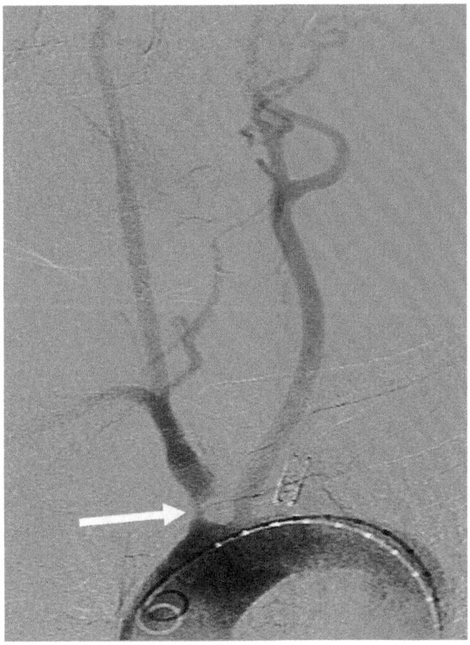

Fig. 20. Left anterior oblique arch aortogram with innominate stenosis (*arrow*).

interventions, which can be done with 2 exchange length wires via femoral artery access, as discussed earlier. As an alternative, right radial or brachial artery access can be used to carefully access the right carotid artery for placement of a distal embolic protection system from the arm via a 6-Fr shuttle sheath (**Figs. 25** and **26**). If a distal protection system is deployed in the right

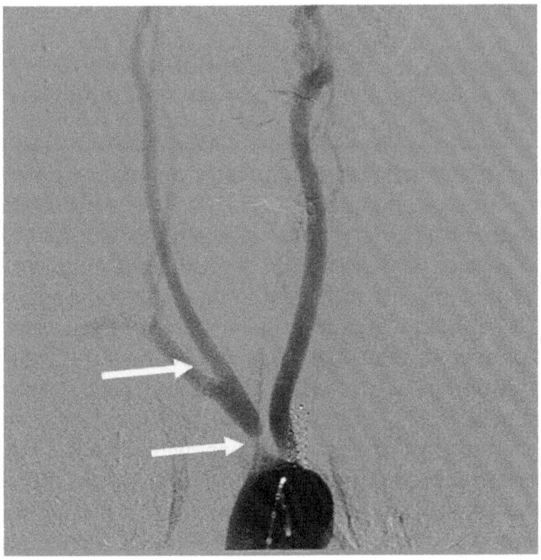

Fig. 21. RAO caudal angiogram showing innominate distal bifurcation. *Arrows* show stenosis of the innominate artery and the distal bifurcation of the innominate artery.

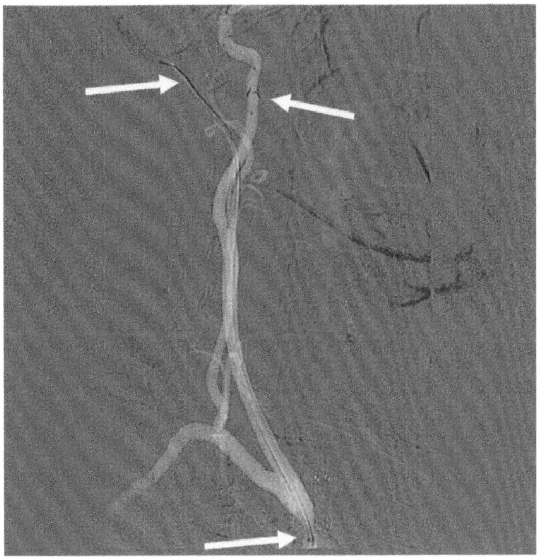

Fig. 22. Roadmap with 8-F shuttle at innominate origin (*arrow*), 0.018 inch wire in the ECA (*arrow*), and distal embolic protection device in the internal carotid artery (*arrow*).

internal carotid artery from an arm approach first, the innominate lesion can be treated from femoral access using 0.035 inch–compatible devices. With this technique, we often wire the innominate lesion with an angled Glidewire into the external carotid artery, exchange for a supportive wire, and then perform angioplasty and stenting with 0.035 inch–compatible balloons and stents.

For innominate interventions, attention should be given to the distal innominate artery using a 20° RAO, 20° caudal angiogram (see **Fig. 21**) with a predilatation balloon in place. We usually use a 6 × 20 or 7 × 20 predilatation balloon, and consider a short rapid exchange scoring balloon if the distal embolic protection is placed from femoral artery access, as discussed earlier. The innominate artery is short and is of larger diameter. Balloon-expandable covered stents are therefore usually not an option, because the shortest available covered stents are 38 mm in length. We use 10 × 25–29 balloon-expandable stents for most innominate interventions. The innominate artery is often subject to even more angulation of the arch than the left common carotid artery, and great care must be taken when placing the stent to ensure coverage of the ostium. This placement can sometimes be better accomplished via a brachial artery approach, but this requires a 7-Fr sheath and also requires concomitant femoral artery access for an imaging catheter for precise ostial positioning and placement.

There are significant limitations to performance of innominate interventions via radial or brachial

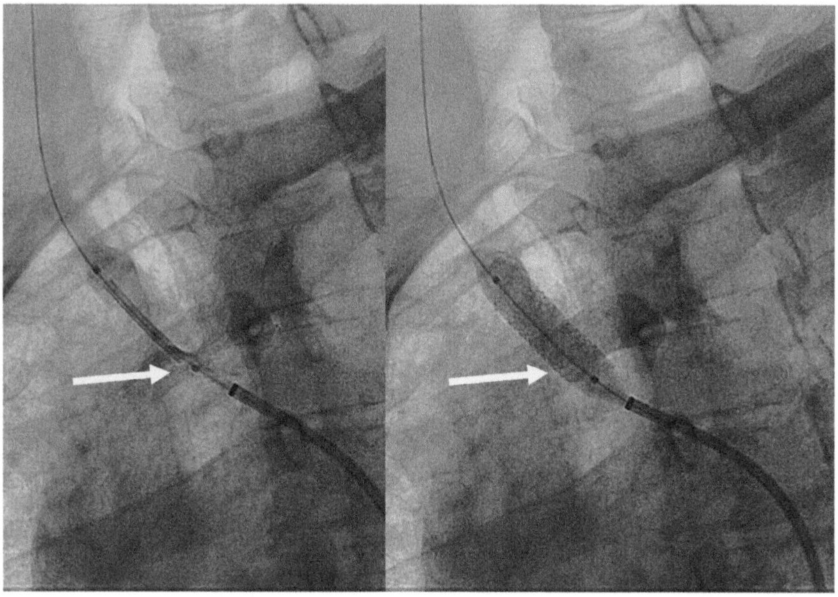

Fig. 23. Positioning and deploying innominate stent after predilatation. *Left arrow* shows proximal end of the stent relative to the aortic arch and *right arrow* shows inflated stent.

access. In general, embolic protection is not an option (both the embolic protection system and the stent cannot be placed via arm access, and the stent placed from arm access would trap an embolic protection wire placed from femoral access, making embolic protection device retrieval impossible). Also, larger sheaths are required, which is less attractive in the smaller radial and brachial arteries. If stenting is performed via arm access (without embolic protection), additional imaging from a second catheter placed in the aortic arch from an additional access site is required for accurate stent placement.

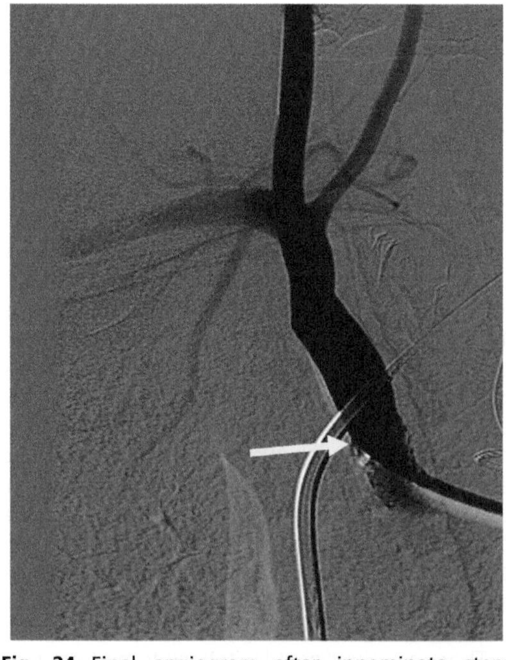

Fig. 24. Final angiogram after innominate stent placement.

In general, innominate interventions are complex with significant inherent risk, and should only be performed by experienced carotid and endovascular operators after a careful, individualized risk/benefit assessment. There are also surgical options of endarterectomy or bypass procedures that should be considered.

Endovascular Treatment of Concomitant Ostial Brachiocephalic Disease and Internal Carotid Artery Disease

In patients who have both ostial common carotid/innominate and internal carotid artery disease with appropriate indication for intervention, we use the following modified approach. After careful discussions and considerations and arch aortography, a 7-Fr shuttle sheath is placed in the descending aorta as discussed previously. We use the most appropriate neurodiagnostic catheter (with as little angulation as possible) to wire both the ostial and internal carotid artery lesions with 2 exchange length wires as previously discussed, and bring the shuttle sheath in close proximity while removing the neurodiagnostic catheter. The ostial lesion is predilated, usually with a 6-mm balloon. After reassessment, the shuttle sheath is advanced (with the dilator in the sheath) over both exchange length guide wires and using road

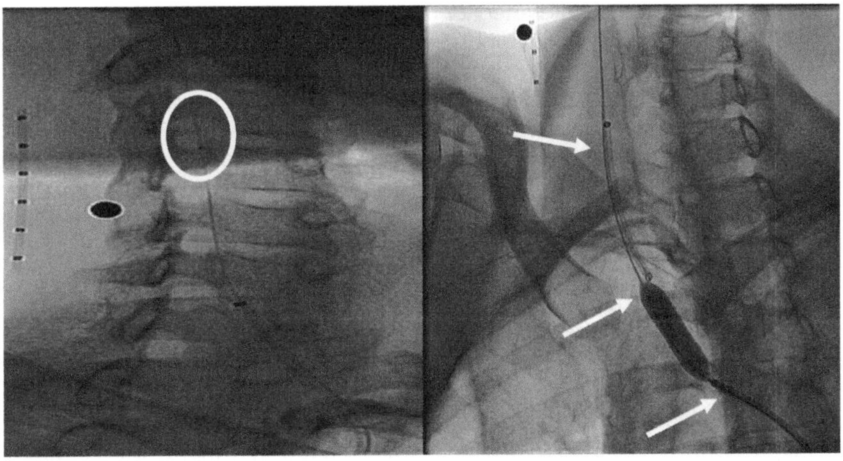

Fig. 25. Distal embolic protection device placed via right brachial access; innominate stented via femoral access.

mapping, with great care to avoid advancing the dilator of the sheath into the internal carotid artery. It is imperative to have all equipment for treatment of the internal carotid artery lesion prepared before advancing the shuttle sheath into the common carotid artery, because there can be diminished inflow even after predilatation of the ostial lesion. The internal carotid artery lesion is then treated per standard of care. After completion of the internal carotid stenting, the ostial 0.035 inch over-the-wire balloon-expandable stent is placed over both exchange length guide wires as discussed earlier. This stent is advanced into position while the shuttle sheath remains in the common carotid artery. With the stent in position, the shuttle sheath is withdrawn carefully, and the stent is unsheathed.

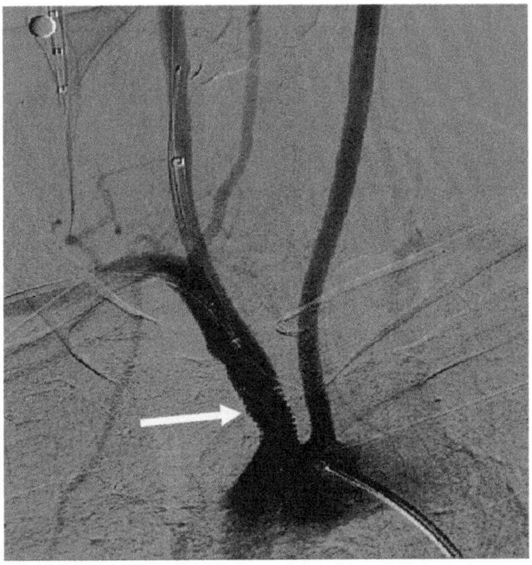

Fig. 26. Final angiogram after innominate stent placement.

The ostial stent is then deployed as the final interventional portion of the procedure as described previously, followed by removal of the embolic protection system.

If the aortic arch is steeply angulated and unfavorable for this technique, and the patient is an appropriate surgical candidate, a hybrid approach can be used. A standard internal carotid artery endarterectomy can be performed. Following successful completion of this, and with the distal clamp serving as embolic protection, a sheath can be placed antegrade into the endarterectomy patch and used to deliver the angioplasty balloon and balloon-expandable stent over an 0.035 inch guidewire. If this technique is used, it is often helpful to have femoral artery access to perform arch aortography for precise ostial positioning, and have adequate angiographic capabilities as defined earlier.

Ostial Vertebral Artery Interventions

This article focuses only on ostial vertebral intervention techniques. It is our opinion that intervention should be performed only in symptomatic lesions after careful discussions and considerations. Operators should be aware that endovascular vertebral intervention is not consistently reimbursed even if there are appropriate indications. In general, unilateral vertebral stenosis is unlikely to be symptomatic in the presence of an intact contralateral vertebral artery, and/or a patent circle of Willis. However, if there are clear-cut vertebrobasilar insufficiency symptoms (it may be helpful to obtain neurologic consultation for borderline symptoms), or if there are posterior strokes or transient ischemic attacks, endovascular intervention by experienced operators is appropriate and indicated.

In contrast with ostial common carotid artery or innominate lesions, we do not use distal embolic protection for most ostial vertebral interventions. For discrete ostial lesions, the embolic risk during intervention is low. In addition, the vertebral arteries are less ideal for the use of embolic protection devices, because they are often prone to spasm and are smaller, tortuous vessels. Furthermore, with ostial stents in these smaller arteries, retrieval of these devices can be technically challenging and lead to spasm and or dissection higher in the vertebral artery, such that the risk of using an embolic protection system usually exceeds its potential benefits.

For vertebral intervention in appropriate patients, we routinely perform 4-vessel cerebral angiography to determine the completeness of the circle of Willis and contributions to the posterior circulation before intervention. After this, and following anticoagulation, multiple access strategies can be considered. Often brachial or radial access is preferable if there is a more favorable angle into the vertebral artery. Either coronary guiding catheters or sheaths may be used depending on the arch and vertebral anatomy (if a sheath is used, it is often beneficial to place a second 0.014 inch or 0.018 inch guidewire into the subclavian artery for additional sheath stability). Our approach is to always predilate the lesion with a conservative 0.014 inch rapid exchange low-profile balloon. After predilatation, we routinely perform intravascular ultrasonography interrogation of the vertebral artery. This interrogation helps with precise selection of an appropriate stent, which is especially important because this vessel has a high rate of restenosis. If the artery is less than 4.5 mm in diameter, we consider a coronary drug-eluting stent in appropriate patients (this is an off-label use). If the vessel is greater than 4.5 mm, we select a rapid exchange, balloon-expandable, low-profile renal artery stent (again, off label). We carefully position this such that the stent clearly covers the ostial lesion, and accept a position slightly into the large lumen of the subclavian artery. Two angiographic views are obtained for positioning, and the contralateral cranial view usually provides the best delineation of the relationship of the vertebral artery origin to the subclavian artery. The patient's neurologic status is assessed throughout the procedure, and baseline and postprocedural cerebral angiograms are performed.

SUMMARY

Brachiocephalic disease can pose important clinical risks and manifestations. Most of these lesions are amenable to endovascular treatment. However, these treatments have significant risks associated with them and require modified procedural techniques. All interventions require a careful preprocedural evaluation and consultation, carefully weighing the risks and benefits of endovascular intervention versus the natural history of the disease with medical therapy or surgical intervention. These endovascular interventions should only be performed by experienced operators with extensive previous carotid and endovascular experience in appropriate adequately equipped venues. Most brachiocephalic disease also has surgical options for treatment, which should be carefully considered in a vascular team approach. It is hoped that the guidelines presented in this article can serve as an additional reference to assist experienced operators to perform these procedures with proper technique after using good clinical judgment.

REFERENCES

1. American Heart Association. Heart disease and stroke statistics. 2004. Available at: http://www.americanheart.org/downloadable/heart/1079736729696HDSStats2004Update REV3-19-04.pdf.
2. Yadav JS, Wholey MH, Kuntz RE, et al. Protected carotid artery stenting versus endarterectomy in high-risk patients. N Engl J Med 2004;351:1493–501.
3. Brott TG, Hobson RW, Roubin GS, et al, CREST Investigators. Stenting versus endarterectomy for treatment of carotid-artery stenosis. N Engl J Med 2010;363:11–23.
4. Myla S, Bacharach JM, Ansel GM, et al. Carotid artery stenting in high surgical risk patients using the FiberNet embolic protection system: the EPIC trial results. Catheter Cardiovasc Interv 2010;75:817–22.
5. The PROTECT Study, presented at 2009 International Stroke Conference at the American Heart Association 02/18/09, San Diego, CA; Chaturedi S, Gray WA, Matsumara J. Safety Outcomes for the PROTECT Carotid Artery Stenting Multicenter Study. Stroke 2009;40:2.
6. Hopkins LN. The EMPIRE trial results. Presented at TCT. Washington, DC, October 17, 2008.
7. Ansel GM, Hopkins LN, Jaff MR, et al. Safety and effectiveness of the Invatec MoMa proximal cerebral protection device during carotid artery stenting: results from the ARMOUR pivotal trial. Catheter Cardiovasc Interv 2010;76:1–8.
8. Bersin RM, Stabile E, Ansel GM, et al. A meta-analysis of proximal occlusion device outcomes in carotid artery stenting. Catheter Cardiovasc Interv 2012;80:1072–8.
9. Metzger DC, Hibbard D, Massop D, et al. Peri-procedural outcomes after carotid artery stenting in

the first 15,000 patients enrolled in SAPPHIRE WW Study. J Am Coll Cardiol 2012;60(Suppl B):17.
10. Massop D, Dave R, Metzger C, et al. Stenting and angioplasty with protection in patients at high risk for endarterectomy: SAPPHIRE World-Wide Registry in the first 2001 patients. Catheter Cardiovasc Interv 2009;73:129–36.
11. White CJ, Metzger DC, Ansel GM, et al. Safety and efficacy of carotid stenting in the very elderly. Catheter Cardiovasc Interv 2010;75(5):651–5.
12. Roubin GS, Iyer S, Halkin A, et al. Realizing the potential of carotid artery stenting proposed paradigms for patient selection and procedural technique. Circulation 2006;113:2021–30.
13. Montorsi P, Caputi L, Gali S, et al. Microembolization during carotid artery stenting in patients with high-risk, lipid-rich plaque. A randomized trial of proximal versus distal cerebral protection. J Am Coll Cardiol 2011;58:1656–63.
14. Birjuklic K, Wandler A, Hazizi F, et al. The PROFI Study (Prevention of Cerebral Embolization by Proximal Balloon Occlusion Compared to Filter Protection During Carotid Artery Stenting): a prospective, randomized trial. J Am Coll Cardiol 2012;59:1383–9.
15. Metzger DC. Skin to skin transfemoral carotid angiography and stenting. Intervent Cardiol Clin 2014;3(1):37–49.

Management of Mesenteric Ischemia

Anvar Babaev, MD, PhD*, David W. Lee, MD, Louai Razzouk, MD

KEYWORDS

• Mesenteric ischemia • Management • Endovascular therapy

KEY POINTS

- Acute mesenteric ischemia has a high mortality rate, and should be diagnosed early and managed surgically.
- Chronic mesenteric ischemia also has significant mortality and morbidity rates.
- Percutaneous or surgical revascularization for chronic mesenteric ischemia is indicated in symptomatic patients, with tailoring of the appropriate therapy based on patients' comorbidities, vascular anatomy, life expectancy, and goals of care.

INTRODUCTION

Mesenteric ischemia is an uncommon clinical condition that manifests in the chronic form as postprandial abdominal pain with weight loss and emaciation, and in the acute form as sudden onset of abdominal pain, lower gastrointestinal bleeding, and intestinal necrosis. Both forms are fatal if left untreated. Despite major developments in noninvasive and invasive modalities, the diagnosis of chronic mesenteric ischemia remains challenging. Occlusive disease of the mesenteric arteries occurs frequently in the elderly population, especially those with established atherosclerotic disease. In asymptomatic patients with abdominal aortic aneurysms, 40% have evidence of mesenteric stenosis on angiography.[1] In patients with renal artery stenosis, the reported prevalence of severe mesenteric artery stenosis exceeds 50%.[1]

ANATOMY

The mesenteric arterial vasculature includes the following anterior branches of the abdominal aorta: the celiac artery, the superior mesenteric artery (SMA), and the inferior mesenteric artery (IMA) (**Fig. 1**).

Celiac Artery

The first major branch of the abdominal aorta is the celiac artery, which usually arises at the level of the twelfth thoracic vertebra and courses anteriorly and slightly inferiorly. In most patients, the celiac artery gives off the left gastric artery and then bifurcates into the splenic artery to the left and the common hepatic artery to the right.

Superior Mesenteric Artery

The second major branch of the abdominal aorta is the SMA, which typically arises at the level of the first lumbar vertebra, just inferior to the celiac trunk. It initially gives off the inferior pancreaticoduodenal artery to the right and then courses inferiorly to the right. Along the left surface of the SMA, 4 to 6 jejunal arteries arise, followed by 8 to 12 ileal arteries. Along the right surface of the SMA, the middle colic artery arises followed by the right colic artery and the ileocolic artery, supplying the ascending and transverse colon.

Inferior Mesenteric Artery

The third major branch of the abdominal aorta is the IMA, which typically arises at the level of the

Relationship with Industry: Drs L. Razzouk and D.W. Lee have no conflicts of interest to report. Dr A. Babaev has received honoraria for physician training courses from: Abbott, CSI, Medtronic, and Cook Medical.
Division of Cardiology, NYU Langone Medical Center, New York, NY 10069, USA
* Corresponding author. NYU Langone Medical Center, 530 First Avenue, HCC14, New York, NY 10069.
E-mail address: anvar.babaev@nyumc.org

Intervent Cardiol Clin 3 (2014) 493–500
http://dx.doi.org/10.1016/j.iccl.2014.06.005

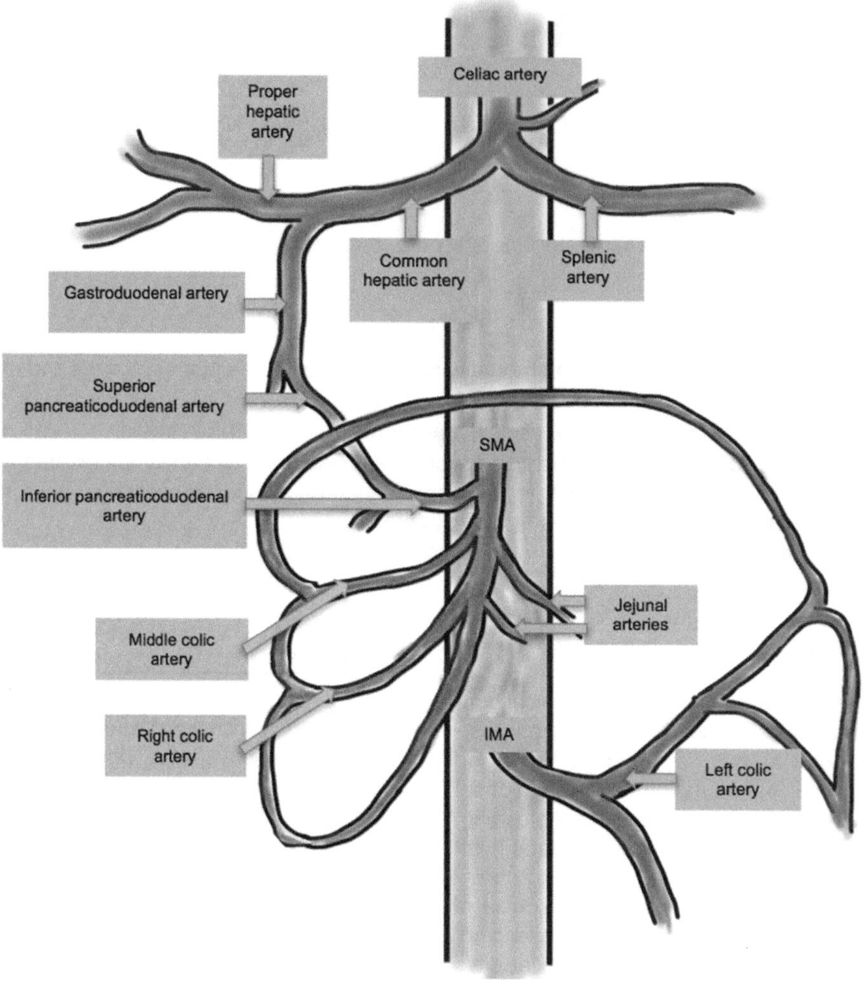

Fig. 1. Abdominal aorta and mesenteric vascular anatomy.

third lumbar vertebra and courses inferiorly to the left. Branches of the IMA typically supply the descending colon, sigmoid, and rectum; these branches include the left colic artery, the marginal artery, the sigmoid artery, and superior hemorrhoidal arteries.

Collateral Circulation

Several important collateral pathways exist among the 3 major branches. The branches of the superior and inferior pancreaticoduodenal arteries anastomose, providing collateral circulation between the celiac artery and the SMA. The arc of Riolan and the marginal artery of Drummond run along the colon and connect the right, middle, and left colic arteries, providing collateral circulation between the SMA and IMA. In addition, multiple hemorrhoidal arteries provide collateral circulation between the IMA and internal iliac arteries.

ACUTE MESENTERIC ISCHEMIA

Acute mesenteric ischemia (AMI) is a surgical emergency with a reported mortality rate ranging from 60% to 80%.[2–4] AMI results from an abrupt interruption in mesenteric perfusion, which leads to bowel ischemia and eventually infarction. It can be caused by arterial embolism in 50% of cases, arterial thrombosis in 20%, nonocclusive arterial disease in 20%, and venous thrombosis in 10% (**Table 1**).[5] The clinical presentation of patients with AMI varies based on the cause. Patients with occlusive AMI in the setting of embolism or thrombosis usually present with acute abdominal pain that does not worsen with palpation and is, classically, out of proportion to physical

Table 1
Risk factors in acute mesenteric ischemia

Etiology	Arterial Embolism	Arterial Thrombosis	Nonocclusive Disease	Venous Thrombosis
Risk factors	• Arrhythmia • Myocardial ischemia • Myocardial infarction • Cardiomyopathy • Valvular disease • Ventricular aneurysm • Aortic aneurysm • Recent aortic catheterization ○ Coronary angiography ○ Cerebral angiography	• Atherosclerosis • Hypercoagulable state ○ Smoking ○ Pregnancy ○ Oral contraceptives ○ Malignancy ○ Cirrhosis ○ Antithrombin III deficiency ○ Protein C deficiency ○ Protein S deficiency ○ Factor V Leiden mutation ○ Lupus anticoagulant	• Hypotension • Hypovolemia • Cardiogenic shock • Vasoconstrictors ○ Epinephrine ○ Norepinephrine ○ Phenylephrine ○ Vasopressin • Vasoactive drugs ○ Digoxin ○ Cocaine ○ Ergots • Recent aortic coarctation repair	• Hypercoagulable state ○ Smoking ○ Pregnancy ○ Oral contraceptives ○ Malignancy ○ Cirrhosis ○ Antithrombin III deficiency ○ Protein C deficiency ○ Protein S deficiency ○ Factor V Leiden mutation ○ Lupus anticoagulant • Sepsis • Pancreatitis • Intra-abdominal infection • Abdominal trauma • Abdominal surgery

examination findings. Diarrhea and vomiting may also occur but are nonspecific symptoms. The abdominal pain tends to be diffuse initially and then localizes with progression of ischemia. Patients with acute nonocclusive disease typically have vague abdominal symptoms in the setting of critical illness. Finally, patients with acute mesenteric venous thrombosis usually present with gradually worsening diffuse abdominal discomfort. In all cases, bloody stools are usually a sign of progressive bowel ischemia and infarction.

Given its high mortality rate, patients with a suspicious clinical presentation should undergo emergent evaluation. Computed tomography angiography (CTA) with 3-dimensional (3D) reconstruction is the gold standard for diagnosing AMI, with 96% sensitivity and 94% specificity.[2,6,7] Patients diagnosed with acute occlusive mesenteric ischemia or with suspected bowel infarction, regardless of cause, should undergo emergent exploratory laparotomy with subsequent revascularization, assessment for bowel viability, and resection of necrotic bowel (**Table 2**).[8,9] Initial management before surgery includes volume resuscitation with isotonic fluids, broad-spectrum antibiotics, and systemic anticoagulation with heparin infusion if no contraindication exists. Acute mesenteric arterial occlusion can be surgically managed by embolectomy, endarterectomy, arterial bypass, or retrograde open mesenteric stenting.[2,5]

Patients with acute nonocclusive mesenteric ischemia can initially be managed medically by treating the underlying cause of hypoperfusion.[9] In more than 60% of cases, acute nonocclusive mesenteric ischemia has been successfully managed nonsurgically through fluid resuscitation, antibiotics, and bowel rest.[5] Likewise, patients with acute mesenteric venous thrombosis can also be managed medically by starting an unfractionated heparin bolus followed by a continuous infusion. Exploratory laparotomy is indicated in patients who are initially medically managed and whose symptoms do not improve after initial treatment.[9]

Angiography, which was previously considered the gold standard in diagnosis, has become popular for percutaneous endovascular therapy. Although open laparotomy with surgical or endovascular revascularization remains the standard in management of AMI, increasing evidence shows that primary endovascular therapy reduces mortality and complications.[10–12]

CHRONIC MESENTERIC ISCHEMIA

Chronic mesenteric ischemia (CMI) is most commonly caused by progressive atherosclerotic

Table 2
Current treatment guidelines for acute and chronic mesenteric ischemia

Presentation		Therapy
Acute mesenteric ischemia	Arterial obstruction	Surgical treatment includes revascularization, resection of necrotic bowel, and a second-look operation 24–48 h after the revascularization (class I, level of evidence B). Percutaneous interventions are appropriate in selected patients. Patients may still require laparotomy (class IIb, level of evidence C).
	Nonocclusive ischemia	Treatment of the underlying shock state is the most important initial step (class I, level of evidence C). Patients with persistent symptoms despite initial treatment should undergo laparotomy and resection of nonviable bowel in (class I, level of evidence B).
Chronic mesenteric ischemia		Percutaneous endovascular treatment of intestinal arterial stenosis is indicated (class I, level of evidence B). Surgical treatment is indicated in patients with chronic intestinal ischemia (class I, level of evidence B). Revascularization of asymptomatic intestinal arterial obstructions may be considered in patients undergoing aortic/renal artery surgery for other indications (class IIb, level of evidence B). Surgical revascularization is not indicated for patients with asymptomatic intestinal arterial obstruction, except in patients undergoing aortic/renal artery surgery for other indications (class III, level of evidence B).

Adapted from Hirsch AT, Haskal ZJ, Hertzer NR, et al. ACC/AHA 2005 Practice guidelines for the management of patients with peripheral arterial disease (lower extremity, renal, mesenteric, and abdominal aortic): a collaborative report from the American Association for Vascular Surgery/Society for Vascular Surgery, Society for Cardiovascular Angiography and Interventions, Society for Vascular Medicine and Biology, Society of Interventional Radiology, and the ACC/AHA Task Force on Practice Guidelines (Writing Committee to Develop Guidelines for the Management of Patients With Peripheral Arterial Disease): endorsed by the American Association of Cardiovascular and Pulmonary Rehabilitation;

stenosis or occlusion of the mesenteric arterial circulation.[13] Because of the presence of extensive collateral network between arteries, patients usually remain asymptomatic until at least 2 major mesenteric arteries develop a critical level of stenosis or total occlusion. A systematic review showed that, although only 14% of patients with CMI undergoing revascularization had single-vessel disease, 42% had 2-vessel disease and 44% had 3-vessel disease.[14] Less common causes include superior mesenteric vein thrombosis, fibromuscular dysplasia, Takayasu arteritis, and external compression from mesenteric tumors or the median arcuate ligament.[13]

In contrast to those with AMI, patients with CMI have a more insidious clinical presentation. Patients classically present with recurrent postprandial abdominal pain. Also known as *intestinal angina*, the abdominal pain usually occurs within the first hour after eating and persists for several hours. Patients can become reluctant to eat and develop sitophobia, the fear of food, which can lead to significant weight loss. Similar to the acute presentation, the abdominal pain tends to be out of proportion to physical examination findings.

Abdominal Doppler ultrasound is the best initial diagnostic screening modality, and allows for calculation of peak systolic velocity (PSV). Studies have shown that a PSV greater than 200 cm/s in the celiac artery is 87% sensitive and 80% specific for an angiographic stenosis greater than 70%.[15] A PSV greater than 275 cm/s in the SMA is 92% sensitive and 96% specific for an angiographic stenosis of greater than 70%.[15] Both CTA and magnetic resonance angiography can be used to confirm the diagnosis of CMI with excellent sensitivity and specificity. In patients with indeterminate results on noninvasive imaging, both nonselective and selective invasive angiography are indicated for further diagnostic evaluation of CMI.

MANAGEMENT OF CHRONIC MESENTERIC ISCHEMIA

Surgical revascularization (SR) for symptomatic CMI has been the gold standard of therapy since its introduction in 1958.[16] Endovascular revascularization (ER) with percutaneous angioplasty and stenting of the mesenteric arteries was introduced in 1980.[17] Over the past 20 years, a surge has occurred in the total number of revascularization procedures performed, predominantly driven by an increase in the number of ERs (**Fig. 2**).[10] Because of the low prevalence of symptomatic patients, no large-scale randomized controlled trials have compared outcomes between SR and ER.

In a meta-analysis published in 2010, Gupta and colleagues[18] collected data from 25 studies between 1990 and 2009 that included 1163 patients who underwent SR and 776 patients who underwent ER. The meta-analysis showed no difference in mortality comparing these groups.[18] From 2000 to 2009, patients who underwent SR had a higher 5-year primary patency rate (odds ratio [OR], 3.8; $P<.001$), but a higher complication rate (OR, 3.2; $P<.001$).[18] Because significant differences were seen in the baseline characteristics between the groups, this meta-analysis was found to have significant selection bias in the choice of revascularization. A more recent meta-analysis published in 2013 collected data from 43 studies between 1986 and 2010 that included 1795 patients.[19] In this analysis, perioperative mortality and perioperative morbidity rates were lower in the ER group than in the SR group (perioperative mortality 3.6% vs 7.2%, $P<.001$; perioperative morbidity 13.2% vs 33.1%, $P<.001$).[19] However, if the patient survived open surgery, the survival rate at 5 years was the same for both groups.[19] Primary and secondary patency rates at 5 years were superior in the surgical group (primary patency 49.12% vs 80.9%, $P<.001$; secondary patency 87.9% vs 97.9%, $P<.001$).[19] In a large retrospective study of 5583 patients with CMI from 2000 to 2006, Schermerhorn and colleagues[10] found a lower mortality rate after ER compared with SR (**Table 3**).

In the American College of Cardiology/American Heart Association (ACC/AHA) 2005 practice guidelines for peripheral artery disease, both percutaneous and surgical revascularization approaches have a class I indication for the treatment of symptomatic CMI (see **Table 2**).[9] Important factors that should be considered when determining the method of revascularization for CMI include patient preference, vascular anatomy, comorbidities, nutritional status, and predicted life expectancy. The fact that ER carries a lower risk of mortality and complications may explain the substantial increase in ER procedures but the flat rate of surgeries over the past 10 years (see **Fig. 2**).

ENDOVASCULAR TECHNIQUES

Access and Angiography

Access can be obtained via the femoral artery, the radial artery, or the brachial artery, with each access site having its inherent limitations. Arteriography is performed with a pigtail catheter placed at the twelfth level of the thoracic vertebra. To visualize the origins of the celiac artery and the SMA, steep lateral angles and anteroposterior views are necessary. Selective catheterization of the individual visceral arteries is then obtained to assess for the presence of stenosis and for collateral flow. Commonly used diagnostic catheters (5 or 6 Fr) are similar to the ones used to engage the renal arteries (IMA catheter, Judkins Right, Cobra, Renal double curve, Simmons, and the multipurpose when using brachial access).

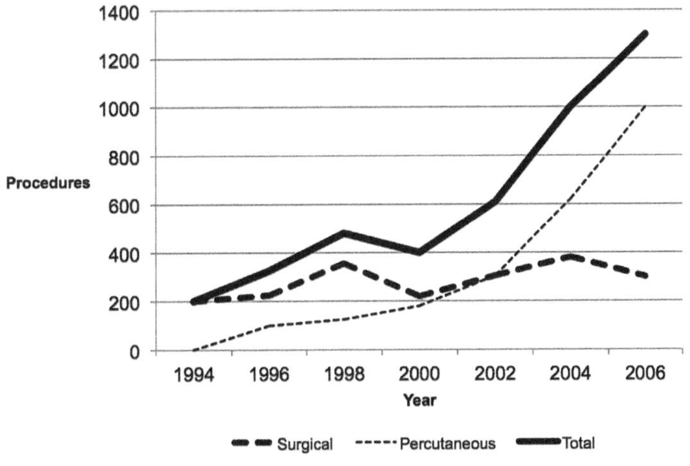

Fig. 2. Trends in revascularization of chronic mesenteric ischemia from 1994 to 2006. (*Adapted from* Schermerhorn ML, Giles KA, Hamdan AD, et al. Mesenteric revascularization: management and outcomes in the United States, 1988-2006. J Vasc Surg 2009;50(2):341–8.e1.)

Table 3
Comparison of mortality and periprocedural complications between surgical and endovascular revascularization for chronic mesenteric ischemia from 2000 to 2006

	Surgical Revascularization	Endovascular Revascularization	*P* Value
Patients, n	2128	3455	
All-cause mortality	15.4%	3.7%	<.001
Mortality by age group			
Age <60 y	8.8%	0.7%	<.01
Age 60–70 y	14.8%	2.4%	<.001
Age 70–80 y	14.1%	3.8%	<.001
Age >80 y	39.2%	6.8%	<.001
All complications	39.7%	20.2%	<.001
Type of complication			
Acute myocardial infarction	4.8%	3.0%	.13
Cardiac	5.9%	0.7%	<.001
Pulmonary	5.3%	0.3%	<.001
Stroke	0.7%	0%	<.05
Bowel resection	8.0%	3.0%	<.001

Data from Schermerhorn ML, Giles KA, Hamdan AD, et al. Mesenteric revascularization: management and outcomes in the United States, 1988–2006. J Vasc Surg 2009;50(2):341–8.e1.

After placement of a guiding catheter (typically 6 or 7 Fr), a 0.014" or 0.018" guidewire is used to cross the lesion and balloon angioplasty is performed. A guidewire with a good shaft support is recommended. After careful measurement of the reference vessel diameter (RVD) with quantitative angiography, an angioplasty is performed. Typical ostial diameters of the arteries are 3 to 6 mm for the IMA, 4 to 7 mm for the SMA, and 6 to 8 mm for the celiac artery. The lesion is then dilated with a

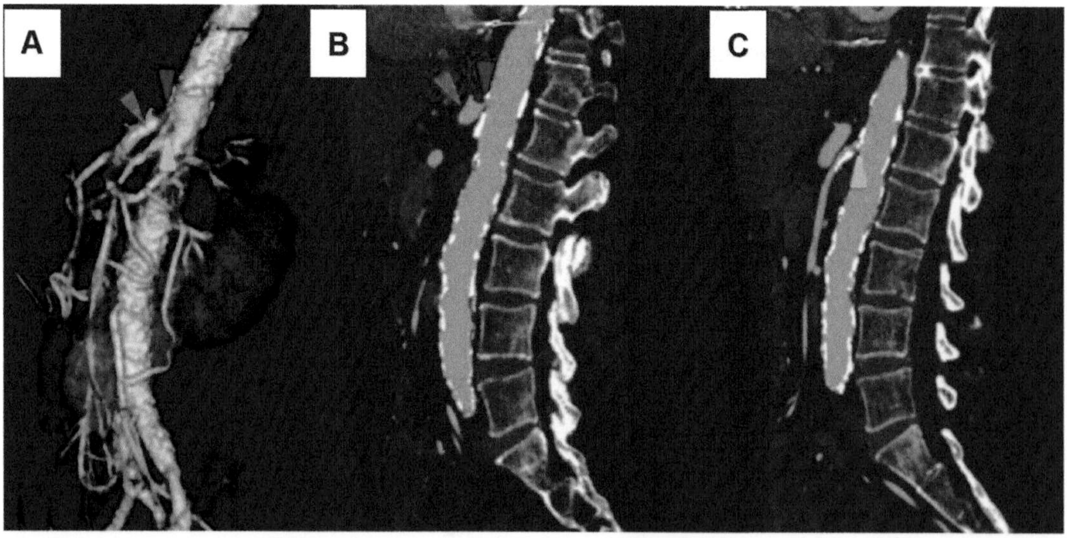

Fig. 3. (*A*) Three-dimensional reconstruction on CTA of a 75-year-old man with ischemic colitis with a high-grade stenosis in the superior mesenteric artery (*green arrowhead*) and a high-grade stenosis in the celiac artery (*red arrowhead*) with downstream poststenotic dilatation (*blue arrowhead*). (*B*) Slice of CTA showing the high-grade stenosis in the celiac artery (*red arrowhead*) with downstream poststenotic dilatation (*blue arrowhead*). (*C*) Slice of CTA showing the high-grade stenosis in the superior mesenteric artery (*green arrowhead*).

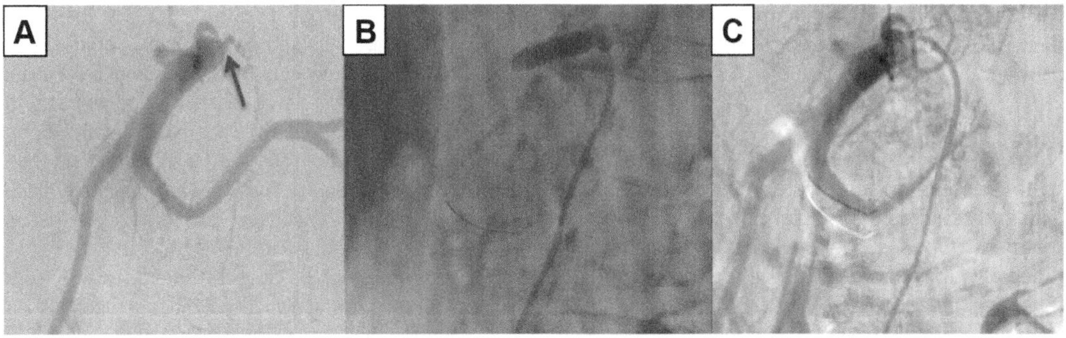

Fig. 4. (*A*) Severe ostial celiac artery stenosis (*arrow*) shown on digital-subtraction angiography (DSA) in the same 75-year-old man with ischemic colitis. (*B*) Balloon-expandable stent (Herculink 7.0 × 18 mm) deployment at ostium of celiac artery under fluoroscopy after balloon angioplasty. (*C*) DSA after stent deployment showing good stent apposition and widely patent flow down the celiac artery.

balloon matching the size 1:1 with the RVD, using the lowest pressure that will fully expand the balloon.

When choosing the type of noncovered bare metal stents needed for intervention, balloon-expandable stents (BES) are thought to be superior to self-expanding stents because of the typical aorto-ostial nature of mesenteric atherosclerosis and the need for significant radial force and precise positioning. When treating ostial lesions, it is also important to protrude the stent about 1 mm into the aorta to ensure complete coverage of the ostium of the artery. Self-expanding stents can be safely used for more distal or longer lesions of arterial trunk.

In patients who undergo ER with stents, recent data suggest superiority of covered stents compared with noncovered bare metal stents. This finding was confirmed in a study of 225 patients who were treated at 2 academic centers for CMI between 2000 and 2010, and showed higher freedom from restenosis in the polytetrafluoroethylene-covered stents group compared with the bare metal stents group (92% vs 56%; *P* = .005).[20]

To prevent thrombosis, patients are typically started on antiplatelet therapy with aspirin and clopidogrel before the procedure and on systemic anticoagulation with intravenous heparin administration after vascular access is obtained.

Sample Case

A 75-year-old man with past medical history of severe congestive heart failure, coronary artery disease, and atrial fibrillation presented with typical symptoms of CMI. He underwent CTA of the abdomen (**Fig. 3**), which showed severe ostial stenoses of the celiac artery, SMA, and IMA. Given the patient's age and significant comorbidities, the decision was made to proceed with ER as a primary approach. Digital-subtraction angiography confirmed the CTA findings and the patient underwent successful placement of 2 BES in the celiac and SMA (**Figs. 4** and **5**). The patient

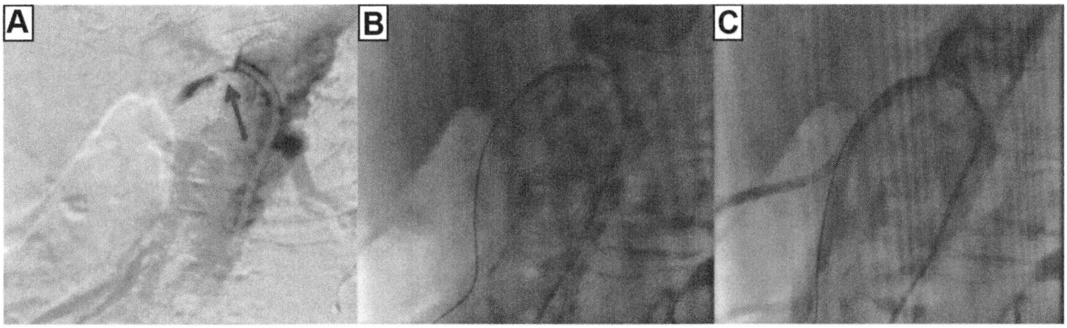

Fig. 5. (*A*) Severe ostial superior mesenteric artery (SMA) stenosis (*arrow*) shown on digital-subtraction angiography in the same 75-year-old man with ischemic colitis shown in **Figs. 3** and **4**. (*B*) Initial angioplasty of ostial stenosis with a small-diameter noncompliant balloon (Quantum 3.0 × 20 mm) under fluoroscopy. (*C*) Fluoroscopy and angiogram after deployment of a balloon-expandable stent (Herculink 6.0 × 18 mm) show good stent apposition and widely patent flow down the SMA.

was discharged home the same day of the procedure, and was asymptomatic on outpatient clinic follow-up.

SUMMARY

Acute mesenteric ischemia can lead to high mortality and requires early diagnostic evaluation and treatment. Open surgery allows for assessment of bowel viability and remains the primary method of revascularization in AMI. Chronic mesenteric ischemia can also lead to significant mortality and poor quality of life. Patients with CMI can undergo either endovascular or surgical revascularization. In recent studies, ER has been shown to have lower mortality and morbidity rates compared with SR, and could be considered as a preferable first-line revascularization approach.

REFERENCES

1. Valentine RJ, Martin JD, Myers SI, et al. Asymptomatic celiac and superior mesenteric artery stenoses are more prevalent among patients with unsuspected renal artery stenoses. J Vasc Surg 1991;14(2):195–9.
2. Wyers MC. Acute mesenteric ischemia: diagnostic approach and surgical treatment. Semin Vasc Surg 2010;23(1):9–20.
3. Oldenburg WA, Lau LL, Rodenberg TJ, et al. Acute mesenteric ischemia: a clinical review. Arch Intern Med 2004;164(10):1054–62.
4. Kassahun WT, Schulz T, Richter O, et al. Unchanged high mortality rates from acute occlusive intestinal ischemia: six year review. Langenbecks Arch Surg 2008;393(2):163–71.
5. Sise MJ. Acute mesenteric ischemia. Surg Clin North Am 2014;94(1):165–81.
6. Oliva IB, Davarpanah AH, Rybicki FJ, et al. ACR Appropriateness Criteria (R) imaging of mesenteric ischemia. Abdom Imaging 2013;38(4):714–9.
7. Menke J. Diagnostic accuracy of multidetector CT in acute mesenteric ischemia: systematic review and meta-analysis. Radiology 2010;256(1):93–101.
8. American Gastroenterological Association Medical Position Statement: guidelines on intestinal ischemia. Gastroenterology 2000;118(5):951–3.
9. Hirsch AT, Haskal ZJ, Hertzer NR, et al. ACC/AHA 2005 Practice Guidelines for the management of patients with peripheral arterial disease (lower extremity, renal, mesenteric, and abdominal aortic): a collaborative report from the American Association for Vascular Surgery/Society for Vascular Surgery, Society for Cardiovascular Angiography and Interventions, Society for Vascular Medicine and Biology, Society of Interventional Radiology, and the ACC/AHA Task Force on Practice Guidelines (Writing Committee to Develop Guidelines for the Management of Patients With Peripheral Arterial Disease): endorsed by the American Association of Cardiovascular and Pulmonary Rehabilitation; National Heart, Lung, and Blood Institute; Society for Vascular Nursing; TransAtlantic Inter-Society Consensus; and Vascular Disease Foundation. Circulation 2006;113(11):e463–654.
10. Schermerhorn ML, Giles KA, Hamdan AD, et al. Mesenteric revascularization: management and outcomes in the United States, 1988-2006. J Vasc Surg 2009;50(2):341–8.e1.
11. Beaulieu RJ, Arnaoutakis KD, Abularrage CJ, et al. Comparison of open and endovascular treatment of acute mesenteric ischemia. J Vasc Surg 2014; 59(1):159–64.
12. Arthurs ZM, Titus J, Bannazadeh M, et al. A comparison of endovascular revascularization with traditional therapy for the treatment of acute mesenteric ischemia. J Vasc Surg 2011; 53(3):698–704 [discussion: 704–5].
13. Chandra A, Quinones-Baldrich WJ. Chronic mesenteric ischemia: how to select patients for invasive treatment. Semin Vasc Surg 2010;23(1):21–8.
14. Oderich GS, Malgor RD, Ricotta JJ 2nd. Open and endovascular revascularization for chronic mesenteric ischemia: tabular review of the literature. Ann Vasc Surg 2009;23(5):700–12.
15. Moneta GL, Lee RW, Yeager RA, et al. Mesenteric duplex scanning: a blinded prospective study. J Vasc Surg 1993;17(1):79–84 [discussion: 85–6].
16. Shaw RS, Maynard EP 3rd. Acute and chronic thrombosis of the mesenteric arteries associated with malabsorption; a report of two cases successfully treated by thromboendarterectomy. N Engl J Med 1958;258(18):874–8.
17. Furrer J, Gruntzig A, Kugelmeier J, et al. Treatment of abdominal angina with percutaneous dilatation of an arteria mesenterica superior stenosis. Preliminary communication. Cardiovasc Intervent Radiol 1980;3(1):43–4.
18. Gupta PK, Horan SM, Turaga KK, et al. Chronic mesenteric ischemia: endovascular versus open revascularization. J Endovasc Ther 2010;17(4): 540–9.
19. Pecoraro F, Rancic Z, Lachat M, et al. Chronic mesenteric ischemia: critical review and guidelines for management. Ann Vasc Surg 2013; 27(1):113–22.
20. Oderich GS, Erdoes LS, Lesar C, et al. Comparison of covered stents versus bare metal stents for treatment of chronic atherosclerotic mesenteric arterial disease. J Vasc Surg 2013;58(5):1316–23.

Management of Renal Arterial Disease

Jun Li, MD[a,b], Sahil A. Parikh, MD[b,c,*]

KEYWORDS

- Atherosclerotic renal artery stenosis • Renal artery stenting • Resistant hypertension
- Ischemic nephropathy • Cardiac disturbance syndrome

KEY POINTS

- Noninvasive testing can be used for screening for renal artery stenosis in the patient presenting with symptoms consistent with renovascular disease.
- Invasive testing and intervention can be performed safely by the experienced operator, with a high success rate.
- Patient history and workup are vital to determine the appropriate candidate for revascularization.
- Revascularization is appropriate in patients with cardiac disturbance syndromes (recurrent flash pulmonary edema, heart failure, and unstable angina), refractory or malignant hypertension, and ongoing renal ischemia.
- Contemporary randomized controlled trials affirm that optimal medical therapy should be first implemented before pursuing revascularization in most cases.

INTRODUCTION

The influences of the renal system on cardiovascular health have been described as early as 1836 by Richard Bright.[1] In 1934, Goldblatt, working in the Western Reserve of Cleveland, described a method by which sequential, partial constriction of both renal arteries in a dog reliably produced hypertension.[2] During the next 25 years, investigators sought the pathway that would later become the enzymatic relationship between renin and angiotensin.[1]

It is now well established that renal artery stenosis activates the renin-angiotensin-aldosterone system (RAAS), causing systemic hypertension. The most common cause of renal artery stenosis is atherosclerosis. Other less prominent causes include fibromuscular dysplasia (FMD), vasculitis, embolic phenomenon, and trauma. Owing to the prevalence of atherosclerotic renal artery stenosis (ARAS) and the continued debate on its clinical management, this review addresses the pathophysiology and management of the condition.

ARAS is defined as stenosis 50% or more in the proximal one-third of a renal artery.[3] ARAS has been estimated to affect 1% to 5% of patients with essential hypertension.[4] The prevalence increases to 20% to 40% in certain patient populations, for example, in patients with severe or refractory hypertension, with documented multivessel coronary artery disease, and with newly

Disclosures: Dr J. Li reports no disclosures. Dr S.A. Parikh serves as a consultant for Abbott Vascular, Boston Scientific, and Medtronic and receives research support from Atrium Medical, Boston Scientific and Medtronic.
[a] Department of Medicine, Case Western Reserve University School of Medicine, 11100 Euclid Avenue, Cleveland, OH 44106, USA; [b] Division of Cardiovascular Medicine, Harrington Heart and Vascular Institute, University Hospitals Case Medical Center, 11100 Euclid Avenue, Cleveland, OH 44106, USA; [c] Interventional Cardiology Fellowship Program, Experimental Interventional Cardiology Laboratory, Department of Medicine, Case Western Reserve University School of Medicine, 11100 Euclid Avenue, Cleveland, OH 44106, USA
* Corresponding author. Division of Cardiovascular Medicine, Harrington Heart and Vascular Institute, University Hospitals Case Medical Center, 11100 Euclid Avenue, Cleveland, OH 44106.
E-mail address: Sahil.Parikh@UHhospitals.org

Intervent Cardiol Clin 3 (2014) 501–516
http://dx.doi.org/10.1016/j.iccl.2014.06.002

initiated hemodialysis.[5–7] The presence of ARAS is associated with atherosclerotic disease in other vascular beds, which renders it an important surrogate for coronary, carotid, and peripheral arterial disease.[4,8,9]

The common clinical scenarios that prompt a clinician to consider the diagnosis of ARAS include the following:

1. A patient with poorly controlled hypertension despite the use of multiple antihypertensives
2. A patient with chronic kidney disease whose kidney function worsens with initiation of an RAAS blocking agent
3. A patient with recurrent flash pulmonary edema despite a normal left ventricular systolic function (**Box 1**)[10–12]

The diagnosing clinician must exercise vigilance, as it is feasible that the presence of ARAS is simply a bystander of an underlying medical renal disease from another cause, such as diabetic nephropathy. Similarly, the concomitant presence of hypertension and renal artery stenosis in a patient does not always imply the diagnosis of renovascular hypertension, as hypertension is known to result in increased systemic atherosclerotic burden and may in fact lead to ARAS.[13]

Appropriate patient selection for referral for renal artery revascularization is vital for procedural success and adequate clinical response. The favorable patient profile includes hemodynamically significant stenoses in bilateral renal arteries or in a solitary kidney, cardiac disturbance syndromes consisting of flash pulmonary edema or exacerbation of coronary ischemia in setting of peripheral arterial vasoconstriction, and ischemic nephropathy resulting in a rapid decline of renal function.[14–16] These characteristics are highlighted in the most up-to-date American College of Cardiology/American Heart Association (ACC/AHA) Practice Guidelines and reflect class I and II recommendations for renal artery revascularization (**Table 1**).

Box 1
Common clinical scenarios to prompt workup for renal artery stenosis

Indications for noninvasive testing for atherosclerotic renal artery stenosis

- Cardiac disturbance syndromes
  - Recurrent flash pulmonary edema
  - Refractory heart failure
  - Refractory unstable angina
- Hypertension
  - Accelerated, defined as sudden and persistent worsening of previously well-controlled hypertension
  - Resistant, defined as inability to achieve goal blood pressure with greater than or equal to 3 antihypertensive agents
  - Malignant, defined as coexistence with end-organ damage
  - Onset of hypertension at a young age (<30 years old)
- Rapidly progressive renal dysfunction
  - Acute worsening of kidney dysfunction with initiation of an RAAS blocking agent
  - New initiation of renal replacement therapy
- Asymmetric atrophic kidney with greater than 1.5 cm discrepancy in size
- Evaluation of a prior renal artery stent

Data from Hirsch AT, Haskal ZJ, Hertzer NR, et al. ACC/AHA 2005 guidelines for the management of patients with peripheral arterial disease (lower extremity, renal, mesenteric, and abdominal aortic): executive summary a collaborative report from the American Association for Vascular Surgery/Society for Vascular Surgery, Society for Cardiovascular Angiography and Interventions, Society for Vascular Medicine and Biology, Society of Interventional Radiology, and the ACC/AHA Task Force on Practice Guidelines (writing committee to develop guidelines for the management of patients with peripheral arterial disease) endorsed by the American Association of Cardiovascular and Pulmonary Rehabilitation; National Heart, Lung, and Blood Institute; Society for Vascular Nursing; TransAtlantic Inter-Society Consensus; and Vascular Disease Foundation. J Am Coll Cardiol 2006;47(6):1239–312; and Gerhard-Herman M, Gardin JM, Jaff M, et al. Guidelines for noninvasive vascular laboratory testing: a report from the American Society of Echocardiography and the Society of Vascular Medicine and Biology. J Am Soc Echocardiogr 2006;19(8):955–72.

PATHOPHYSIOLOGY

The presence of renal artery stenosis results in decreased perfusion pressure to the juxtaglomerular apparatus (JGA), prompting the release of renin. Activation of the RAAS results in subsequent retention of salt and water to create a hypertensive milieu and increased perfusion back to normal in the poststenotic JGA and its associated nephron (**Fig. 1**). Unilateral ARAS creates a concomitant increase in flow to the nonstenotic kidney. Pressure natriuresis occurs in the contralateral and unaffected kidney, ultimately resulting in a decrease in systemic blood pressure back to normal. In bilateral ARAS, RAAS activation increases the perfusion pressure of the poststenotic JGA back to normal. However, the lack of natriuresis causes

Table 1
The most recent ACC/AHA guidelines on indications for renal artery revascularization

Indication	Recommendation	Level of Evidence
Hemodynamically significant RAS with		
Recurrent and unexplained heart failure	Class I	B
Recurrent and unexplained pulmonary edema	Class I	B
Accelerated, resistant, or malignant hypertension	Class IIa	B
Inability to tolerate antihypertensives	Class IIa	B
Unstable angina	Class IIa	B
Chronic renal insufficiency and worsening renal function	Class IIa	B
Asymptomatic bilateral or solitary kidney ARAS with viable kidneys	Class IIb	C
Asymptomatic unilateral ARAS in a viable kidney	Class IIb	C
Chronic renal insufficiency in unilateral ARAS (with 2 kidneys present)	Class IIb	C

Data from Hirsch AT, Haskal ZJ, Hertzer NR, et al. ACC/AHA 2005 guidelines for the management of patients with peripheral arterial disease (lower extremity, renal, mesenteric, and abdominal aortic): executive summary a collaborative report from the American Association for Vascular Surgery/Society for Vascular Surgery, Society for Cardiovascular Angiography and Interventions, Society for Vascular Medicine and Biology, Society of Interventional Radiology, and the ACC/AHA Task Force on Practice Guidelines (writing committee to develop guidelines for the management of patients with peripheral arterial disease) endorsed by the American Association of Cardiovascular and Pulmonary Rehabilitation; National Heart, Lung, and Blood Institute; Society for Vascular Nursing; TransAtlantic Inter-Society Consensus; and Vascular Disease Foundation. J Am Coll Cardiol 2006;47(6):1239–312; and Rooke TW, Hirsch AT, Misra S, et al. 2011 ACCF/AHA focused update of the guideline for the management of patients with peripheral artery disease (updating the 2005 guideline): a report of the American College of Cardiology Foundation/American Heart Association task force on practice guidelines. J Am Coll Cardiol 2011;58(19):2020–45.

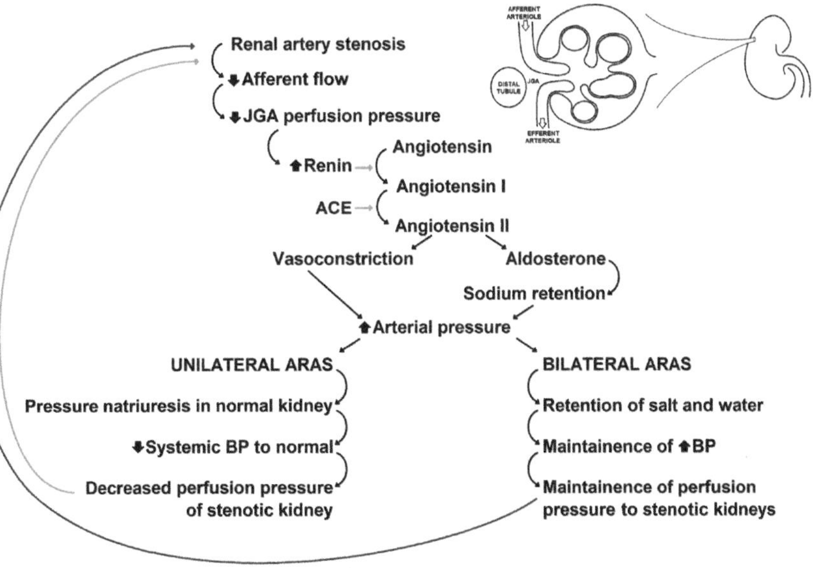

Fig. 1. The cascade of effects due to decreased renal perfusion in ARAS in unilateral and bilateral disease. In the affected kidney, decreased perfusion pressure results in the release of renin, which activates the downstream angiotensin and aldosterone, resulting in increased systemic arterial blood pressure (BP). In the unilateral ARAS system, a compensatory pressure natriuresis occurs in the contralateral normal kidney, which decreases the systemic BP back to normal and again decreases perfusion pressure to the stenotic kidney; this prompts a vicious cycle of feedback stimulation. In the bilateral ARAS system, there is a lack of pressure natriuresis, with maintenance of an elevated systemic BP and adequate perfusion to the stenotic kidneys. With preservation of adequate nephron perfusion pressure, RAAS is ultimately downregulated in the bilateral stenosis system. ACE, angiotensin converting enzyme.

the host to retain salt and water, with persistent hypertensive response.[3]

In the patient with 2 kidneys, the response to initiation of RAAS blockade such as angiotensin converting enzyme (ACE) inhibitors or angiotensin receptor blockers depends on whether unilateral or bilateral stenosis is present. In the patient with unilateral ARAS, as pressure natriuresis occurs in the nonstenotic kidney and normotension is maintained, RAAS continues to be stimulated by the persistently stenotic kidney and may be halted by use of an RAAS blocking agent. Conversely, in the patient with bilateral ARAS, as the volume-dependent hypertensive response is sustained and perfusion to the poststenotic kidneys is maintained, RAAS is downregulated (see **Fig. 1**). Initiation of an RAAS blocking agent in this situation to further suppress angiotensin and aldosterone may result in decreased perfusion pressure with increased incidence of azotemia.

It has been suggested that oxidative stress is a contributor to vascular and renal dysfunction in ARAS.[17–20] Angiotensin II is thought to contribute to vascular inflammation, and although its exact mechanism of action in vivo is not definitively known, it is suspected to involve activation of reactive oxygen species through intravascular activation of nicotinamide adenine dinucleotide phosphate oxidase.[18,21]

DIAGNOSTIC TESTING

Noninvasive Testing

Renal artery duplex ultrasound

Ultrasound imaging is an easily accessible, noninvasive test that can be performed for screening and follow-up. Renal artery duplex ultrasound (RADUS) scanning can be a technically challenging procedure and requires a high level of expertise.[12,22] These challenges are due to depth of the renal arteries, along with superimposed abdominal gas and respiratory motion that limit windows for evaluation. Patient-dependent factors also include body habitus and the ability to breath-hold and to lay in the lateral decubitus position for flank approach imaging. Nonetheless, with current advancements in sonographic equipment, RADUS scan can be completed successfully in an estimated 90% of patients referred for the procedure.[23]

Hemodynamically significant lesions corresponding to the angiographic finding of greater than or equal to 60% stenosis are based on the finding of a peak systolic velocity (PSV) of greater than or equal to 200 cm/s.[8,23] Presence of an end-diastolic velocity (EDV) of greater than or equal to 150 cm/s is suggestive of a stenosis greater than or equal to 80%.[12] **Fig. 2** illustrates the difference in PSV and EDV measurements of a patient with severe renal artery stenosis versus a patient with moderate renal artery stenosis. Factors affecting renal artery PSV include intrinsically increased velocities due to underlying hypertension, as well as poor flow due to severe renal impairment resulting in a falsely low PSV.[23] An alternative technique is to normalize PSV of the renal artery to that of the aorta to optimize the specificity and sensitivity of testing. The renal-aortic ratio uses the PSV of the renal artery of interest compared with the prerenal abdominal aorta PSV, with a ratio of greater than or equal to 3.5 suggestive of a hemodynamically significant lesion.[23]

The resistive index (RI) is used to assess for intrinsic parenchymal disease due to causes such as diabetes, hypertension, and tubulointerstitial disease. RI is the measurement of intrarenal arterial impedance based on the calculation of (PSV − EDV)/PSV, with a normal value of less than 0.7.[23] In small prospective studies, there has been mixed evidence as to whether RI can be used as a predictor for clinical response to stenting, with a threshold of greater than 0.8 being used to predict less benefit.[12,24,25] It has also been suggested that lateralization of the RI (with the contralateral side serving as a control and a difference between the 2 kidneys of >0.05) may indicate severe stenosis.[22] The predictive value of this index in clinical outcomes remains to be completely elucidated.

Captopril radionuclide renography

The use of captopril during renography offers a glimpse into the functional or hemodynamic significance of a stenotic lesion.[26] Administration of an ACE inhibitor capitalizes on the fact that the stenotic kidney has a glomerular filtration rate (GFR) that highly depends on angiotensin II, and use of captopril increases the asymmetry of perfusion between a stenotic and a normal kidney.

The renogram is a time-activity curve illustrating renal uptake and excretion, which is divided into three phases: (1) flow phase, the upslope of which depends on renal perfusion; (2) cortical function phase, with peak cortical uptake typically occurring within 1 to 3 minutes; and (3) clearance phase, which depends on urine excretion into the collecting system (**Fig. 3**A).[27] Baseline renography and response to captopril administration partially depends on the type of tracer used and whether it is secreted or filtered. The secreted tracer of choice is the tubular agent technetium Tc 99m mercaptoacetyltriglycine (MAG3), whereas the filtered tracer of choice is glomerular agent technetium Tc 99m diethylene triamine pentaacetic

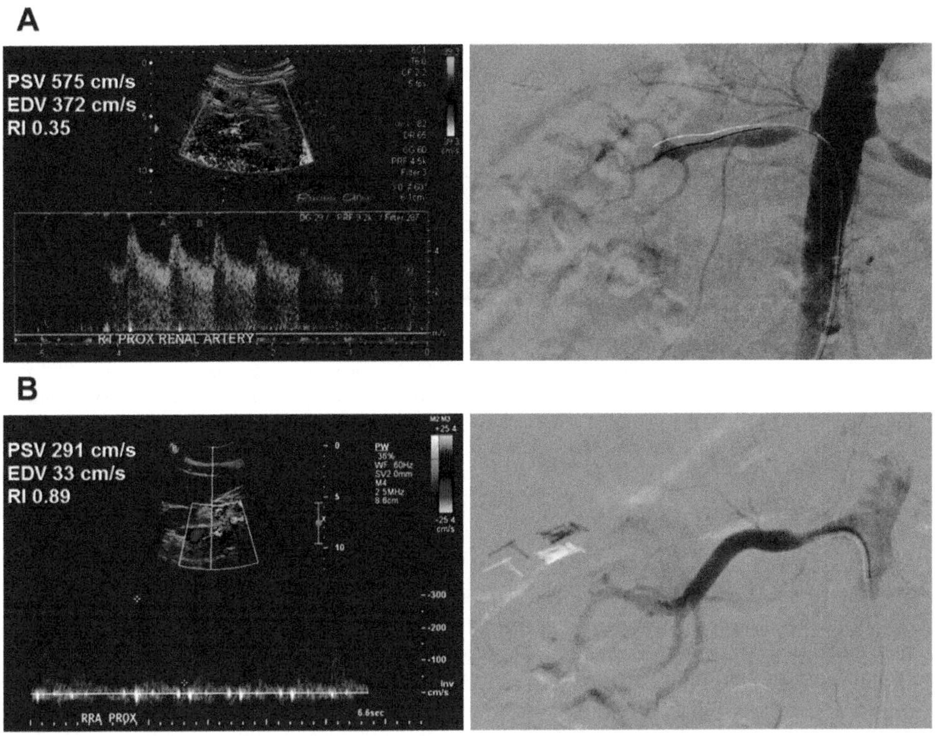

Fig. 2. Renal artery duplex ultrasound findings in (*A*) a patient with severe 90% stenosis of the right renal artery and (*B*) a patient with angiographically moderate stenosis but not hemodynamically significant stenosis of the right renal artery (see **Fig. 4**A for hemodynamic assessment of the right renal artery of patient B). Considerably higher end-diastolic velocity and lower resistive index (RI) are noted in the artery with significant stenosis.

acid (DTPA).[27] DTPA levels may be normal or slightly reduced in the stenotic kidney at baseline and can also be used to measure GFR. MAG3 levels may be normal, decreased, or increased in the stenotic kidney depending on factors of renal plasma flow and extraction fraction of the radiopharmaceutic.[26]

Administration of an ACE inhibitor blocks the conversion of angiotensin I to II, vasodilating the efferent and afferent arterioles and causing a decrease in GFR. The overall effect is a renogram that becomes more abnormal than baseline (see **Fig. 3**B). Based on the renogram findings, patients are categorized as having low, intermediate, or high probability of disease.[28] The reported sensitivity and specificity of predicting a significant response to revascularization are on the order of 85% to 90% and 50%, respectively.[26,29]

Although captopril radionuclide renography (CRR) may assist with providing physiologic data of a poststenotic kidney, it does have some limitations, including decreased accuracy in patients with underlying severe kidney dysfunction, particularly in stage IV–V chronic kidney disease; lack of anatomic information; and lateralization to the more hemodynamically significant side in a patient with bilateral renal artery stenosis.[26,29] For these reasons, CRR is not typically chosen as a first-line screening test in suspected ARAS.

Computed tomography angiography

Computed tomography angiography (CTA) is a sensitive and specific test for the detection of renal artery stenosis, although with the disadvantage of intravenous contrast in a patient population likely to have baseline kidney dysfunction. However, an added advantage of CTA is that a preceding, noncontrasted study can be performed to assess for unsuspected pathophysiology such as nephrolithiasis, intra-arterial calcium deposits, or hemorrhagic renal cysts or adrenal masses.[30] Furthermore, anatomy of other vessels, such as the presence of accessory renal arteries and integrity of the descending aorta with either occlusive or aneurysmal disease, can be clarified.

Magnetic resonance angiography

Magnetic resonance angiography (MRA) is another sensitive and specific imaging modality to detect ostial and proximal renal artery pathology but may miss subtle presentations of FMD.[30,31] Similar to CTA, it can provide additional anatomic information, such

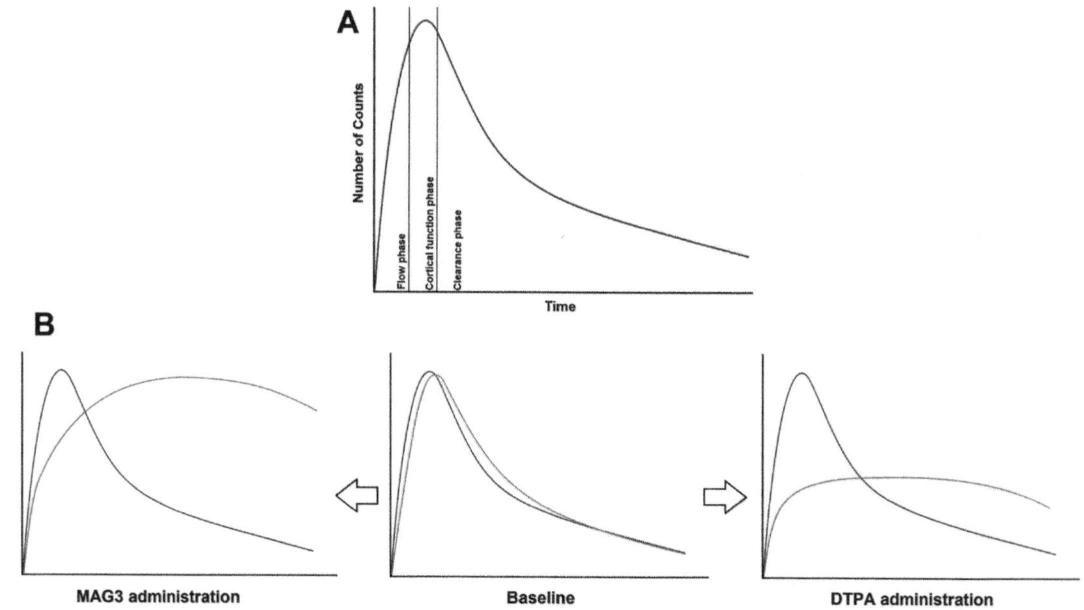

Fig. 3. (*A*) A nuclear renogram illustrating the phases of renal uptake and clearance decay of signal as excretion occurs with a normal examination. Decreased perfusion results in a slow upslope during the flow phase, decreased renal function manifests as delayed peak in the cortical function phase, and hydronephrosis results in the lack of clearance. (*B*) With administration of an ACE inhibitor, the stenotic kidney (*orange tracing*) exhibits an abnormal uptake and excretion. The pattern of abnormality depends on the tracer used; MAG3 is a secreted tubular agent, whereas DTPA is a filtered glomerular agent. With MAG3, flow and cortical phases are generally preserved but delayed; the clearance phase is prolonged because of diminished washout. Conversely, with DTPA, there is decreased uptake and cortical excretion. Interpretation depends on patient pretest probability. (*Data from* Mandell J. Core radiology. New York: Cambridge University Press; 2013; and Taylor AT Jr, Fletcher JW, Nally JV Jr, et al. Procedure guideline for diagnosis of renovascular hypertension. Society of Nuclear Medicine. J Nucl Med 1998;39(7):1297–302.)

as renal size, the presence of masses or cysts, and other intraparenchymal pathologies. Gadolinium-enhanced gradient-echo MRA carries sensitivity and specificity ranging from 97% to 98% and 90% to 100%, respectively.[31] To improve detection of ARAS, fat suppression should be used to remove the competing high signal intensity of fat and 3-dimensional sequence acquisition to achieve a thickness of 1 to 2 mm.[31] Flow sequences hold the potential for providing noninvasive physiologic information.[30] The limitations of MRA include possibility of nephrogenic systemic fibrosis if gadolinium is used in a patient with severe kidney dysfunction, cost, time, patient discomfort with duration of study, and potential false-positive results due to respirations, gut peristalsis, and tortuous renal arteries.[29] In the authors' experience, MRA tends to exaggerate the degree of stenosis at the renal artery ostium.

Invasive Testing

Renal artery angiography carries the advantage of being able to perform a diagnostic and therapeutic intervention simultaneously. The study provides not only anatomic information but also physiologic data. The methodology of performing the renal artery angiogram is detailed in the "Revascularization" section.

MANAGEMENT

Medical Management

As with optimal medical therapy for all vascular diseases, the cornerstone of medical management for ARAS comprises blood pressure control, management of dyslipidemia, and use of antiplatelet therapy. In those patients who do not undergo revascularization, blood pressure management should entail careful titration of medications to avoid decreasing renal perfusion. In patients with bilateral ARAS or ARAS in a solitary kidney, the use of RAAS blocking agents is likely to result in an increase in creatinine levels and lower GFR by mechanisms outlined earlier.

Revascularization

Historically, the primary intervention for ARAS has been surgical bypass with aortorenal, hepatorenal, and splenorenal conduits.[32] Renal artery bypass grafting has significant associated morbidity and mortality, with nationwide mortality rate approaching 10%.[33,34] Percutaneous transluminal renal angioplasty (PTRA) was initially introduced in 1978, when Grüentzig and colleagues[35] used a coaxial balloon catheter to dilate a renal artery stenosis. The use of renal artery stent revascularization (RASR) was introduced in the early 1990s but was used only as a bailout mechanism for patients who had restenosis, acute recoil, or dissection after PTRA.[32] RASR affords more favorable angiographic and hemodynamic results and decreases the occurrence of restenosis (48% vs 14% in balloon angioplasty vs RASR).[36–38] It has been estimated that a provisional stent strategy (ie, bailout stenting) avoids use of a stent approximately 40% of the time, yet 45% of patients require a second procedure for stenting due to restenosis, rendering primary stenting technique more efficient.[14,38] In current practice, RASR is the treatment of choice for revascularization; surgical revascularization is reserved for those with complex anatomy or requiring aortic intervention such as in the case of juxtarenal abdominal aortic aneurysm.

Preparation for angiography

Before pursuing renal angiography, patient evaluation with noninvasive modalities should be performed. Anatomic details to be obtained include presence of aortic or iliac atherosclerosis, aortic aneurysm with or without mural thrombus, accessory renal arteries, angulation of renal arteries, location of the stenosis (eg, aorto-ostial vs body of the renal artery), presence of FMD, and pole-to-pole kidney size. This information influences the choice of access (radial, brachial, or femoral) for diagnostic angiography and revascularization.[8,30,39]

Abdominal aortography followed by selective renal angiography can be performed in a safe and effective fashion. Selective renal angiography is performed to visualize perfusion of the kidney. A segmental defect may suggest the presence of an accessory artery, infarcted segment, or renal mass or cyst; preprocedural noninvasive imaging can assist with this differentiation.

The minimization of contrast dye with a goal of renal preservation is particularly important for patients with ARAS. Diluted contrast or carbon dioxide, along with digital subtraction angiography, can be used to reduce the amount of iodinated contrast used.

Hemodynamic assessment and advanced imaging

Fractional flow reserve (FFR) and intravascular ultrasound (IVUS) are well-validated methods commonly used in the coronary circulation to obtain details pertaining to lesion hemodynamics or quantification of intraluminal area and plaque characteristics, respectively. These assessments allow the interventionalist to further categorize moderate-sized (50–70%) lesions into hemodynamically significant or nonsignificant lesions. This can help determine the appropriateness of intervention.[40]

Hemodynamic measurements of the renal artery are made in the form of translesional pressure gradients (TPGs), which can be further subdivided into resting systolic gradient, hyperemic systolic gradient (HSG), hyperemic mean gradient (HMG), and renal FFR (P_d/P_a, the ratio of distal renal artery to aortic pressure).[40] De Bruyne and colleagues[41] have shown that sequential increase of an intra-arterial balloon inflation results in a decreasing P_d/P_a. The direct effect of progressive occlusion of a renal artery is an increase in ipsilateral renal vein levels of renin; this is a recapitulation of the Goldblatt model, albeit in a transient and refined fashion, but provides inferential support for the use of renal FFR to assess the hemodynamic significance of ARAS.

Compared with coronary hemodynamic measurements, hyperemia is not induced by adenosine, as it is a renal vasoconstrictor. Alternatively, intrarenal boluses of nitroglycerin, 30 mg papaverine, or 50 μg/kg of dopamine can be used.[42,43] Hemodynamically significant lesions that may benefit from revascularization are characterized by FFR less than 0.8, resting mean gradient of greater than 10 mm Hg, or HSG greater than or equal to 20 mm Hg.[40,42] **Fig. 4** shows the angiogram of a patient with bilateral renal artery stenosis of moderate caliber. Hemodynamic assessment with HSG and other types of TPGs help to avoid unnecessary revascularization of lesions that are not clearly hemodynamically significant.

IVUS can provide details on lesion size (plaque burden, minimal luminal area, and reference vessel diameter) and plaque characteristics including calcification and assess quality of stent apposition. IVUS has not been shown to improve outcomes in patients undergoing renal stenting and therefore cannot be recommended for routine use.[40] Nonetheless, it can be used at the operator's discretion to help improve anatomic assessment and stent deployment.

Stenting technique

Before introduction of a wire selectively into the renal artery, anticoagulation is typically initiated. Unfractionated heparin is the preferred anticoagulant, with an activated clotting time goal of greater than 250 seconds. Alternatives to unfractionated

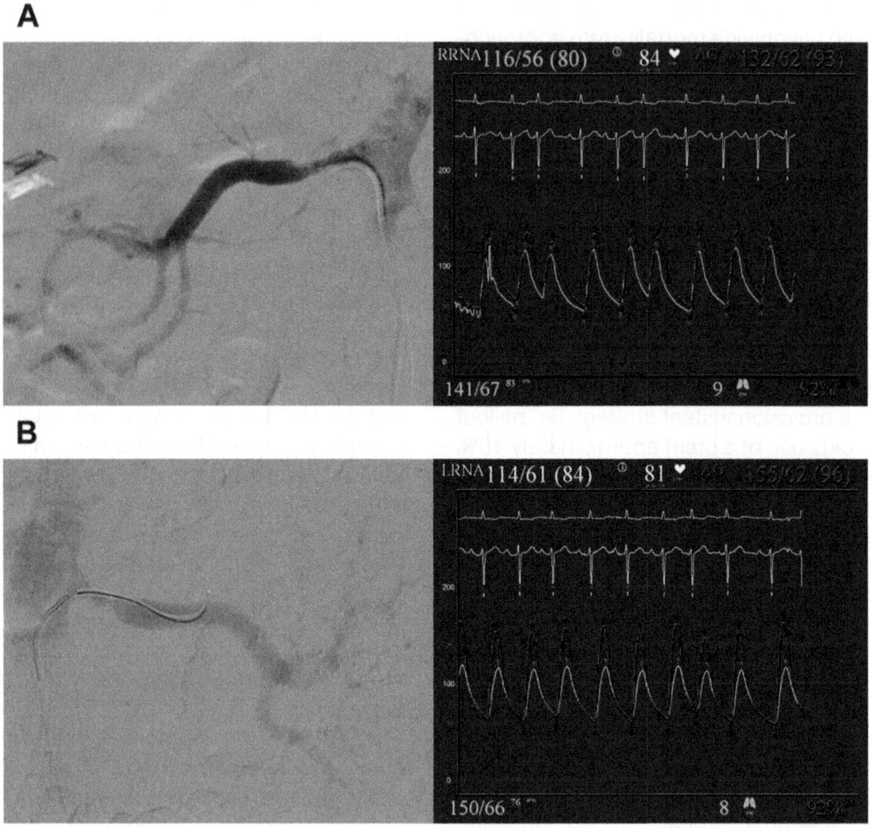

Fig. 4. A patient found to have bilateral renal artery stenosis by renal artery duplex ultrasound imaging. Angiographically, the right side (*A*) and left side (*B*) are both modestly narrowed at approximately 70%. On hemodynamic assessment using nitroglycerin to induce hyperemia, the right and left renal arteries were found to have HSG of 16 mm Hg and 41 mm Hg, respectively. Due to significant hemodynamic changes in the left renal artery, renal artery stent revascularization was pursued for that side.

heparin (low-molecular-weight heparin and bivalirudin) are not currently recommended and lack data to claim superiority over heparin.[14,44,45]

As manipulation within the aorta may lead to disruption of the intima and atheroembolism, operators should attempt to minimize trauma and scraping of the perirenal aorta. The authors recommend the use of a guide catheter with a primary and secondary curve. Specific renal length guides are available for transfemoral renal artery intervention. Atraumatic engagement with either the no-touch or telescoping technique is advised to reduce distal embolization.[44,46] The no-touch technique uses an intra-aortic 0.035-in J-wire or stiff 0.014-in soft-tip wire to guide the catheter near the area of the renal ostium without coming into direct contact. Then, a 0.014-in steerable guidewire is advanced into the distal renal artery, and withdrawal of the intra-aortic wire allows for selective, coaxial renal artery engagement.[46] The telescoping technique entails placement of a 4F diagnostic catheter within a 6F guiding catheter. The catheter-in-catheter system is advanced into the level of the renal artery with a 0.035-in guidewire, the soft-tipped diagnostic 4F catheter is used to engage the ostium, a 0.014-in guidewire is advanced into the distal renal artery, and the 6F guide catheter is then telescoped over the 4F diagnostic catheter for atraumatic engagement.[44]

Radial artery access has increasingly been used to decrease access-site complications and to improve patient comfort. A multipurpose guiding catheter provides excellent alignment with the renal ostia. Some patients may require a 110- or 125-cm-length guide to reach the renal artery, along with balloons and stents with longer shafts. Left radial access may shorten the distance to the renal ostia when catheter length is a concern.

At present, there are three 0.014-in platform US Food and Drug Administration–approved balloon expandable stents available for renal artery stenting (Express SD, Boston Scientific, Natick, MA, USA; Formula, Cook Incorporated, Bloomington, IN, USA; and Herculink Elite, Abbott Vascular,

Santa Clara, CA, USA). Planning for an appropriate-sized stent incorporates use of preprocedural imaging with CTA or MRA, semiquantitative angiography, and IVUS if necessary. Appropriate stent sizing is important to reduce restenosis rates and procedural complications as consequences of undersizing and oversizing, respectively. The poststenotic, dilated segment should not be used as a reference, as this results in oversizing. Rather, the reference point ought to be the most proximal, normal-appearing segment beyond the stenosis (**Fig. 5**). The goal of stenting is to achieve appearance residual stenosis of less than or equal to 30% and to reduce the TPG to zero. Pain during balloon inflation may indicate impending vascular rupture due to adventitial stretching, at which point the balloon should be immediately deflated. This deflation may result in incomplete expansion of the stent, and further postdilation should be done with great care.

As with stenting in other vascular beds, distal embolization of atherosclerotic plaque can occur. Occasionally, RASR may come with the cost of worsening renal failure, a phenomenon most pronounced in patients with baseline severe renal dysfunction.[32] The cause is likely due to a component of distal plaque embolization as well as contrast-induced nephropathy.[14] Embolic protection devices (EPDs) are widely used in other interventional applications such coronary saphenous vein graft intervention and carotid intervention. However, there remains no consensus on the use of EPDs in renal artery intervention. Risks of using EPDs include distal artery injury or spasm, suboptimal support for stent delivery, and lack of the requisite distance for delivering a stent, particularly when using filter-based EPDs.[14] Despite the conceptual benefits of using EPDs, current data do not support their routine use.[45] Selected patients with significant baseline renal dysfunction at risk of worsening GFR with atheromatous embolization who have appropriate anatomy may be considered for EPD use.

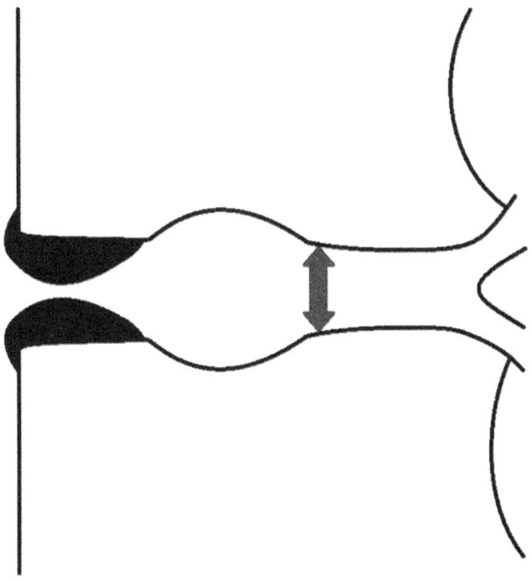

Fig. 5. Ostial and proximal stenosis, with poststenotic dilation. Arrows denote the most proximal, normal-appearing segment of the renal artery, which should be used for sizing of stent. Typical stent sizes range from a diameter of 4 to 7 mm and length of 12 to 18 mm.

Complications

RASR is a safe procedure, with a major complication rate of less than or equal to 2.3%.[44] The most common complications are due to access of the femoral artery, such as hematoma, pseudoaneurysm, arteriovenous fistula, or localized deep venous thrombosis. Less common complications that have been reported include retroperitoneal bleeding, renal artery perforation or dissection, aortic dissection, renal or lower extremity atheromatous embolization, renal infarct, and death. To minimize complication rates, one should use techniques of atraumatic target vessel engagement, appropriate 1:1 stent sizing, conservative balloon sizing for predilation and postdilation inflations, awareness of patient complaints of periprocedural pain, and radial artery access if anatomy is favorable.

The Evolution of Interventional Clinical Trials

Debate over the appropriateness of percutaneous renal artery revascularization continues despite more than 5 decades of experience. The crux of the debate hinges on seemingly contradictory findings in nonrandomized and registry data compared with randomized controlled trials. Nonrandomized trials and device registry data reaffirm positive clinical response to RASR in the appropriately selected patient population.[47–52] As shown previously, **Table 1** outlines the current multisociety guideline-based recommendations in accordance with patient characteristics that favor beneficial results after revascularization.

On the other hand, randomized trials to date have been unable to demonstrate a clear clinical benefit from RASR. The discrepancy is primarily due to flawed study designs in the first-generation trials and inadequate inclusion criteria in the most recent studies. These imperfections beget biased patient recruitment and results.

Clinical trials from the early era of PTRA and RASR were plagued by several shortcomings. First, trials were neither randomized nor controlled

Table 2
Study characteristics of contemporary trials

Study	Years	*n*	Design	Enrollment Criteria	Exclusion Criteria[a]	Run-in Period	Mean Stenosis[g]	Core Laboratory	Crossover	End Points	Results
EMMA	1992–1995	49	• Unblinded RCT • Balloon angioplasty +/−RASR vs OMT • 6 mo follow-up	• DBP >95 mm Hg on 3 occasions and/or on anti-HTN • eGFR ≥50 mL/min • Unilateral ARAS • ≥75% without thrombus or ≥60% with positive lateralization without prior dilation	• Malignant HTN • Pulmonary edema, MI, or stroke in last 6 mo • DBP >109 after run-in	• 2–6 wk • Goal DBP <110 mm Hg	• Not stated • Study arm: 65% (60%–74%) 35% (>75%) • Control arm: 50% (60%–74%) 50% (>75%)	Not specified	• 7/26 control patients	• 1⁰: BP at termination of study • 2⁰: Number of anti-HTN, complications	• Trend toward ↓BP in treatment arm • Significant reduction in number of anti-HTN
DRASTIC	1993–1998	106	• Unblinded RCT • Balloon angioplasty vs OMT • 12 mo follow-up	• Ostial or nonostial lesion ≥50% • Difficult to treat HTN	• Unstable CAD or CHF • Cr >1.7 mg/dL • Single kidney • AAA	• Not specified • Goal DBP <95 mm Hg	• Study arm: 76% • Control arm: 72%	Yes	• 22/50 control patients	• 1⁰: SBP/DBP at 3 and 12 mo • 2⁰: anti-HTN, Cr, CrCl, results of nuclear renogram, stent patency, complications	• No significant difference in BP • anti-HTN, Cr, CrCl better in study arm at 3 mo[b] • Renograms better in study arm at 3 and 12 mo

STAR	2000–2005	140	• Unblinded RCT • RASR vs OMT • 2 y follow-up	• eGFR <80 mL/min • Ostial lesion ≥50% in ≥1 artery • Stable BP during run-in	• eGFR <15 mL/min • Malignant HTN • DM • Proteinuria • Renal size <8 cm	• 1 mo • Stable BP <140/90	• Not stated • Study arm: 34% (50%–70%) 31% (70%–90%) 34% (>90%) • Control arm: 32% (50%–70%) 46% (70%–90%) 22% (>90%)	Yes	• 1/76 control patients • 12/64 study patients[d]	• 1^0: ≥20% decrease in eGFR[c] • 2^0: Change in BP, refractory or malignant HTN, pulmonary edema, CV mortality and morbidity, total mortality, complications	• Trend toward improvement in study arm in all 1^0 and 2^0 outcomes (exception of CAD and procedural complications)
ASTRAL	2000–2007	806	• Unblinded RCT • RASR vs OMT • 5 y follow-up	• Uncontrolled/refractory HTN • Substantial stenosis in ≥1 renal artery • Physician uncertain of benefit of revascularization	• High likelihood of requiring revascularization in 6 mo • Nonatheromatous CV disease • Prior revascularization	• Not specified	• Study arm: 76% • Control arm: 75%	Not specified	• 24/403 control patients • 33/403 study patients[e]	• 1^0: Change in renal function in 5 y follow-up • 2^0: BP, time to first renal or CV event, mortality	• Trend toward favoring RASR in 1^0 end point • No difference in 2^0 outcomes
CORAL	2005–2010	947	• Unblinded RCT • RASR vs OMT • 43 mo follow-up	• ARAS 60%–99% If 60%–80%, SPG ≥20 mm Hg • HTN (≥2 anti-HTN)[f] or • eGFR <60 mL/min	• Hospitalization for CHF in preceding 30 d • Cr >4.0 mg/dL	• Not specified	• Study arm: 67% • Control arm: 67%	Yes	• 19/480 control patients	• 1^0: Major CV or renal event: Includes CHF, MI, stroke, ↓ eGFR ≥30% for >60 d • 2^0: Individual results	• Trend toward favoring RASR in 1^0 end point • Modest reduction in SBP at 5 y with RASR

Abbreviations: BP, blood pressure; CAD, coronary artery disease; CHF, congestive heart failure; Cr, creatinine; CrCl, creatinine clearance; CV, cardiovascular; DBP, diastolic blood pressure; DM, diabetes mellitus; eGFR, estimated glomerular filtration rate; HTN, hypertension; OMT, medical therapy; RASR, renal artery stent revascularization; RCT, randomized controlled trial; SBP, systolic blood pressure; SPG, systolic pressure gradient; 1^0, primary; 2^0, secondary.

[a] Not all exclusion criteria are listed; see primary article and supplemental data for full exclusion criteria.

[b] No difference was noted between the 2 arms at 12-month follow-up; note that after 3 months, 22 of 50 patients in the control arm were crossed over to angioplasty.

[c] For patients in the revascularization arm, a drop in eGFR ≥20% prompted evaluation for restenosis. If no restenosis is present, then primary end point is met. If restenosis is present, repeat revascularization was performed; if there was persistently low eGFR 1 month after repeat revascularization for restenosis, patient was then considered to have met the primary end point.

[d] A total of 18 patients in the study group did not undergo RASR, 12 of which were due to severity of lesion less than 50%.

[e] A total of 68 patients in the study group did not undergo an attempt at revascularization, 33 of which were due to severity of lesion less than 50%.

[f] During enrollment period, criteria for BP was changed to no longer specifying a threshold of greater than 155 mm Hg.

[g] For studies without a published degree of mean stenosis for each arm, the total percentage of patients within each category of stenosis is listed.

Data from Refs.[55–58,61,65]

and included patients with FMD, an entity with unreliable angiographic and clinical response to intervention.[53] Second, in its infancy, technical success of PTRA was widely variable and operator dependent, with failure rates ranging from 3% to 24% (average failure rate of 12%).[53] The rate of technical success did improve after the introduction of RASR to 96% to 100%.[32,38] Consequently, RASR is now the preferred technique for renal intervention. Third, patient selection and management were variable, with a lack of uniformity in the severity of disease treated and nonstandardized antihypertensive regimens.[32,53] Finally, the end points in the early interventional trials focused on the ability to cure hypertension or improve blood pressure, with the former defined as complete cessation of antihypertensive drugs and latter with varying definitions. Renal function was not routinely assessed in the PTRA trials of the 1980s.[53] Meta-analyses of trials in the 1980s and the 1990s suggest that there is neither benefit nor harm on renal function after PTRA or stenting.[32,53] Given the natural history of progressive renal dysfunction in patients with ARAS, these findings may indicate that the renal function was in fact preserved by the intervention.[32,54]

In the late 1990s into the 2000s, several randomized trials compared medical therapy with percutaneous intervention; **Table 2** reviews characteristics of these contemporary trials. Despite lessons learned from early interventional trials, several technical problems remain unresolved: (1) the use of renal artery stenting became ubiquitous only in trials conducted after 2001, (2) enrollment indications were varied and may entail resistant hypertension and/or chronic kidney failure yet may not necessarily include patients with clinical manifestations of severe stenosis, (3) crossover rates varied and were as high as 44%, and (4) patients who did not have significant stenosis by angiographic findings and did not undergo revascularization remained in the study arm as part of the intention-to-treat analysis.[55–59]

Bearing in mind the aforementioned criticisms of the included trials, a contemporary meta-analysis reveals no statistically significant difference in end points of hypertension, reduction of antihypertensives, creatinine level, mortality, congestive heart failure, and progressive renal dysfunction, although there was a trend to suggest that revascularization is better in all categories.[58] As such, the appropriate management of ARAS is contingent on individualized patient care. The 2011 update of ACC/AHA guidelines for renal artery stenting remained optimistic that ongoing renal artery trials, including Cardiovascular Outcomes in Renal Atherosclerotic Lesions (CORAL), would help elucidate the role of RASR.[11]

Despite efforts for an unbiased assessment of efficacy of RASR, the highly anticipated CORAL trial was also notable for limitations in methodology.[60] The patient selection bias noted in the Angioplasty and Stenting for Renal Artery Lesions (ASTRAL) trial persisted in CORAL. Although not a specific exclusion criterion, those patients with severe stenoses were more likely to be diverted to stenting over trial enrollment given the referring clinician's assumption that they are likely to benefit from revascularization.[61] Of the screened 5322 patients, a total of 82% of patients were excluded; 57% of these were based on anatomic or clinical reasons, with the remaining 43% based on either patient declining, clinician withdrawal, or other unspecified reason.[61] This method introduces unintentional selection bias toward patients with less severe stenosis and antihypertensive needs (with a baseline mean number of 2 antihypertensive medications), which results in a mean angiographic stenosis of only 67% in the final study population.[61] Furthermore, 2 important exclusion criteria to consider are recent hospitalization for heart failure within 30 days and a high creatinine level greater than 4.0, both of which are indications of a high-risk patient who is likely to benefit from revascularization.[61]

In this patient population of moderate renal artery stenosis and mild chronic renal insufficiency (mean estimated GFR 57–58 mL/min), the CORAL trial noted no difference in the combined primary end point or its individual components between RASR and medical therapy.[61] The primary end point was composed of death from cardiovascular or renal causes, stroke, myocardial infarction, hospitalization for heart failure, progressive renal insufficiency, and permanent renal replacement therapy. However, there are clinical findings to suggest a benefit from RASR even in this modestly diseased population, with slight reduction in systolic blood pressure (2 mm Hg, $P = .03$) and a trend toward reduced progressive renal insufficiency during the course of 5 years with revascularization.[61]

The conclusions of the CORAL trial mirror other contemporary trials in that there are trends toward benefit in RASR in patients with moderate disease. It has been suggested that with the patient population recruited in these contemporary trials, close to 6000 participants would be needed to find a significant difference in an end point of death, heart failure, and stroke and nearly 28,000 participants would be needed to achieve significant improvement in renal function, which are substantial numbers of patients to recruit in this population.[58]

Patient Selection

Registry and nonrandomized data suggest that patients with severe bilateral ARAS or unilateral ARAS in a solitary functioning kidney with (1) recurrent flash pulmonary edema, (2) accelerated or resistant hypertension defined as failure of 3 or more maximally tolerated medications including one diuretic, and (3) rapid decline of kidney function benefit from RASR.[15,16,50] Contemporary randomized trials suggest that patients without hemodynamically significant ARAS or without truly symptomatic severe renal stenosis likely have similar long-term outcomes when treated with optimal medical therapy versus RASR.

For asymptomatic patients with anatomically and hemodynamically significant lesions, an individualized decision should be made for each patient. The ideal predictor for clinical response to stenting remains elusive to date. Currently available but imperfect predictors can be subdivided into noninvasive imaging (ACE-protocol renography, RI), biomarkers (brain natriuretic peptide), or intraprocedural testing (TPG, IVUS).[44,49] The clinical decision should take into account multiple factors, including patient characteristics, available preprocedural testing, and severity of lesions based on intraprocedural assessment.

Follow-up

After renal artery stenting, the authors recommend dual antiplatelet therapy with aspirin and a P2Y12 inhibitor for 1 to 3 months, then aspirin 81 mg daily indefinitely. Medical management of blood pressure should continue as before revascularization and titrating off antihypertensives as needed.

There are no current guidelines for routine follow-up imaging to assess stent patency. In general, RADUS is the preferred modality for follow-up assessment. The most recent appropriate use criteria for peripheral vascular ultrasound imaging affirm that it is appropriate to obtain a baseline ultrasound image within 1 month of revascularization and yearly thereafter for surveillance in an asymptomatic patient.[62] Recurrence of symptoms may also prompt a clinician to assess for restenosis.

Although renal artery stenting is superior to balloon angioplasty for patency rates, it is associated with a restenosis rate on the order of 16% to 17% (can vary from 12% to 29%).[14,63] This process is likely a consequence of smooth muscle proliferation and neointimal hyperplasia and tends to occur less often in large vessels (>4.5 mm) or those with larger acute gain from stenting.[14,63,64] The appropriate management of clinically significant restenosis in RASR is not yet known, although it may entail the use of cutting balloon angioplasty, stent-in-stent technique, drug-eluting stents, covered stents, or endovascular brachytherapy.[64]

SUMMARY

Renal artery stenosis constitutes an important cause of (1) cardiac disturbance syndromes manifesting as recurrent flash pulmonary edema, refractory heart failure, and unstable angina; (2) renovascular hypertension; and (3) ischemic nephropathy. Renal artery stenting is the contemporary revascularization method of choice for ARAS because of its high technical success rate, low complication rate in experienced hands, and minimally invasive nature compared with open surgical bypass. Patients with global renal ischemia (ie, those with bilateral ARAS or unilateral ARAS in a solitary kidney) that is documented via hemodynamic assessment are likely to benefit most from renal artery stenting. However, such patients have frequently been excluded from large randomized clinical trials. Therefore, a data gap remains in the evidence base for treatment of these patients. On the other hand, patients with hemodynamically insignificant lesions (ie, mild stenosis <50% or moderate stenosis 50%–70% with negative hemodynamic testing) are unlikely to benefit from revascularization compared with optimal medical therapy. Patients who fall in between these 2 ends of the spectrum ought to have a tailored management strategy whereby a trial of optimal medical therapy is provided first with careful, serial assessment of clinical symptoms and renal function. In all cases, optimal medical therapy should include appropriate cardiovascular risk factor management and ongoing clinical follow-up.

REFERENCES

1. Basso N, Terragno NA. History about the discovery of the renin-angiotensin system. Hypertension 2001;38(6):1246–9.
2. Goldblatt H, Lynch J, Hanzal RF, et al. Studies on experimental hypertension: I. The production of persistent elevation of systolic blood pressure by means of renal ischemia. J Exp Med 1934;59(3):347–79.
3. Chrysant SG. The current status of angioplasty of atherosclerotic renal artery stenosis for the treatment of hypertension. J Clin Hypertens 2013;15(9):694–8.
4. Dworkin LD. Controversial treatment of atherosclerotic renal vascular disease: the cardiovascular outcomes in renal atherosclerotic lesions trial. Hypertension 2006;48(3):350–6.

5. Radermacher J, Haller H. The right diagnostic work-up: investigating renal and renovascular disorders. J Hypertens Suppl 2003;21(2):S19–24.
6. Balk E, Raman G, Chung M, et al. Effectiveness of management strategies for renal artery stenosis: a systematic review. Ann Intern Med 2006;145(12): 901–12.
7. van Ampting JM, Penne EL, Beek FJ, et al. Prevalence of atherosclerotic renal artery stenosis in patients starting dialysis. Nephrol Dial Transplant 2003;18(6):1147–51.
8. Heuser RR, Henry M. Textbook of peripheral vascular interventions. 2nd edition. United Kingdom: Taylor & Francis; 2008.
9. Kuroda S, Nishida N, Uzu T, et al. Prevalence of renal artery stenosis in autopsy patients with stroke. Stroke 2000;31(1):61–5.
10. Hirsch AT, Haskal ZJ, Hertzer NR, et al. ACC/AHA 2005 guidelines for the management of patients with peripheral arterial disease (lower extremity, renal, mesenteric, and abdominal aortic): executive summary a collaborative report from the American Association for Vascular Surgery/Society for Vascular Surgery, Society for Cardiovascular Angiography and Interventions, Society for Vascular Medicine and Biology, Society of Interventional Radiology, and the ACC/AHA Task Force on practice guidelines (writing committee to develop guidelines for the management of patients with peripheral arterial disease) endorsed by the American Association of Cardiovascular and Pulmonary Rehabilitation; National Heart, Lung, and Blood Institute; Society for Vascular Nursing; TransAtlantic Inter-Society Consensus; and Vascular Disease Foundation. J Am Coll Cardiol 2006;47(6):1239–312.
11. Rooke TW, Hirsch AT, Misra S, et al. 2011 ACCF/AHA focused update of the guideline for the management of patients with peripheral artery disease (updating the 2005 guideline): a report of the American College of Cardiology Foundation/American Heart Association Task Force on practice guidelines. J Am Coll Cardiol 2011;58(19):2020–45.
12. Gerhard-Herman M, Gardin JM, Jaff M, et al. Guidelines for noninvasive vascular laboratory testing: a report from the American Society of Echocardiography and the Society of Vascular Medicine and Biology. J Am Soc Echocardiogr 2006;19(8):955–72.
13. Derkx FH, Schalekamp MA. Renal artery stenosis and hypertension. Lancet 1994;344(8917):237–9.
14. White CJ. Catheter-based therapy for atherosclerotic renal artery stenosis. Circulation 2006; 113(11):1464–73.
15. Gray BH, Olin JW, Childs MB, et al. Clinical benefit of renal artery angioplasty with stenting for the control of recurrent and refractory congestive heart failure. Vasc Med 2002;7(4):275–9.
16. Muray S, Martín M, Amoedo ML, et al. Rapid decline in renal function reflects reversibility and predicts the outcome after angioplasty in renal artery stenosis. Am J Kidney Dis 2002;39(1):60–6.
17. Metra M, Cotter G, Gheorghiade M, et al. The role of the kidney in heart failure. Eur Heart J 2012; 33(17):2135–42.
18. Saeed A, Herlitz H, Nowakowska-Fortuna E, et al. Oxidative stress and endothelin-1 in atherosclerotic renal artery stenosis and effects of renal angioplasty. Kidney Blood Press Res 2011;34(6):396–403.
19. Textor SC, Lerman L. Renovascular hypertension and ischemic nephropathy. Am J Hypertens 2010; 23(11):1159–69.
20. Lerman LO, Textor SC, Grande JP. Mechanisms of tissue injury in renal artery stenosis: ischemia and beyond. Prog Cardiovasc Dis 2009;52(3): 196–203.
21. Montezano AC, Nguyen Dinh Cat A, Rios FJ, et al. Angiotensin II and vascular injury. Curr Hypertens Rep 2014;16(6):431.
22. Meola M, Petrucci I. Color Doppler sonography in the study of chronic ischemic nephropathy. J Ultrasound 2008;11(2):55–73.
23. Granata A, Fiorini F, Andrulli S, et al. Doppler ultrasound and renal artery stenosis: an overview. J Ultrasound 2009;12(4):133–43.
24. Radermacher J, Chavan A, Bleck J, et al. Use of Doppler ultrasonography to predict the outcome of therapy for renal-artery stenosis. N Engl J Med 2001;344(6):410–7.
25. Garcia-Criado A, Gilabert R, Nicolau C, et al. Value of Doppler sonography for predicting clinical outcome after renal artery revascularization in atherosclerotic renal artery stenosis. J Ultrasound Med 2005;24(12):1641–7.
26. Prigent A, Chaumet-Riffaud P. Clinical problems in renovascular disease and the role of nuclear medicine. Semin Nucl Med 2014;44(2):110–22.
27. Mandell J. Core radiology. New York: Cambridge University Press; 2013.
28. Taylor AT Jr, Fletcher JW, Nally JV Jr, et al. Procedure guideline for diagnosis of renovascular hypertension. Society of nuclear medicine. J Nucl Med 1998;39(7):1297–302.
29. Vashist A, Heller EN, Brown EJ, et al. Renal artery stenosis: a cardiovascular perspective. Am Heart J 2002;143(4):559–64.
30. Kaufman JA, Lee MJ. Vascular & interventional radiology. St. Louis (MO): Mosby; 2004.
31. Semelka RC. Abdominal-pelvic MRI. Hoboken (NJ): Wiley; 2010.
32. Isles CG, Robertson S, Hill D. Management of renovascular disease: a review of renal artery stenting in ten studies. QJM 1999;92(3):159–67.
33. Pradhan N, Rossi NF. Interactions between the sympathetic nervous system and angiotensin

system in renovascular hypertension. Curr Hypertens Rev 2013;9(2):121–9.
34. Modrall JG, Rosero EB, Smith ST, et al. Operative mortality for renal artery bypass in the United States: results from the National Inpatient Sample. J Vasc Surg 2008;48(2):317–22.
35. Grüntzig A, Kuhlmann U, Vetter W, et al. Treatment of renovascular hypertension with percutaneous transluminal dilatation of a renal-artery stenosis. Lancet 1978;1:801–2.
36. White CJ, Ramee SR, Collins TJ, et al. Renal artery stent placement: utility in lesions difficult to treat with balloon angioplasty. J Am Coll Cardiol 1997; 30(6):1445–50.
37. Dorros G, Prince C, Mathiak L. Stenting of a renal artery stenosis achieves better relief of the obstructive lesion than balloon angioplasty. Cathet Cardiovasc Diagn 1993;29(3):191–8.
38. van de Ven PJ, Kaatee R, Beutler JJ, et al. Arterial stenting and balloon angioplasty in ostial atherosclerotic renovascular disease: a randomised trial. Lancet 1999;353(9149):282–6.
39. Rutherford RB. Review of vascular surgery: companion to vascular surgery. 6th edition. Philadelphia: Elsevier Science Health Science Division; 2005.
40. Leesar MA, Varma J, Shapira A, et al. Prediction of hypertension improvement after stenting of renal artery stenosis: comparative accuracy of translesional pressure gradients, intravascular ultrasound, and angiography. J Am Coll Cardiol 2009;53(25): 2363–71.
41. De Bruyne B, Manoharan G, Pijls NH, et al. Assessment of renal artery stenosis severity by pressure gradient measurements. J Am Coll Cardiol 2006; 48(9):1851–5.
42. Mitchell JA, Subramanian R, White CJ, et al. Predicting blood pressure improvement in hypertensive patients after renal artery stent placement: renal fractional flow reserve. Catheter Cardiovasc Interv 2007;69(5):685–9.
43. Mangiacapra F, Trana C, Sarno G, et al. Translesional pressure gradients to predict blood pressure response after renal artery stenting in patients with renovascular hypertension. Circ Cardiovasc Interv 2010;3(6):537–42.
44. White CJ. Optimizing outcomes for renal artery intervention. Circ Cardiovasc Interv 2010;3(2):184–92.
45. Cooper CJ, Haller ST, Colyer W, et al. Embolic protection and platelet inhibition during renal artery stenting. Circulation 2008;117(21):2752–60.
46. Feldman RL, Wargovich TJ, Bittl JA. No-touch technique for reducing aortic wall trauma during renal artery stenting. Catheter Cardiovasc Interv 1999; 46(2):245–8.
47. Messerli FH, Bangalore S, Makani H, et al. Flash pulmonary oedema and bilateral renal artery stenosis: the Pickering syndrome. Eur Heart J 2011;32(18):2231–5.
48. Rocha-Singh K, Jaff MR, Lynne Kelley E, et al. Renal artery stenting with noninvasive duplex ultrasound follow-up: 3-year results from the RENAISSANCE renal stent trial. Catheter Cardiovasc Interv 2008; 72(6):853–62.
49. Jaff MR, Bates M, Sullivan T, et al. Significant reduction in systolic blood pressure following renal artery stenting in patients with uncontrolled hypertension: results from the HERCULES trial. Catheter Cardiovasc Interv 2012;80(3):343–50.
50. Weinberg I, Keyes MJ, Giri J, et al. Blood pressure response to renal artery stenting in 901 patients from five prospective multicenter FDA-approved trials. Catheter Cardiovasc Interv 2014;83(4):603–9.
51. Laird JR, Rundback J, Zierler RE, et al. Safety and efficacy of renal artery stenting following suboptimal renal angioplasty for de novo and restenotic ostial lesions: results from a nonrandomized, prospective multicenter registry. J Vasc Interv Radiol 2010;21(5):627–37.
52. Rocha-Singh K, Jaff MR, Rosenfield K, et al. Evaluation of the safety and effectiveness of renal artery stenting after unsuccessful balloon angioplasty: the ASPIRE-2 study. J Am Coll Cardiol 2005; 46(5):776–83.
53. Ramsay LE, Waller PC. Blood pressure response to percutaneous transluminal angioplasty for renovascular hypertension: an overview of published series. BMJ 1990;300(6724):569–72.
54. Caps MT, Perissinotto C, Zierler RE, et al. Prospective study of atherosclerotic disease progression in the renal artery. Circulation 1998;98(25): 2866–72.
55. Investigators A, Wheatley K, Ives N, et al. Revascularization versus medical therapy for renal-artery stenosis. N Engl J Med 2009;361(20):1953–62.
56. van Jaarsveld BC, Krijnen P, Pieterman H, et al. The effect of balloon angioplasty on hypertension in atherosclerotic renal-artery stenosis. Dutch Renal Artery Stenosis Intervention Cooperative Study Group. N Engl J Med 2000;342(14):1007–14.
57. Plouin PF, Chatellier G, Darne B, et al. Blood pressure outcome of angioplasty in atherosclerotic renal artery stenosis: a randomized trial. Essai Multicentrique Medicaments vs Angioplastie (EMMA) Study Group. Hypertension 1998;31(3):823–9.
58. Kumbhani DJ, Bavry AA, Harvey JE, et al. Clinical outcomes after percutaneous revascularization versus medical management in patients with significant renal artery stenosis: a meta-analysis of randomized controlled trials. Am Heart J 2011; 161(3):622–30.e1.
59. White CJ. Kiss my astral: one seriously flawed study of renal stenting after another. Catheter Cardiovasc Interv 2010;75(2):305–7.

60. White CJ. The "chicken little" of renal stent trials: the CORAL trial in perspective. JACC Cardiovasc Interv 2014;7(1):111–3.
61. Cooper CJ, Murphy TP, Cutlip DE, et al. Stenting and medical therapy for atherosclerotic renal-artery stenosis. N Engl J Med 2014; 370(1):13–22.
62. American College of Cardiology Foundation (ACCF), American College of Radiology (ACR), American Institute of Ultrasound in Medicine (AIUM), et al. ACCF/ACR/AIUM/ASE/ASN/ICAVL/SCAI/SCCT/SIR/SVM/SVS/SVU [corrected] 2012 appropriate use criteria for peripheral vascular ultrasound and physiological testing part I: arterial ultrasound and physiological testing: a report of the American College of Cardiology Foundation appropriate use criteria task force, American College of Radiology, American Institute of Ultrasound in Medicine, American Society of Echocardiography, American Society of Nephrology, Intersocietal Commission for the Accreditation of Vascular Laboratories, Society for Cardiovascular Angiography and Interventions, Society of Cardiovascular Computed Tomography, Society for Interventional Radiology, Society for Vascular Medicine, Society for Vascular Surgery, [corrected] and Society for Vascular Ultrasound [corrected]. J Am Coll Cardiol 2012;60(3):242–76.
63. Shammas NW, Kapalis MJ, Dippel EJ, et al. Clinical and angiographic predictors of restenosis following renal artery stenting. J Invasive Cardiol 2004;16(1): 10–3.
64. Zeller T, Rastan A, Schwarzwalder U, et al. Treatment of in-stent restenosis following stent-supported renal artery angioplasty. Catheter Cardiovasc Interv 2007; 70(3):454–9.
65. Bax L, Woittiez AJ, Kouwenberg HJ, et al. Stent placement in patients with atherosclerotic renal artery stenosis and impaired renal function: a randomized trial. Ann Intern Med 2009;150(12):840–8. W150–841.

Contemporary Management of Femoral Popliteal Revascularization

Phillip A. Erwin, MD, PhD,
Mehdi H. Shishehbor, DO, MPH, PhD*

KEYWORDS

- Peripheral artery disease • Femoral popliteal revascularization • Intermittent claudication
- Critical limb ischemia • Endovascular revascularization • Infrainguinal bypass

KEY POINTS

- Peripheral artery disease of the femoral popliteal segment can manifest as claudication and critical limb ischemia.
- Revascularization can alleviate symptoms, but controversy exists over whether a surgical or endovascular approach is superior.
- Infrainguinal bypass surgery is effective and durable but, is associated with significantly greater morbidity and mortality than endovascular therapy.
- Endovascular revascularization has less morbidity than bypass surgery and has a high success rate, but restenosis is common.
- Advances in endovascular techniques have increased the success of the percutaneous approach and may increase the durability of endovascular revascularization of femoral popliteal occlusive disease.
- The decision to pursue surgical, endovascular, or combined approaches to revascularization should be tailored to the patient, the lesion, and the goals of care.

INTRODUCTION

Atherosclerotic peripheral arterial disease (PAD) affects nearly 30 million people in North America and has a prevalence of almost 30% in persons older than 70 years,[1–3] with significant implications for quality of life and health care–related expenditures.[4,5] Clinical manifestations of PAD of the femoral popliteal (FP) segment can span from intermittent claudication to critical limb ischemia (CLI).[2] Although revascularization of FP occlusive disease is an accepted treatment for short-distance claudication or CLI, the optimal approaches to revascularization of the FP segment remain controversial.

Endovascular revascularization is minimally invasive and is technically successful more than 95% of the time,[6] but the restenosis rate can be as high as 40% to 60% at 1 year.[7–9] Durable endovascular revascularization of the FP segment is exceptionally challenging because of the vessel's unique anatomy and biomechanics. The FP segment is the longest vessel in the body and its atherosclerotic burden is typically diffuse, with multiple foci of calcified disease, and in 20% to 50% of cases, chronic total occlusions.[10,11] These long lesions can often be treated successfully, but the constant flexion, torsion, and compression of the FP segment can cause stents to fracture and

The authors have no relevant disclosures.
Department of Cardiovascular Medicine, Heart & Vascular Institute, Cleveland Clinic, 9500 Euclid Avenue, Cleveland, OH 44195, USA
* Corresponding author. Interventional Cardiology, Department of Cardiovascular Medicine, Cleveland Clinic, 9500 Euclid Avenue, J3-5, Cleveland, OH 44195.
E-mail address: shishem@ccf.org

Intervent Cardiol Clin 3 (2014) 517–530
http://dx.doi.org/10.1016/j.iccl.2014.06.004
2211-7458/14/$ – see front matter

fail.[12,13] Endovascular revascularization of FP disease is further complicated by the pronounced inflammatory response of the vessel's smooth muscle cells to injury from angioplasty and stenting, which may explain why this segment has greater propensity for restenosis than other vascular beds.[14]

By contrast, surgical bypass of the FP segment with saphenous vein is a durable treatment that has greater patency[15] and less symptom recurrence than endovascular treatment.[16] But, surgery also requires general anesthesia, has a longer convalescence, and has more frequent complications than endovascular treatment.[16] Given the morbidity and mortality risks of surgery,[2,17–19] not all patients have acceptable surgical risk. Even for patients who are good surgical candidates, the morbidity of surgery may make it unpalatable compared with endovascular treatment.

PRINCIPLES OF MEDICAL MANAGEMENT

All patients with symptomatic PAD should be treated with statins,[2,20] angiotensin-converting enzyme inhibitors,[21] and aspirin, or preferably, clopidogrel.[22] These medications are known to mitigate the considerable cardiovascular risk associated with PAD.[2,20] Smoking cessation should also be emphasized.[2,20] Some clinicians recommend dual antiplatelet therapy with both aspirin and clopidogrel to prevent adverse cardiovascular outcomes in patients with PAD, and there is some support for this practice in the guideline recommendations.[20] Supervised exercise therapy should be prescribed for all patients with intermittent claudication, whether or not they are undergoing revascularization.[23,24] Cilostazol also can be considered for claudicants without heart failure,[20] but its utility in severe short-distance claudicants is limited.

For patients who undergo surgical bypass of PAD, aspirin promotes graft patency, particularly when synthetic grafts are used.[25] In patients at high risk of graft thrombosis (ie, prior failed graft, poor vein conduit or runoff), addition of warfarin to aspirin may improve patency.[26,27] But, for patients who are not at high risk of graft thrombosis, combining aspirin and warfarin increases only the risk of major bleeding and of death.[26,27]

CHOOSING A REVASCULARIZATION STRATEGY

In our opinion, the most important question in FP revascularization is whether to intervene at all. Factors to consider include the goals of revascularization (ie, treatment of claudication vs CLI), vascular anatomy, comorbid conditions, life expectancy, patient preferences, and local expertise. The patient's baseline mobility and functional status before the procedure are perhaps the best predictors of functional outcomes for both open surgical and endovascular procedures,[28] and should always be considered. In patients with CLI, the answer is relatively straightforward, because revascularization will treat the patient's pain, prevent amputation, and improve quality of life.[29,30] As such, the threshold to revascularize is lower than for claudication, and immediate symptom management with revascularization takes precedence over long-term patency.[30,31] Given the high mortality and operative risk of these patients, an endovascular approach is preferable.

In claudicants, the question of when to revascularize is more nuanced because most nondiabetic patients with intermittent claudication do not progress to CLI.[32] Accordingly, control of symptoms and avoidance of repeat interventions are probably the most important goals. Our practice for claudication is to intervene only for patients with lifestyle-limiting claudication who have exhausted noninvasive therapy (ie, supervised exercise and cilostazol). This is particularly true if revascularization appears high risk or is not likely to be durable. Once the decision to revascularize for claudication has been made, bypass surgery-first with autologous vein is a reasonable choice for patients with good operative risk and a high propensity for restenosis after endovascular treatment. Risk factors for restenosis are summarized in **Box 1**.

Once the decision to revascularize has been made, one must determine whether traditional open surgery, endovascular therapy, or some combination of the two (ie, "hybrid" revascularization) is the best approach. The Inter-Society

Box 1
Predictors of restenosis after endovascular revascularization

- Critical limb ischemia
- Diabetes
- Diffuse disease
- Female sex
- Lesion complexity (TASC II C/D)
- Number of runoff vessels
- Number of stents
- Stent fracture

Data from Refs.[41,51,74]

Consensus for the Management of Peripheral Arterial Disease (TASC II)[2] recommends using anatomic criteria to decide on therapy. As shown in **Fig. 1**, the TASC II guidelines classify lesions of the FP segment according to anatomic complexity (types A–D).[2] The guidelines recommend endovascular therapy as the treatment of choice for relatively short and uncomplicated type A and type B lesions. Type C lesions are recommended for surgery in suitable patients, but endovascular therapy can be considered. Surgery is described as the preferred therapy for the long chronic total occlusions of the common femoral artery, superficial femoral artery (SFA), and

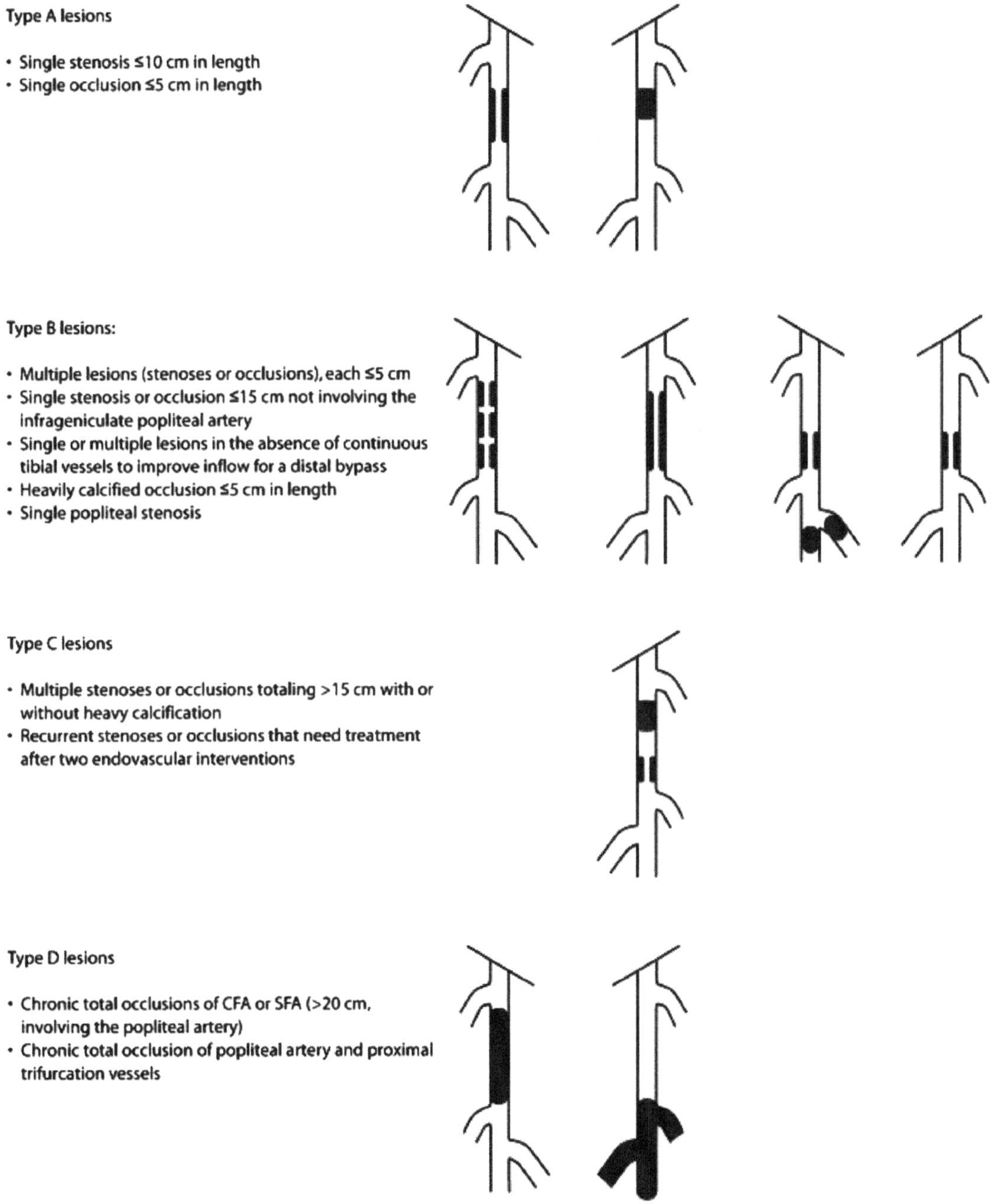

Type A lesions
• Single stenosis ≤10 cm in length
• Single occlusion ≤5 cm in length
Type B lesions:
• Multiple lesions (stenoses or occlusions), each ≤5 cm
• Single stenosis or occlusion ≤15 cm not involving the infrageniculate popliteal artery
• Single or multiple lesions in the absence of continuous tibial vessels to improve inflow for a distal bypass
• Heavily calcified occlusion ≤5 cm in length
• Single popliteal stenosis
Type C lesions
• Multiple stenoses or occlusions totaling >15 cm with or without heavy calcification
• Recurrent stenoses or occlusions that need treatment after two endovascular interventions
Type D lesions
• Chronic total occlusions of CFA or SFA (>20 cm, involving the popliteal artery)
• Chronic total occlusion of popliteal artery and proximal trifurcation vessels

Fig. 1. TASC II anatomic classification of FP disease. CFA, common femoral artery. (*From* Norgren L, Hiatt WR, Dormandy JA, et al, on behalf of the TASC II Working Group. Inter-Society Consensus for the Management of Peripheral Arterial Disease (TASC II). Eur J Vasc Endovasc Surg 2007;33(Suppl 1):S58; with permission.)

popliteal arteries that comprise type D lesions.[2] However, the utility of these guidelines is limited: they do not incorporate patient characteristics or the indication for revascularization (eg, claudication, rest pain, tissue loss). Furthermore, these guidelines were developed before the current era of endovascular technology.

The largest randomized trial comparing an endovascular-first versus surgery-first strategy for PAD of the FP segment was performed in patients with severe limb ischemia (a term for patients with symptoms consistent with CLI, but who might not meet ankle-brachial index criteria).[33] The Bypass versus Angioplasty in Severe Ischemia of the Leg (BASIL) trial randomized 452 patients at 27 hospitals in the United Kingdom to either conventional bypass surgery or to percutaneous transluminal angioplasty (PTA).[34] Intention-to-treat analysis showed that amputation-free survival was not significantly different between the 2 treatment arms at 6 months.[34] However, for patients surviving more than 2 years, bypass surgery–first was associated with increased overall mean survival (7.3 months) and a trend toward greater amputation-free survival.[33] As such, the investigators concluded that a bypass surgery–first strategy may be preferred for patients with life expectancy of more than 2 years.[33] However, this trial had many limitations, as described in the next paragraph. Clinical risk scores have been developed to help identify patients who might benefit from surgery over PTA, but determining a priori who those patients are remains a challenge.[35]

Although the BASIL data are suggestive, patients who have severe limb ischemia and clinical equipoise between endovascular and bypass revascularization of infrainguinal disease are not common. For example, in the BASIL audit, only about a third of patients who were eligible for revascularization were considered suitable for randomization to either bypass or PTA.[34] Furthermore, whereas BASIL used simple PTA (no stents) as the endovascular approach, the proliferation of technologies that facilitate endovascular revascularization, even of highly complex lesions and of totally occluded segments,[10] has increased the feasibility of an endovascular-first approach in patients for whom there is not a clear reason to perform bypass surgery. Finally, the generalizability of the BASIL data is further limited by the high crossover rate between groups and by the absence of claudicants without severe limb ischemia in the trial.

Contemporary clinical experience shows that nearly all FP lesions (TASC II A–D) can be successfully approached endovascularly first, albeit with less durability in the most complex lesions.[16,36–40] Importantly, an endovascular approach that is respectful of sites of potential bypass inflow and outflow will not preclude future bypass surgery.[41–43] It also should be recognized that endovascular and bypass techniques are not mutually exclusive. Combined revascularization procedures composed of endovascular therapy for inflow and outflow disease coupled with conventional bypass surgery for complex or totally occluded portions of the FP segment are safe and effective.[42,44,45] Taken together, rather than following strict anatomic criteria, it is reasonable to tailor an approach to the patient and the patient's clinical condition using both conventional surgical and endovascular therapies.

ENDOVASCULAR TOOLS AND TECHNIQUES FOR COMPLEX ANATOMY

Historically, percutaneous revascularization was limited by the ability to cross total occlusions and/or suboptimal results after angioplasty and stenting. The development of crossing catheters and reentry devices[10,11] has facilitated crossing of totally occluded segments that might have once been prohibitive. Furthermore, tibial-pedal access and combined antegrade/retrograde recanalization of total occlusions also has expanded the application of endovascular approaches to even the 25% to 40% of infrainguinal chronic total occlusions that cannot be recanalized antegrade.[46,47] Once lesions are crossed, atherectomy devices can be used to modify complex lesions and facilitate angioplasty and stenting.[48,49] Unfortunately, there are few data to suggest that any of these approaches produces better long-term patency, nor have the various technologies been evaluated head-to-head in a randomized fashion. Nonetheless, technical advances in percutaneous technology have increased the feasibility of an endovascular-first approach. For example, **Fig. 2** shows an exemplary case of a long chronic total occlusion that was successfully revascularized using endovascular techniques.

ENDOVASCULAR REVASCULARIZATION OF FEMORAL POPLITEAL DISEASE: ANGIOPLASTY AND STENTS

The mainstay of endovascular therapy for FP segment atherosclerosis is PTA.[2,20] Although PTA has a high rate of acute success and low rate of complications, its durability remains suboptimal, with some studies quoting a patency rate of only 33% at 1 year.[2,6,7,50] Risk factors for poor long-term patency after PTA include diabetes,

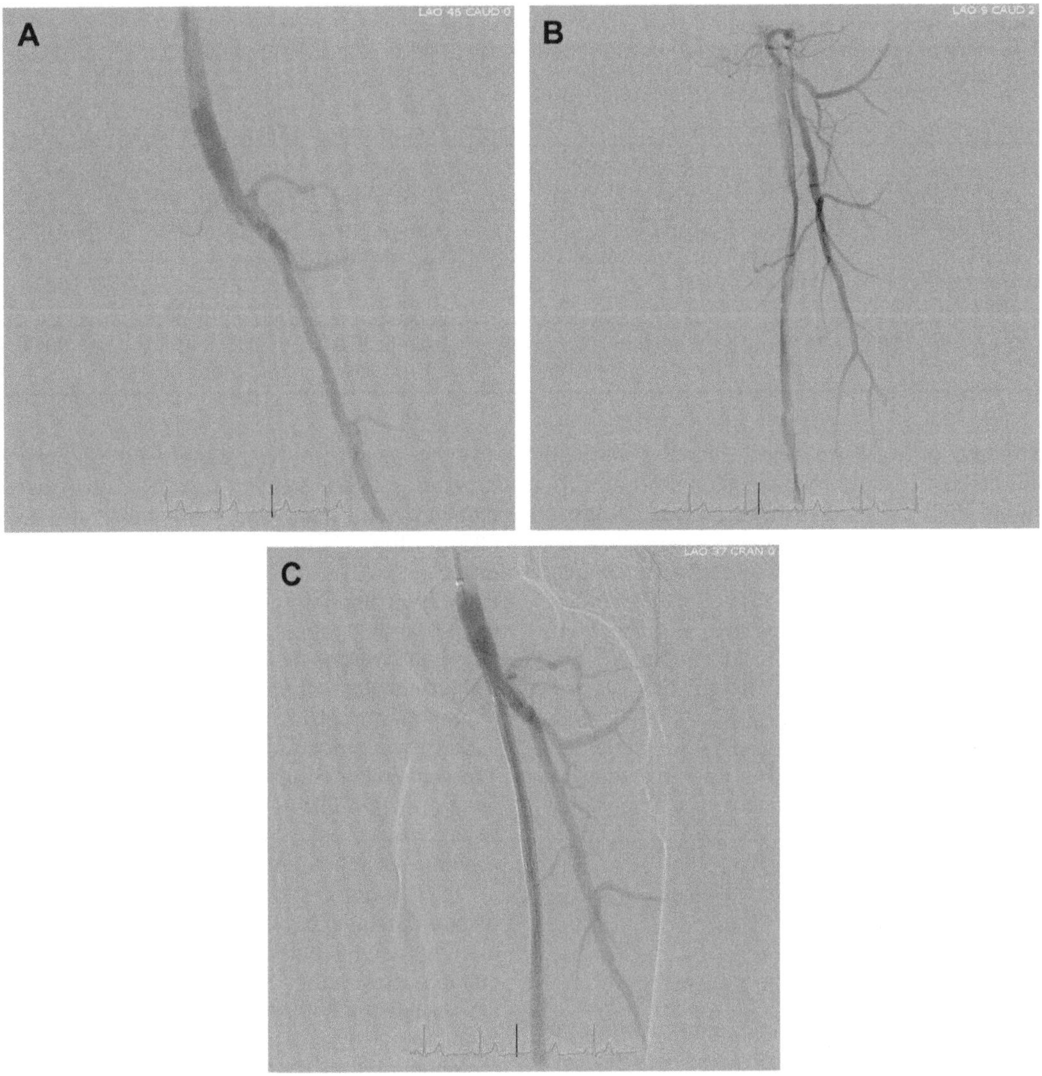

Fig. 2. Endovascular revascularization of a TASC D FP total occlusion (350 mm) in a 55-year-old man with Rutherford 4 claudication symptoms who had failed medical management and refused bypass surgery. (*A*) The angiogram shows a completely occluded SFA. (*B*) Angiogram of the vessel after antegrade subintimal recanalization, laser atherectomy, and balloon angioplasty. A dissection is evident and the angioplasty result was suboptimal. (*C*) Angiographic appearance of the vessel after deployment of 3 overlapping self-expanding nitinol stents.

diffuse disease (particularly lesions >100 mm in length), disease complexity, CLI, and number of runoff vessels.[41,51]

When PTA results are suboptimal, stenting of the FP segment can be used to mitigate acute recoil, flow-limiting dissection, or flow-limiting residual stenosis by scaffolding the vessel open. The long-term patency of FP stenting depends on the type of stent used. For example, when balloon-expandable bare-metal stents are used in the FP segment, restenosis outcomes are no better than PTA alone.[52–55] This is probably because the balloon-expandable stents are not well-suited to the mechanical stresses of the FP segment. By contrast, self-expanding nitinol stents are highly elastic and resistant to kinking and fracturing.[41] As summarized in **Table 1**, self-expanding nitinol stents can improve the patency of FP interventions in moderate and long lesions (>50 mm and >100 mm, respectively), but at the risk of in-stent restenosis (ISR).[56,57]

Endovascular stent-grafts (also known as covered stents) are stents covered with prosthetic graft material.[58] In the United States, the Viabahn stent-graft (W.L. Gore & Associates, Newark, DE, USA) is approved for use in the iliacs and SFA. It is

Table 1
Summary of randomized controlled trials of angioplasty (PTA) versus stenting in the femoral popliteal segment

First Author, Year	Stent Platform	Patients	Lesion Length	Restenosis Rate (%)	*P* Value
Krankenberg et al,[63] 2007	Luminexx (Bard Peripheral Vascular, Tempe, AZ, USA)	244	44 mm PTA 45 mm stent	38.6 PTA at 1 y 31.7 Stent at 1 y	.377
Schillinger et al,[57] 2006	Dynalink or Absolute (Abbott Vascular, Santa Clara, CA, USA)	104	127 mm PTA 132 mm stent	63 PTA at 1 y 37 Stent at 1 y	.01
Schillinger et al,[65] 2007		98		69.2 PTA at 2 y 45.7 Stent at 2 y	.031
Laird et al,[124] 2010	Lifestent (Bard Peripheral Vascular, Tempe, AZ, USA)	206	64 mm PTA 71 mm stent	63.3 PTA at 1 y 18.7 Stent at 1 y	.0001

composed of a self-expanding nitinol stent lined with heparin-bonded expanded polytetrafluoroethylene (PTFE) on its luminal surface.[58] Saxon and colleagues[59] randomized 197 cases with symptomatic SFA occlusive disease (mostly claudicants) and lesions of 13 cm or shorter to either PTA alone or to PTA followed by deployment Viabahn stent grafts. Mean lesion length was 70 ± 40 mm.[59] Primary patency at 1 year was 65% versus 40% for Viabahn and PTA, respectively (*P* = .0003). But, although Viabahn is better than PTA for moderate-length lesions in the SFA, it is not clear that the covered stents in the FP segment have a significant clinical or patency benefit over bare-metal nitinol stents.[60,61] They do, however, have their own attendant complications, including stent edge stenosis and acute stent thrombosis.[58,62]

WHEN TO STENT THE FP SEGMENT

The role of stenting with nitinol stents in the FP segment depends on the lesion length and the indication for revascularization. As summarized in **Table 1**, for short lesions (<45 mm), data from the Femoral Artery Stenting Trial (FAST) support PTA alone over primary stenting.[63] FAST randomized 244 mainly claudicants to either PTA (with bailout stenting) or to primary stenting with a single stent. Mean lesion length was 45 mm. At 1 year, there was no significant difference between the groups for restenosis, target lesion revascularization rate, or improvement in Rutherford class.[64] Of interest, a subset study showed that patients who received stents showed greater improvement in median walking distance (20 m and 52 m, respectively).[63]

For moderate (50–100 mm) and long (>100 mm) lesions, randomized trials of PTA versus primary stenting with nitinol stents show that primary stenting increases long-term patency (see **Table 1**). For example, the Balloon Angioplasty versus Stenting with Nitinol Stents in the Superficial Femoral Artery (ABSOLUTE) trial randomized 104 mostly severe claudicants with long lesions to either primary stenting or to PTA with bailout stenting. At 1 year, the restenosis rates were 63% for the PTA group and 37% for the stenting group (*P* = .01). Walking distance at 6 months and 1 year also was better in the stented group.[57] However, at 2 years, the benefits of stenting with respect to walking distance or need for revascularization were lost, despite a lower restenosis rate in the stented group.[65]

Despite advocates of primary stenting at first intervention,[66] current guideline recommendations are to reserve FP stenting for suboptimal angioplasty results (ie, "bailout" stenting),[20,50] which are not rare in the complex lesions characteristic of the FP segment. For patients with CLI, the acute gains of stenting may be sufficiently important to merit primary stenting.[2] For claudicants, it is difficult to know whether transient increases in walking time outweigh the risks of in-stent restenosis.[67,68] Stent fracture[69] and/or ISR can transform a simple restenosis into a more complex lesion requiring repeat stenting or more invasive therapies.[70] Stenting of a lesion that has restenosed after PTA has the same patency as primary stenting,[71] so it is reasonable to consider a PTA-first approach with bailout stenting if acute results are hemodynamically acceptable. Then, if there is symptomatic restenosis, stenting can be considered.

ISR

Femoral popliteal ISR is divided into 3 classes: class I corresponds to segments of 50 mm or less, class II is diffuse ISR greater than 50 mm, and class III is totally occluded.[72] With respect to outcomes, patients with class I and II ISR appear to do relatively well after repeat balloon angioplasty, with repeat ISR rates of 49.9% (*P*<.0001) and 53.3% (*P* = .0003) at 2 years, respectively. By contrast, patients with ISR leading to total occlusion (class III) have a recurrent ISR rate of

84.8% ($P<.0001$) and a recurrent occlusion rate of 64.6% ($P<.0001$) at 2 years.[72] Importantly, patients with Class III ISR have a greater need for subsequent bypass.[72] Because of the challenges posed by totally occlusive ISR, some operators argue for an aggressive plan of assisted patency, treating ISR, even when asymptomatic, so as to prevent total occlusion. However, the most optimal schedule of surveillance for ISR remains uncertain.[73]

Risk factors for early ISR (within 1 year) include severe lower extremity ischemia, diabetes, lesion complexity (TASCII C and D lesions), female sex, and number of stents implanted. Predictors of late ISR include female sex, TASC II C and D lesions, and chronic total occlusions.[74] Stent design itself also appears to be associated with ISR risk, so each stent technology should be closely examined before implementing its use.[74] Although recent developments in stent technology promise to deliver stents with greater radial strength and fracture resistance than in the past,[75] there are unfortunately few head-to-head comparisons to guide stent selection.

The best treatment strategies for ISR remain undetermined, although class II and III ISR often require adjunctive atherectomy in addition to PTA to get an adequate acute result.[76] Traditional treatment options for ISR have included balloon angioplasty, cutting balloon angioplasty, directional atherectomy, laser atherectomy, brachytherapy, and restenting, but there is no evidence that one is superior to the others for preventing restenosis or need for repeat revascularization.[77–79] The role of laser atherectomy may be delineated by the results of the EXCITE ISR trial, a randomized trial of laser plus balloon angioplasty versus PTA alone for treatment of ISR.[80]

The decision to perform repeat stenting of ISR is challenging because the risk of restenosis is not obviated by another stent. Moreover, repeat stenting increases the technical difficulty of future interventions. Not surprisingly, despite a high rate of technical success, the long-term patency rates of repeat stenting are worse than for primary stenting.[81] Treating ISR with stent grafts has the theoretic benefit of excluding the neointima with the expanded PTFE surface, but there are relatively few data on its efficacy.[82] Laird and colleagues[83] published a series of 27 patients with ISR who were treated with Viabahn stent-grafts after pretreatment with excimer laser and PTA. Their series demonstrated the safety of such an approach, but primary patency at 1 year was only 48%.[83] The introduction of drug-eluting stents (ie, stents coated with antiproliferative medicines) to the FP segment has elicited interest in their use to prevent and treat ISR, and is discussed in the next section.[84]

PREVENTING AND TREATING ISR: DRUG-ELUTING STENTS

Given the success of drug-eluting stents (DES) at preventing ISR in the coronary vasculature, their application to the FP segment is intuitive. Although initial experience with sirolimus-eluting stents in the FP segment was disappointing (summarized in **Table 2**),[85] the Zilver PTX paclitaxel-coated stent showed itself to be superior to PTA and to bare-metal self-expanding nitinol stents (BMS) in a trial of 479 patients with moderate-length lesions.[86] Primary patency was 83.1% in patients treated with Zilver PTX versus 32.8% in those treated with optimal PTA ($P<.001$). Furthermore, head-to-head testing of DES against BMS in the provisional stent groups (ie, patients who were randomized to DES vs BMS after suboptimal PTA) showed 89.9% primary patency for DES versus 73.0% for BMS ($P = .01$).[86] Importantly, there was also greater clinical benefit (defined as freedom from persistent or worsening claudication, rest pain, ulcer, or tissue loss after the initial treatment) in the provisional DES versus the provisional BMS group (90.5% vs 72.3%, $P = .009$).[86] At 2-year follow-up, the DES group continued to have greater primary patency and persistent clinical benefit.[87] The Zilver PTX is currently the only DES approved in the United States for use in the FP segment. Further follow-up studies are needed to determine whether it

Table 2
Summary of randomized controlled trials of drug-eluting stents (DES) versus angioplasty (PTA) and bare-metal stents (BMS) in the femoral popliteal segment

First Author, Year	Stent Platform	Patients	Lesion Length	Restenosis Rate (%)	*P* Value
Duda et al,[85] 2006	SMART (Cordis Corporation, Miami, FL, USA)	93	81 mm BMS 85 mm DES	21.1 BMS at 2 y 22.9 DES at 2 y	>.05
Dake et al,[86] 2011	Zilver (Cook Medical, Bloomington, IN, USA)	474	63 mm PTA 66 mm DES	67.2 PTA at 1 y 16.9 DES at 1 y	<.001
Dake et al,[87] 2013				73.5 PTA at 2 y 25.2 DES at 2 y	<.01

will be cost-effective to use DES (which are more expensive than BMS) for primary stenting, although some argue that decreased ISR from DES may lead to cost savings over time, particularly in patients with high risk for ISR after endovascular intervention (see **Table 1**).[88,89]

In addition to increasing long-term patency, one potential application of DES is to treat FP ISR. In a study of 108 patients with 119 ISR lesions (mean lesion length 133 mm, 33.1% were total occlusions) and Rutherford category of 2 or higher, restenting of ISR lesions with Zilver PTX (2.1 stents per lesion, on average) yielded primary patency rates of 78.8% at 1 year and freedom from target lesion revascularization of 81% and 60.8% at 1 and 2 years, respectively.[84] Importantly, all patients enjoyed improvement in the walking speed and distance up to 2 years after the procedure.[84]

Future directions in DES technology may include bioabsorbable DES, which could provide the temporary scaffold needed to prevent acute recoil or vessel closure, deliver antiproliferative drugs to counteract neointimal hyperplasia produced in response to the intervention, and then, over time, dissolve.[90] So far, evidence for utility of absorbable stents comes from the coronary and infragenicular vasculatures.[91–93] Given the unique challenges of the FP segment, it will be interesting to see whether bioabsorbable stents are able to address the current limits of FP stenting.

PREVENTING AND TREATING ISR: DRUG-COATED BALLOONS

Drug-coated balloons (DCBs) are a means by which the same antiproliferative drugs eluted from DES can be delivered to the site of intervention (either de novo lesions or ISR) without the vascular injury and inflammation associated with deploying a stent.[94] When considering DCBs, it is important to appreciate that the effects of the drug on neointimal proliferation exceed the short time of exposure that occurs during balloon inflation. For example, administration of paclitaxel during balloon inflation appears to be sufficient to prevent subsequent restenosis to a degree comparable with DES.[95]

As summarized in **Table 3**, trials of different balloon technologies coated with paclitaxel (the preferred agent at present) have shown significantly decreased late lumen loss compared with regular PTA.[8,95–98] For example, the Local Taxane with Short Exposure for Reduction of Restenosis in Distal Arteries (THUNDER) trial was a prospective, randomized, multicenter trial of 154 patients with Rutherford class 1 to 5 symptoms and FP lesions.[8] Patients were randomized to either standard PTA, PTA with paclitaxel-coated balloons, or to PTA with uncoated balloons and paclitaxel dissolved in the contrast medium. Mean lesion length was 74 mm. The primary outcome was late lumen loss at 6 months: 1.7 ± 1.8 mm for the control group compared with 0.4 ± 1.2 mm in the paclitaxel-coated balloon group ($P<.001$) and 2.2 ± 1.6 in the group with the paclitaxel in the contrast ($P = .11$). More clinically relevant was that target lesion revascularization at 24 months was 52% in the control group versus 15% in the DCB group ($P<.001$), versus 40% in the group with paclitaxel in the contrast medium ($P = .25$).[8] DCBs have also shown promise to reduce ISR before BMS stenting.[99] Whether decreased late lumen loss will translate into decreased need for revascularization in larger trials remains a question, however. For example, 6-month data from the Levant 2 trial of 476 patients randomized to angioplasty with the Moxy paclitaxel-coated balloon (Bard Peripheral Vascular, Tempe, AZ, USA)

Table 3
Summary of randomized controlled trials of angioplasty (PTA) versus drug-coated balloon (DCB) angioplasty in the femoral popliteal segment

First Author, Year	Trial	Patients	Lesion Length	Lumen Loss at 6 mo, mm	*P* Value
Tepe et al,[8] 2008	THUNDER	154	74 mm PTA 75 mm DCB	1.7 mm PTA 0.4 mm DCB	<.001
Werk et al,[95] 2008	Not applicable	87	57 mm PTA 61 mm DCB	1 mm PTA 0.5 mm DCB	.031
Werk et al,[96] 2012	PACIFIER	85	66 mm PTA 70 mm DCB	0.65 mm PTA −0.01 mm DCB	.001
Scheinert et al,[97] 2013	LEVANT I	101	80.2 mm PTA 80.8 mm DCB	1.09 mm PTA 0.46 mm DCB	.016

Abbreviations: LEVANT, Lutonix Paclitaxel-Coated Balloon for the Prevention of Femoropopliteal Restenosis; PACIFIER, Paclitaxel-coated Balloons in Femoral Indication to Defeat Restenosis; THUNDER, Local Taxane with Short Exposure for Reduction of Restenosis in Distal Arteries.

versus PTA alone in FP occlusive disease showed no significant difference between the 2 groups with respect to need for revascularization, despite superior patency in the DCB group.[100]

One major limitation of current DCB technology is that the balloons deliver paclitaxel at effective concentrations only on first inflation. Accordingly, long lesions may require multiple balloons, with implications for cost. Avoidance of geographic miss also will be important,[97] particularly if lesions are predilated with a conventional balloon before DCB use. Potential applications of DCBs continue to be explored, including treatment of ISR, or the use of DCBs in conjunction with atherectomy.[101] But, given the prevalence of FP disease that is refractory to PTA alone, the solo use of DCBs without adjunctive stenting in long and calcified de novo lesions is improbable.

BYPASS SURGERY FOR FP DISEASE

Bypass of FP atherosclerotic disease is typically infrainguinal, with the common femoral, superficial femoral, or deep femoral arteries serving as inflow vessels. Good inflow to the bypass segment can be ensured by performing endarterectomy of the common femoral artery and femoral bifurcation, with or without a patch of vein or bovine pericardium at the arteriotomy site.[102] The outflow vessel is typically the most proximal distal vessel that supplies in-line flow to the foot. In patients with CLI whose outflow vessel is below the trifurcation, direct revascularization of the affected angiosome may be important for effective wound healing.[103–105]

With respect to the bypass conduit, the saphenous vein has significantly better patency over prosthetic conduits for FP bypass (approximately 70% for above-the-knee vein vs approximately 50% for above-the-knee PTFE at 5 years).[15,106] In the absence of appropriate saphenous vein (estimated to occur in approximately 20% of patients),[107] other veins, such as long arm veins and spliced segments of arm veins, can be used as an alternative, with greater patency than PTFE,[107–110] but still less than saphenous vein.[111–113] For operative candidates with limited vein length, endovascular treatment of stenotic inflow disease combined with autologous vein bypass of a relatively short completely occluded segment can avoid having to use synthetic conduit.[114,115] Such combined procedures, known as hybrid revascularization, can be a viable option in patients with suitable anatomy and can decrease the amount of open surgery needed to accomplish revascularization.[116]

When no autologous single segment or spliced autologous vein of suitable size (3–4 mm) and quality is available for bypass, prosthetic grafts (usually PTFE) or composites of vein spliced with synthetic grafts can be used.[117,118] But, given the relatively poor patency of prosthetic grafts,[15,106] their benefit over endovascular revascularization is uncertain. For example, a prospective trial of 86 patients with occlusive SFA disease randomized to either percutaneous therapy with Viabahn endovascular stent-grafts (mean stented length of 25 $\pm$ 15 cm) or to above-the-knee FP bypass graft with prosthetic conduit found no significant difference between the groups with respect to primary and secondary patency.[119] At 4-year follow-up, primary patency was 59% in the stented group versus 58% in the bypass group ($P = .807$).[120] Secondary patency was 74% versus 71% in the stent versus surgery group, respectively ($P = .891$).[120] These data suggest a role for endovascular therapy when no autologous vein is present for bypass. When prosthetic graft bypasses are performed, addition of a vein cuff to the distal anastomosis may decrease intimal hyperplasia at the outflow site and improve patency.[121,122] The mechanism is believed to improved anastomotic hemodynamics.[123]

TAILORED APPROACHES TO FP REVASCULARIZATION

Despite advances in both endovascular and surgical techniques, procedural complications, graft thrombosis, stent fracture, and recurrent restenosis all have the potential to make a patient more symptomatic than before the index procedure. For this reason, the clinician should be careful in selecting patients for revascularization, particularly when the goal of therapy is relief of claudication symptoms and not treatment of CLI. Once the decision to intervene has been made, the optimal approach is controversial. Developments in endovascular therapy, particularly technologies that increase the durability of percutaneous interventions, will allow the application of endovascular-first approaches to complex lesions that historically could have been treated only with open surgery. That said, the durability of surgical bypass with autologous vein will continue to have an important role in FP revascularization, particularly for lesions that are high risk for restenosis or at high risk for adverse outcomes from endovascular approaches (eg, femoral bifurcation). Given the evidence, we argue that it is reasonable to consider endovascular approaches first, as long as the procedure does not jeopardize the patient's bypass options. But, when bypass surgery–first is the best choice, consideration of a hybrid strategy that synergizes the patency benefits of open surgery with the decreased morbidity of endovascular therapy may optimize outcomes.[116]

REFERENCES

1. Henry TD, Schwartz RS, Hirsch AT. "POBA Plus": will the balloon regain its luster? Circulation 2008; 118(13):1309–11.
2. Norgren L, Hiatt WR, Dormandy JA, et al. Inter-Society Consensus for the Management of Peripheral Arterial Disease (TASC II). J Vasc Surg 2007; 45(Suppl S):S5–67.
3. Hirsch AT, Criqui MH, Treat-Jacobson D, et al. Peripheral arterial disease detection, awareness, and treatment in primary care. JAMA 2001; 286(11):1317–24.
4. Regensteiner JG, Hiatt WR, Coll JR, et al. The impact of peripheral arterial disease on health-related quality of life in the Peripheral Arterial Disease Awareness, Risk, and Treatment: New Resources for Survival (PARTNERS) Program. Vasc Med 2008;13(1):15–24.
5. Hirsch AT, Hartman L, Town RJ, et al. National health care costs of peripheral arterial disease in the Medicare population. Vasc Med 2008;13(3): 209–15.
6. Dorrucci V. Treatment of superficial femoral artery occlusive disease. J Cardiovasc Surg (Torino) 2004;45(3):193–201.
7. Rocha-Singh KJ, Jaff MR, Crabtree TR, et al. Performance goals and endpoint assessments for clinical trials of femoropopliteal bare nitinol stents in patients with symptomatic peripheral arterial disease. Catheter Cardiovasc Interv 2007;69(6):910–9.
8. Tepe G, Zeller T, Albrecht T, et al. Local delivery of paclitaxel to inhibit restenosis during angioplasty of the leg. N Engl J Med 2008;358(7):689–99.
9. Schillinger M, Minar E. Percutaneous treatment of peripheral artery disease: novel techniques. Circulation 2012;126(20):2433–40.
10. Rogers JH, Laird JR. Overview of new technologies for lower extremity revascularization. Circulation 2007;116(18):2072–85.
11. Murarka S, Heuser RR. Chronic total occlusions in peripheral vasculature: techniques and devices. Expert Rev Cardiovasc Ther 2009;7(10):1283–95.
12. Schillinger M, Minar E. Claudication: treatment options for femoropopliteal disease. Prog Cardiovasc Dis 2011;54(1):41–6.
13. Davies MG, Waldman DL, Pearson TA. Comprehensive endovascular therapy for femoropopliteal arterial atherosclerotic occlusive disease. J Am Coll Surg 2005;201(2):275–96.
14. Schillinger M, Exner M, Mlekusch W, et al. Inflammatory response to stent implantation: differences in femoropopliteal, iliac, and carotid arteries. Radiology 2002;224(2):529–35.
15. Pereira CE, Albers M, Romiti M, et al. Meta-analysis of femoropopliteal bypass grafts for lower extremity arterial insufficiency. J Vasc Surg 2006;44(3):510–7.
16. Siracuse JJ, Giles KA, Pomposelli FB, et al. Results for primary bypass versus primary angioplasty/stent for intermittent claudication due to superficial femoral artery occlusive disease. J Vasc Surg 2012;55(4):1001–7.
17. Hunink MG, Wong JB, Donaldson MC, et al. Revascularization for femoropopliteal disease. A decision and cost-effectiveness analysis. JAMA 1995; 274(2):165–71.
18. van der Zaag ES, Legemate DA, Prins MH, et al. Angioplasty or bypass for superficial femoral artery disease? A randomised controlled trial. Eur J Vasc Endovasc Surg 2004;28(2):132–7.
19. Kudo T, Chandra FA, Kwun WH, et al. Changing pattern of surgical revascularization for critical limb ischemia over 12 years: endovascular vs. open bypass surgery. J Vasc Surg 2006;44(2): 304–13.
20. Anderson JL, Halperin JL, Albert NM, et al. Management of patients with peripheral artery disease (compilation of 2005 and 2011 ACCF/AHA guideline recommendations): a report of the American College of Cardiology Foundation/American Heart Association Task Force on Practice Guidelines. Circulation 2013;127(13):1425–43.
21. Yusuf S, Sleight P, Pogue J, et al. Effects of an angiotensin-converting-enzyme inhibitor, ramipril, on cardiovascular events in high-risk patients. The Heart Outcomes Prevention Evaluation Study Investigators. N Engl J Med 2000;342(3):145–53.
22. CAPRIE Steering Committee. A randomised, blinded, trial of clopidogrel versus aspirin in patients at risk of ischaemic events (CAPRIE). CAPRIE Steering Committee. Lancet 1996;348(9038): 1329–39.
23. Mazari FA, Khan JA, Carradice D, et al. Randomized clinical trial of percutaneous transluminal angioplasty, supervised exercise and combined treatment for intermittent claudication due to femoropopliteal arterial disease. Br J Surg 2012;99(1): 39–48.
24. McDermott MM. Functional impairment in peripheral artery disease and how to improve it in 2013. Curr Cardiol Rep 2013;15(4):347.
25. Brown J, Lethaby A, Maxwell H, et al. Antiplatelet agents for preventing thrombosis after peripheral arterial bypass surgery. Cochrane Database Syst Rev 2008;(4):CD000535.
26. Sarac TP, Huber TS, Back MR, et al. Warfarin improves the outcome of infrainguinal vein bypass grafting at high risk for failure. J Vasc Surg 1998; 28(3):446–57.
27. Johnson WC, Williford WO. Benefits, morbidity, and mortality associated with long-term administration

of oral anticoagulant therapy to patients with peripheral arterial bypass procedures: a prospective randomized study. J Vasc Surg 2002;35(3):413–21.
28. Taylor SM, Kalbaugh CA, Blackhurst DW, et al. Determinants of functional outcome after revascularization for critical limb ischemia: an analysis of 1000 consecutive vascular interventions. J Vasc Surg 2006;44(4):747–55 [discussion: 755–6].
29. Marston WA, Davies SW, Armstrong B, et al. Natural history of limbs with arterial insufficiency and chronic ulceration treated without revascularization. J Vasc Surg 2006;44(1):108–14.
30. Slovut DP, Sullivan TM. Critical limb ischemia: medical and surgical management. Vasc Med 2008; 13(3):281–91.
31. Lumsden AB, Davies MG, Peden EK. Medical and endovascular management of critical limb ischemia. J Endovasc Ther 2009;16(2 Suppl 2):II31–62.
32. Hirsch AT, Haskal ZJ, Hertzer NR, et al. ACC/AHA 2005 Practice Guidelines for the management of patients with peripheral arterial disease (lower extremity, renal, mesenteric, and abdominal aortic): a collaborative report from the American Association for Vascular Surgery/Society for Vascular Surgery, Society for Cardiovascular Angiography and Interventions, Society for Vascular Medicine and Biology, Society of Interventional Radiology, and the ACC/AHA Task Force on Practice Guidelines (Writing Committee to Develop Guidelines for the Management of Patients With Peripheral Arterial Disease): endorsed by the American Association of Cardiovascular and Pulmonary Rehabilitation; National Heart, Lung, and Blood Institute; Society for Vascular Nursing; TransAtlantic Inter-Society Consensus; and Vascular Disease Foundation. Circulation 2006;113(11):e463–654.
33. Bradbury AW, Adam DJ, Bell J, et al. Bypass versus Angioplasty in Severe Ischaemia of the Leg (BASIL) trial: an intention-to-treat analysis of amputation-free and overall survival in patients randomized to a bypass surgery-first or a balloon angioplasty-first revascularization strategy. J Vasc Surg 2010;51(Suppl 5):5S–17S.
34. Adam DJ, Beard JD, Cleveland T, et al. Bypass versus angioplasty in severe ischaemia of the leg (BASIL): multicentre, randomised controlled trial. Lancet 2005;366(9501):1925–34.
35. Bradbury AW, Adam DJ, Bell J, et al. Bypass versus Angioplasty in Severe Ischaemia of the Leg (BASIL) trial: a survival prediction model to facilitate clinical decision making. J Vasc Surg 2010;51(Suppl 5):52S–68S.
36. Surowiec SM, Davies MG, Eberly SW, et al. Percutaneous angioplasty and stenting of the superficial femoral artery. J Vasc Surg 2005;41(2):269–78.
37. DeRubertis BG, Faries PL, McKinsey JF, et al. Shifting paradigms in the treatment of lower extremity vascular disease: a report of 1000 percutaneous interventions. Ann Surg 2007;246(3):415–22 [discussion: 422–4].
38. Rabellino M, Zander T, Baldi S, et al. Clinical follow-up in endovascular treatment for TASC C-D lesions in femoro-popliteal segment. Catheter Cardiovasc Interv 2009;73(5):701–5.
39. Lyden SP, Smouse HB. TASC II and the endovascular management of infrainguinal disease. J Endovasc Ther 2009;16(2 Suppl 2):II5–18.
40. Han DK, Shah TR, Ellozy SH, et al. The success of endovascular therapy for all TransAtlantic Society Consensus graded femoropopliteal lesions. Ann Vasc Surg 2011;25(1):15–24.
41. Mewissen MW. Primary nitinol stenting for femoropopliteal disease. J Endovasc Ther 2009;16(2 Suppl 2):II63–81.
42. Setacci C, Galzerano G, Sirignano P, et al. The role of hybrid procedures in the treatment of critical limb ischemia. J Cardiovasc Surg (Torino) 2013; 54(6):729–36.
43. Santo VJ, Dargon P, Azarbal AF, et al. Lower extremity autologous vein bypass for critical limb ischemia is not adversely affected by prior endovascular procedure. J Vasc Surg 2014;60(1):129–35.
44. Ebaugh JL, Gagnon D, Owens CD, et al. Comparison of costs of staged versus simultaneous lower extremity arterial hybrid procedures. Am J Surg 2008;196(5):634–40.
45. Piazza M, Ricotta JJ 2nd, Bower TC, et al. Iliac artery stenting combined with open femoral endarterectomy is as effective as open surgical reconstruction for severe iliac and common femoral occlusive disease. J Vasc Surg 2011;54(2):402–11.
46. Montero-Baker M, Schmidt A, Braunlich S, et al. Retrograde approach for complex popliteal and tibioperoneal occlusions. J Endovasc Ther 2008; 15(5):594–604.
47. Venkatachalam S, Bunte M, Monteleone P, et al. Combined antegrade-retrograde intervention to improve chronic total occlusion recanalization in high-risk critical limb ischemia. Ann Vasc Surg 2014. [Epub ahead of print].
48. Shrikhande GV, McKinsey JF. Use and abuse of atherectomy: where should it be used? Semin Vasc Surg 2008;21(4):204–9.
49. Quevedo HC, Arain SA, Ali G, et al. A critical view of the peripheral atherectomy data in the treatment of infrainguinal arterial disease. J Invasive Cardiol 2014;26(1):22–9.
50. Dormandy JA, Rutherford RB. Management of peripheral arterial disease (PAD). TASC Working Group. TransAtlantic Inter-Society Consensus (TASC). J Vasc Surg 2000;31(1 Pt 2):S1–296.
51. Capek P, McLean GK, Berkowitz HD. Femoropopliteal angioplasty. Factors influencing long-term success. Circulation 1991;83(Suppl 2):I70–80.

52. Zdanowski Z, Albrechtsson U, Lundin A, et al. Percutaneous transluminal angioplasty with or without stenting for femoropopliteal occlusions? A randomized controlled study. Int Angiol 1999; 18(4):251–5.
53. Grimm J, Muller-Hulsbeck S, Jahnke T, et al. Randomized study to compare PTA alone versus PTA with Palmaz stent placement for femoropopliteal lesions. J Vasc Interv Radiol 2001;12(8):935–42.
54. Muradin GS, Bosch JL, Stijnen T, et al. Balloon dilation and stent implantation for treatment of femoropopliteal arterial disease: meta-analysis. Radiology 2001;221(1):137–45.
55. Becquemin JP, Favre JP, Marzelle J, et al. Systematic versus selective stent placement after superficial femoral artery balloon angioplasty: a multicenter prospective randomized study. J Vasc Surg 2003;37(3):487–94.
56. Dick P, Wallner H, Sabeti S, et al. Balloon angioplasty versus stenting with nitinol stents in intermediate length superficial femoral artery lesions. Catheter Cardiovasc Interv 2009;74(7):1090–5.
57. Schillinger M, Sabeti S, Loewe C, et al. Balloon angioplasty versus implantation of nitinol stents in the superficial femoral artery. N Engl J Med 2006; 354(18):1879–88.
58. Kwa AT, Yeo KK, Laird JR. The role of stent-grafts for prevention and treatment of restenosis. J Cardiovasc Surg (Torino) 2010;51(4):579–89.
59. Saxon RR, Dake MD, Volgelzang RL, et al. Randomized, multicenter study comparing expanded polytetrafluoroethylene-covered endoprosthesis placement with percutaneous transluminal angioplasty in the treatment of superficial femoral artery occlusive disease. J Vasc Interv Radiol 2008;19(6): 823–32.
60. Geraghty PJ, Mewissen MW, Jaff MR, et al. Three-year results of the VIBRANT trial of VIABAHN endoprosthesis versus bare nitinol stent implantation for complex superficial femoral artery occlusive disease. J Vasc Surg 2013;58(2):386–95.e4.
61. Lammer J, Zeller T, Hausegger KA, et al. Heparin-bonded covered stents versus bare-metal stents for complex femoropopliteal artery lesions: the randomized VIASTAR trial (Viabahn endoprosthesis with PROPATEN bioactive surface [VIA] versus bare nitinol stent in the treatment of long lesions in superficial femoral artery occlusive disease). J Am Coll Cardiol 2013;62(15):1320–7.
62. Fischer M, Schwabe C, Schulte KL. Value of the hemobahn/viabahn endoprosthesis in the treatment of long chronic lesions of the superficial femoral artery: 6 years of experience. J Endovasc Ther 2006; 13(3):281–90.
63. Krankenberg H, Schluter M, Steinkamp HJ, et al. Nitinol stent implantation versus percutaneous transluminal angioplasty in superficial femoral artery lesions up to 10 cm in length: the Femoral Artery Stenting Trial (FAST). Circulation 2007;116(3): 285–92.
64. Rutherford RB, Baker JD, Ernst C, et al. Recommended standards for reports dealing with lower extremity ischemia: revised version. J Vasc Surg 1997;26(3):517–38.
65. Schillinger M, Sabeti S, Dick P, et al. Sustained benefit at 2 years of primary femoropopliteal stenting compared with balloon angioplasty with optional stenting. Circulation 2007;115(21):2745–9.
66. Acin F, de Haro J, Bleda S, et al. Primary nitinol stenting in femoropopliteal occlusive disease: a meta-analysis of randomized controlled trials. J Endovasc Ther 2012;19(5):585–95.
67. Kasapis C, Henke PK, Chetcuti SJ, et al. Routine stent implantation vs. percutaneous transluminal angioplasty in femoropopliteal artery disease: a meta-analysis of randomized controlled trials. Eur Heart J 2009;30(1):44–55.
68. Twine CP, Coulston J, Shandall A, et al. Angioplasty versus stenting for superficial femoral artery lesions. Cochrane Database Syst Rev 2009;(2): CD006767.
69. Scheinert D, Scheinert S, Sax J, et al. Prevalence and clinical impact of stent fractures after femoropopliteal stenting. J Am Coll Cardiol 2005;45(2): 312–5.
70. Dalainas I, Nano G. Balloon angioplasty or nitinol stents for peripheral-artery disease. N Engl J Med 2006;355(5):521 [author reply: 523–4].
71. Schillinger M, Mlekusch W, Haumer M, et al. Angioplasty and elective stenting of de novo versus recurrent femoropopliteal lesions: 1-year follow-up. J Endovasc Ther 2003;10(2):288–97.
72. Tosaka A, Soga Y, Iida O, et al. Classification and clinical impact of restenosis after femoropopliteal stenting. J Am Coll Cardiol 2012;59(1):16–23.
73. Mohler ER 3rd, Gornik HL, Gerhard-Herman M, et al. ACCF/ACR/AIUM/ASE/ASN/ICAVL/SCAI/SCCT/SIR/SVM/SVS 2012 appropriate use criteria for peripheral vascular ultrasound and physiological testing part I: arterial ultrasound and physiological testing: a report of the American College of Cardiology Foundation Appropriate Use Criteria Task Force, American College of Radiology, American Institute of Ultrasound in Medicine, American Society of Echocardiography, American Society of Nephrology, Intersocietal Commission for the Accreditation of Vascular Laboratories, Society for Cardiovascular Angiography and Interventions, Society of Cardiovascular Computed Tomography, Society for Interventional Radiology, Society for Vascular Medicine, and Society for Vascular Surgery. J Vasc Surg 2012;56(1):e17–51.
74. Iida O, Uematsu M, Soga Y, et al. Timing of the restenosis following nitinol stenting in the

superficial femoral artery and the factors associated with early and late restenoses. Catheter Cardiovasc Interv 2011;78(4):611–7.
75. Werner M, Paetzold A, Banning-Eichenseer U, et al. Treatment of complex atherosclerotic femoropopliteal artery disease with a self-expanding interwoven nitinol stent: midterm results from the Leipzig SUPERA 500 registry. EuroIntervention 2014. [Epub ahead of print].
76. Armstrong EJ, Singh S, Singh GD, et al. Angiographic characteristics of femoropopliteal in-stent restenosis: association with long-term outcomes after endovascular intervention. Catheter Cardiovasc Interv 2013;82(7):1168–74.
77. Dick P, Sabeti S, Mlekusch W, et al. Conventional balloon angioplasty versus peripheral cutting balloon angioplasty for treatment of femoropopliteal artery in-stent restenosis: initial experience. Radiology 2008;248(1):297–302.
78. Yeo KK, Malik U, Laird JR. Outcomes following treatment of femoropopliteal in-stent restenosis: a single center experience. Catheter Cardiovasc Interv 2011;78(4):604–8.
79. Mitchell D, O'Callaghan AP, Boyle EM, et al. Endovascular brachytherapy and restenosis following lower limb angioplasty: systematic review and meta-analysis of randomized clinical trials. Int J Surg 2012;10(3):124–8.
80. Clinicaltrials.gov. Randomized Study of Laser and Balloon Angioplasty Versus Balloon Angioplasty to Treat Peripheral In-stent Restenosis (EXCITE ISR). 2013. 2014. Available at: http://clinicaltrials.gov/ct2/show/NCT01330628?term=spectranetics+and+restenosis&rank=3. Accessed March 1, 2014.
81. Robinson WP 3rd, Nguyen LL, Bafford R, et al. Results of second-time angioplasty and stenting for femoropopliteal occlusive disease and factors affecting outcomes. J Vasc Surg 2011;53(3):651–7.
82. Al Shammeri O, Bitar F, Ghitelman J, et al. Viabahn for femoropopliteal in-stent restenosis. Ann Saudi Med 2012;32(6):572–82.
83. Laird JR Jr, Yeo KK, Rocha-Singh K, et al. Excimer laser with adjunctive balloon angioplasty and heparin-coated self-expanding stent grafts for the treatment of femoropopliteal artery in-stent restenosis: twelve-month results from the SALVAGE study. Catheter Cardiovasc Interv 2012;80(5):852–9.
84. Zeller T, Dake MD, Tepe G, et al. Treatment of femoropopliteal in-stent restenosis with paclitaxel-eluting stents. JACC Cardiovasc Interv 2013;6(3):274–81.
85. Duda SH, Bosiers M, Lammer J, et al. Drug-eluting and bare nitinol stents for the treatment of atherosclerotic lesions in the superficial femoral artery: long-term results from the SIROCCO trial. J Endovasc Ther 2006;13(6):701–10.
86. Dake MD, Ansel GM, Jaff MR, et al. Paclitaxel-eluting stents show superiority to balloon angioplasty and bare metal stents in femoropopliteal disease: twelve-month Zilver PTX randomized study results. Circ Cardiovasc Interv 2011;4(5):495–504.
87. Dake MD, Ansel GM, Jaff MR, et al. Sustained safety and effectiveness of paclitaxel-eluting stents for femoropopliteal lesions: 2-year follow-up from the Zilver PTX randomized and single-arm clinical studies. J Am Coll Cardiol 2013;61(24):2417–27.
88. Bosiers M, Deloose K, Keirse K, et al. Are drug-eluting stents the future of SFA treatment? J Cardiovasc Surg (Torino) 2010;51(1):115–9.
89. De Cock E, Sapoval M, Julia P, et al. A budget impact model for paclitaxel-eluting stent in femoropopliteal disease in France. Cardiovasc Intervent Radiol 2013;36(2):362–70.
90. Peeters P, Keirse K, Verbist J, et al. Are bioabsorbable stents the future of SFA treatment? J Cardiovasc Surg (Torino) 2010;51(1):121–4.
91. Karnabatidis D, Katsanos K, Siablis D. Infrapopliteal stents: overview and unresolved issues. J Endovasc Ther 2009;16(Suppl 1):I153–62.
92. Vermassen F, Bouckenooghe I, Moreels N, et al. Role of bioresorbable stents in the superficial femoral artery. J Cardiovasc Surg (Torino) 2013;54(2):225–34.
93. Escarcega RO, Baker NC, Lipinski MJ, et al. Current application and bioavailability of drug-eluting stents. Expert Opin Drug Deliv 2014;11(5):689–709.
94. Scheller B, Speck U, Abramjuk C, et al. Paclitaxel balloon coating, a novel method for prevention and therapy of restenosis. Circulation 2004;110(7):810–4.
95. Werk M, Langner S, Reinkensmeier B, et al. Inhibition of restenosis in femoropopliteal arteries: paclitaxel-coated versus uncoated balloon: femoral paclitaxel randomized pilot trial. Circulation 2008;118(13):1358–65.
96. Werk M, Albrecht T, Meyer DR, et al. Paclitaxel-coated balloons reduce restenosis after femoropopliteal angioplasty: evidence from the randomized PACIFIER trial. Circ Cardiovasc Interv 2012;5(6):831–40.
97. Scheinert D, Duda S, Zeller T, et al. The LEVANT I (Lutonix Paclitaxel-Coated Balloon for the Prevention of Femoropopliteal Restenosis) trial for femoropopliteal revascularization: first-in-human randomized trial of low-dose drug-coated balloon versus uncoated balloon angioplasty. JACC Cardiovasc Interv 2013;7(1):10–9.
98. Cassese S, Byrne RA, Ott I, et al. Paclitaxel-coated versus uncoated balloon angioplasty reduces target lesion revascularization in patients with femoropopliteal arterial disease: a meta-analysis of randomized trials. Circ Cardiovasc Interv 2012;5(4):582–9.
99. Liistro F, Grotti S, Porto I, et al. Drug-eluting balloon in peripheral intervention for the superficial femoral artery: the DEBATE-SFA randomized trial (Drug Eluting Balloon in Peripheral Intervention for the

Superficial Femoral Artery). JACC Cardiovasc Interv 2013;6(12):1295–302.
100. Peck P. TCT: drug-coated balloon overblown? 2013. 2014. Available at: http://www.medpagetoday.com/MeetingCoverage/TCT/42615. Accessed March 12, 2014.
101. Stabile E, Virga V, Salemme L, et al. Drug-eluting balloon for treatment of superficial femoral artery in-stent restenosis. J Am Coll Cardiol 2013; 60(18):1739–42.
102. McBride RS, Al-Jarrah Q, Al-Khaffaf H. Rotated superficial femoral artery patch after common femoral artery endarterectomy. Ann R Coll Surg Engl 2013; 95(5):379.
103. Neville RF, Attinger CE, Bulan EJ, et al. Revascularization of a specific angiosome for limb salvage: does the target artery matter? Ann Vasc Surg 2009;23(3):367–73.
104. Kabra A, Suresh KR, Vivekanand V, et al. Outcomes of angiosome and non-angiosome targeted revascularization in critical lower limb ischemia. J Vasc Surg 2013;57(1):44–9.
105. Kret MR, Cheng D, Azarbal AF, et al. Utility of direct angiosome revascularization and runoff scores in predicting outcomes in patients undergoing revascularization for critical limb ischemia. J Vasc Surg 2014;59(1):121–8.
106. Klinkert P, Post PN, Breslau PJ, et al. Saphenous vein versus PTFE for above-knee femoropopliteal bypass. A review of the literature. Eur J Vasc Endovasc Surg 2004;27(4):357–62.
107. Chew DK, Conte MS, Donaldson MC, et al. Autogenous composite vein bypass graft for infrainguinal arterial reconstruction. J Vasc Surg 2001;33(2): 259–64 [discussion: 264–5].
108. Donaldson MC, Whittemore AD, Mannick JA. Further experience with an all-autogenous tissue policy for infrainguinal reconstruction. J Vasc Surg 1993;18(1):41–8.
109. Gentile AT, Lee RW, Moneta GL, et al. Results of bypass to the popliteal and tibial arteries with alternative sources of autogenous vein. J Vasc Surg 1996;23(2):272–9 [discussion: 279–80].
110. Faries PL, Arora S, Pomposelli FB Jr, et al. The use of arm vein in lower-extremity revascularization: results of 520 procedures performed in eight years. J Vasc Surg 2000;31(1 Pt 1):50–9.
111. Pomposelli FB, Kansal N, Hamdan AD, et al. A decade of experience with dorsalis pedis artery bypass: analysis of outcome in more than 1000 cases. J Vasc Surg 2003;37(2):307–15.
112. Albers M, Romiti M, Brochado-Neto FC, et al. Meta-analysis of alternate autologous vein bypass grafts to infrapopliteal arteries. J Vasc Surg 2005;42(3): 449–55.
113. Hunter GC, Woodside KJ, Naoum JJ. Healing characteristics and complications of prosthetic and biological vascular grafts. In: Hallet JW, Mills JL, Earnshaw JJ, et al, editors. Comprehensive vascular and endovascular surgery. 2nd edition. Philadelphia: Mosby Elsevier; 2009. p. 665–87.
114. Schneider PA, Caps MT, Ogawa DY, et al. Intraoperative superficial femoral artery balloon angioplasty and popliteal to distal bypass graft: an option for combined open and endovascular treatment of diabetic gangrene. J Vasc Surg 2001; 33(5):955–62.
115. Reed AB. Endovascular as an open adjunct: use of hybrid endovascular treatment in the SFA. Semin Vasc Surg 2008;21(4):200–3.
116. Slovut DP, Lipsitz EC. Surgical technique and peripheral artery disease. Circulation 2012;126(9): 1127–38.
117. London NJ. Surgical intervention for lower extremity arterial occlusive disease: femoropopliteal and tibial interventions. In: Hallet JW, Mills JL, Earnshaw JJ, et al, editors. Comprehensive vascular and endovascular surgery. 2nd edition. Philadelphia: Mosby Elsevier; 2009. p. 665–87.
118. Faries PL, Logerfo FW, Arora S, et al. Arm vein conduit is superior to composite prosthetic-autogenous grafts in lower extremity revascularization. J Vasc Surg 2000;31(6):1119–27.
119. Kedora J, Hohmann S, Garrett W, et al. Randomized comparison of percutaneous Viabahn stent grafts vs prosthetic femoral-popliteal bypass in the treatment of superficial femoral arterial occlusive disease. J Vasc Surg 2007;45(1):10–6 [discussion: 16].
120. McQuade K, Gable D, Pearl G, et al. Four-year randomized prospective comparison of percutaneous ePTFE/nitinol self-expanding stent graft versus prosthetic femoral-popliteal bypass in the treatment of superficial femoral artery occlusive disease. J Vasc Surg 2010;52(3):584–90 [discussion: 590–1, 591.e1–e7].
121. Stonebridge PA, Prescott RJ, Ruckley CV. Randomized trial comparing infrainguinal polytetrafluoroethylene bypass grafting with and without vein interposition cuff at the distal anastomosis. The Joint Vascular Research Group. J Vasc Surg 1997;26(4):543–50.
122. Qu Z, Chaikof EL. Prosthetic grafts. In: Cronenwett JL, Johnston KW, editors. Rutherford's vascular surgery. Philadelphia: Saunders Elsevier; 2010. p. 1335–49.
123. Rowe CS, Carpenter TK, How TV, et al. Local haemodynamics of arterial bypass graft anastomoses. Proc Inst Mech Eng H 1999;213(5):401–9.
124. Laird JR, Katzen BT, Scheinert D, et al. Nitinol stent implantation versus balloon angioplasty for lesions in the superficial femoral artery and proximal popliteal artery: twelve-month results from the RESILIENT randomized trial. Circ Cardiovasc Interv 2010;3(3):267–76.

Management of Atherosclerotic Aortoiliac Occlusive Disease

Marcin Bujak, MD, PhD, Jacqueline Gamberdella, MS,
Carlos Mena, MD*

KEYWORDS

• Aortoiliac occlusive disease • Endovascular interventions • Medical management

KEY POINTS

- The prevalence of aortoiliac occlusive disease (AIOD) increases along with presence of atherosclerotic risk factors such as diabetes, hypertension, hyperlipidemia, and cigarette smoking.
- Medical management remains a cornerstone of AIOD management.
- The most important goal of conservative therapy in patients with AIOD is reduction of the risk of cardiovascular events.
- Supervised exercise training is a recommendation with the widest acceptance in initial treatment of intermittent claudication.
- Aortobifemoral bypass still remains the standard treatment of diffuse and complex AIOD.
- Endovascular therapy for AIOD is associated with significantly lower mortality as well as faster recovery times.
- Indications for percutaneous interventions in AIOD are slowly expanding to TransAtlantic Inter-Society Consensus lesions in categories C and D.

INTRODUCTION

Peripheral arterial disease (PAD) affects up to 10% of patients older than 40 years and up to 20% of population older than 70 years.[1,2] The prevalence of PAD increases with presence of atherosclerotic risk factors such as diabetes, hypertension, hyperlipidemia, and cigarette smoking.[2–4] However, it is estimated that at least half of patients with PAD is asymptomatic, and therefore, the true prevalence is likely underestimated. Development of atherosclerotic changes in the abdominal aorta has been reported as early as the second decade of human life.[5] Interestingly, aortoiliac disease tends to occur in younger patients, with up to 30% of patients being younger than 50 years of age.[6–8] Furthermore, aortoiliac atherosclerosis seems to be more rapidly progressive when compared with infrainguinal disease.[9] Although currently we have a wide range of pharmacologic, percutaneous, and surgical interventions available at our disposal, the research supporting its use in aortoiliac occlusive disease (AIOD) is still rather limited. This article presents recent advances in approaches to management of this prevalent and debilitating disease.

RISK FACTORS FOR OCCLUSIVE AORTOILIAC DISEASE

Several studies attempted to compare risk factors for atherosclerosis affecting proximal and distal

Disclosure Statement: The authors report no financial relationships or conflicts of interest regarding the content herein.
Section of Cardiovascular Medicine, Department of Internal Medicine, Yale University School of Medicine, 333 Cedar Street, DANA3 Cardiology, New Haven, CT 06510, USA
* Corresponding author.
E-mail address: carlos.mena-hurtado@yale.edu

Intervent Cardiol Clin 3 (2014) 531–543
http://dx.doi.org/10.1016/j.iccl.2014.06.001
2211-7458/14/$ – see front matter

arteries. Analysis of the data revealed that apart from histologic differences, there are also significant disparities in the levels of sociodemographic and cardiovascular risk factors between large and small peripheral arteries.[10]

Smoking

The relationship between smoking and PAD has been recognized since 1911, when Erb reported intermittent claudication (IC) to be 3 times more common among smokers than nonsmokers. Additionally, smoking appears to have a synergistic effect on other cardiovascular risk factors. Interestingly, tobacco seems to be also a major risk factor differentially associated with proximal and distal PAD. Results of most studies are concordant and indicate smoking as a key risk factor affecting predominantly proximal vessels, especially the aorta and iliac arteries.[7,11–13] Haltmayer and colleagues[11] reported the strongest association between smoking and aortoiliac disease, a lower but still significant association at the femoropopliteal level and no association at the crural level.

Diabetes

Insulin resistance and the metabolic syndrome are other factors with critical roles in the development of PAD. IC is about twice as common among diabetic patients versus nondiabetic patients. Every 1% increase in hemoglobin A1c is associated with a 26% increased risk of atherosclerotic plaques.[14] Using an angiographic score of atherosclerotic burden, van der Feen and colleagues[15] noted a progressive shift from lower scores in proximal arteries in patients without diabetes to higher scores in infrapopliteal arteries in patients with diabetes.

Hyperlipidemia

In the Framingham study, a fasting cholesterol level greater 270 mg/dL was associated with a doubling of the incidence of IC. However, it was not the cholesterol level but the ratio of total cholesterol to high-density lipoprotein that was the best predictor of PAD.[16] In a study including young patients with PAD, dyslipidemia was more prevalent in cases of aortoiliac lesions than PAD in more distal locations.[17] This finding was also reported by Vogelberg and colleagues[18] in their analysis of angiographic series in patients with PAD. Conversely, Haltmayer and colleagues[11] did not find a site-specific relationship between cholesterol levels and localization of PAD. Nevertheless, in their work they did observe an association between elevated triglycerides levels and development of atherosclerotic disease in the femoropopliteal segments.[11]

Hypertension

The relative risk for developing PAD is smaller for hypertension than diabetes or smoking. Data regarding the association between hypertension and PAD according to lesion localization are rather scant. Hansen in 1990s did observe a trend in hypertensive patients with premature PAD to develop more distal lesions.[17] This finding was not confirmed in other reports, and up to date there are no strong data indicating relationship between hypertension and lesion sites.[8]

Inflammation

Nonspecific aortoarteritis (Takayasu arteritis) is a classic example of a nonatherosclerotic cause of occlusive disease in aortoiliac arteries. With a world wide incidence of 2.6/1 million it is still considered a rare disease in Western countries. Inflammation involving the aorta and its main branches is predominantly present in young women. For yet unknown reasons, it has the highest incidence in India, where it frequently involves the abdominal aorta and aortoiliac vessels.

CLASSIFICATION

Three distinct types of atherosclerosis have been described based on atherosclerotic involvement of arterial segments distal to renal arteries (**Fig. 1**).[19]

- Type I atherosclerosis (5%–10%): involvement limited predominantly to infrarenal aorta and common iliac arteries (CIA). More frequent in women.
- Type II atherosclerosis (35%): lesions prevalent in the infrarenal aorta, CIA, and external iliac arteries (EIA). Atherosclerosis may extend into the common femoral arteries (CFA).
- Type III atherosclerosis (55%–60%): diffuse disease in the infrarenal aorta, iliac, femoral, popliteal, and tibial arteries.

This classification has currently more historical rather than clinical value because it has been largely replaced by the newer TransAtlantic Inter-Society Consensus (TASC) classification. TASC is a result of cooperation between 14 medical, surgical, vascular, cardiovascular, vascular radiology, and cardiology societies in Europe and North America. Their cooperation resulted in more thorough classification of atherosclerotic patterns into 4 categories, A to D. TASC classification however, although the most widely used, definitely cannot be

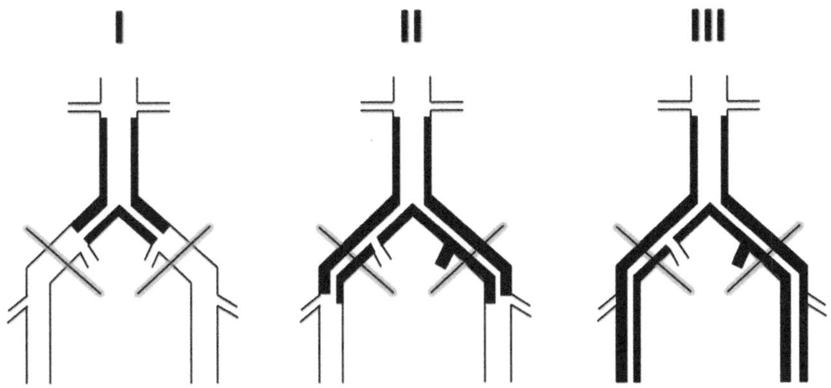

Fig. 1. Patterns of AIOD. (I) type I atherosclerosis, (II) type II atherosclerosis, and (III), type III atherosclerosis.

considered flawless. One of its main negatives is a focus on singular patterns of the disease, whereas obviously most PAD patients tend to have multilevel disease. Its main positive feature, however, is the fact that it was developed based on the nature and distribution of plaques in combination with known outcomes for intervention.[20] Furthermore, its relative simplicity and applicability makes it a great tool, which has been widely used over the last decade. In 2007 TASC classification, schemes were somewhat modified from the original TASC 2000 guidelines to reflect technological advances (examples in **Fig. 2**).

- Type 'A': stenoses of the CIA as well as single and short lesions located in the EIA (<3 cm). Endovascular is a preferred treatment method.
- Type 'B': short stenosis of the infrarenal aorta as well as 3 to 10-cm lesions involving EIA. Unilateral CIA and EIA occlusions not extending to adjacent regions. Endovascular is a preferred method of treatment.
- Type 'C': bilateral occlusions of CIA or EIA. Unilateral lesions in EIA commonly involving origins of internal iliac or CFA.
- Type 'D': complex lesions. This category contains infrarenal occlusions, diffuse unilateral as well as bilateral disease of the iliac arteries. This category also involves iliac disease in patients with abdominal aortic aneurysm not amendable to endograft placement.

Although TASC D and C were considered to have better results with open revascularization, those recommendations are more commonly questioned as discussed later.

MEDICAL MANAGEMENT

Risk Reduction

In recent years, the authors have witnessed a substantial progress in endovascular as well as surgical therapies for PAD. Nevertheless, lifestyle modification and medical treatment still remains

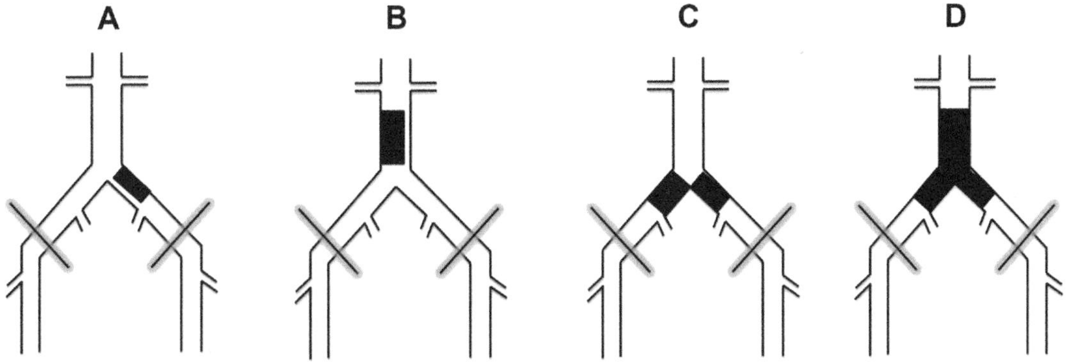

Fig. 2. Examples of different atherosclerotic lesions based on TASC II classification of AIOD. (*A*) Stenoses of the CIA as well as single and short lesions located in the EIA; (*B*) short stenosis of the infrarenal aorta as well as 3 to 10-cm lesions involving EIA; (*C*) bilateral occlusions of CIA or EIA; and (*D*) complex lesions. (*Adapted from* Norgren L, Hiatt WR, Dormandy JA, et al, TASC II Working Group. Inter-Society Consensus for the management of peripheral arterial disease (TASC II). J Vasc Surg 2007;45(Suppl S):S5–67.)

the cornerstone of AIOD management. The most important goal of conservative therapy for claudication is aggressive risk reduction of cardiovascular events. The incidence of myocardial infarction and stroke is significantly elevated in this group of patients. Up to 50% of patients with coronary artery disease may have concomitant PAD. It is estimated that about 30% of PAD patients die within 5 years of diagnosis, and death is usually due to a coronary event. In the Cardiovascular Health Study, the patients with an Ankle Brachial Index of 0.8 were more than twice as likely to suffer from a vascular event such as myocardial infarction, stroke, or transient ischemic attack.[21] Aboyans and colleagues[22] found that patients with aortoiliac disease have significantly worse general prognosis when compared with patients with atherosclerosis located in peripheral segments.

Smoking cessation

Smoking cessation is a condition "sine qua non" when it comes to successful management of patient with AIOD. All patients using any form of tobacco products, even those with early or subclinical signs of PAD, should be strongly and explicitly advised to quit. Current guidelines advise that apart from counseling, all physicians regardless of specialty should be more proactive and offer comprehensive smoking cessation therapies.[23] Most data supporting tobacco cessation are based mostly on observational studies, because randomized clinical trials would likely encounter multiple obstacles of ethical nature. Nevertheless, all available studies clearly and persuasively indicate substantial reduction in death, cardiovascular events, amputations, and also patency rates following revascularization in patients who stop smoking.

Antiplatelet therapy

The protective effects of Aspirin on cardiovascular events in patients with atherosclerosis are very well established. The Antithrombotic Trialists' Collaboration meta-analysis, however, looked specifically at the effects of antiplatelet therapy on patients with PAD. In their analysis, they found that antiplatelet therapy in this group was associated with 22% odds reduction of adverse cardiovascular events.[24] The Critical Leg Ischemia Prevention Study enrolled patients with substantially advanced lower extremity atherosclerosis. This trial was also able to demonstrate a significant reduction in cardiovascular events among subjects randomized to aspirin.[25] Unfortunately, this trial was stopped early due to poor recruitment. The 2009 meta-analysis of aspirin therapy for patients with PAD demonstrated a 34% risk reduction for nonfatal stroke among participants taking aspirin but no statistically significant reduction in overall cardiovascular events.[26] The currently recommended dose of aspirin is between 75 mg and 325 mg per day. Addition of clopidogrel to aspirin is acceptable particularly in high-risk patients.[23]

Statins

Heart Protection Study delivered direct evidence supporting the use of statins to lower low-density lipoprotein levels in PAD patients.[27] Currently high-potency statins are indicated for all patients with PAD regardless of lesion localization.[28]

Symptomatic Treatment

Symptom improvement and amputation prevention are the secondary goals of treatment in PAD. Unfortunately, the evidence supporting symptomatic medical therapy particularly in AIOD is still limited. It is estimated that up to 50% of patients with lower extremity PAD are asymptomatic and only one-third presents with typical claudication. American College of Cardiology (ACC)/American Heart Association (AHA) guidelines on PAD estimate that 70% to 80% of patients with claudication will have stable symptoms at 5 years of follow-up, 10% to 20% of patients will have worsening claudication, and 1% to 2% will progress to critical limb ischemia.[29]

Supervised exercise therapy

Up to date, supervised exercise training is the recommendation with the widest acceptance in the initial treatment of IC. Even relatively short sessions adding to total of 90 min per week (3 × 30 min) for 3 months have been proven effective. Fokkenrood and colleagues[30] in their recently published analysis showed a significant improvement in maximal treadmill walking distance with supervised versus nonsupervised exercise therapy regimens. Watson and colleagues[31] also noticed significantly improved maximal walking time in patients enrolled in exercise programs. In their analysis, mean difference in walking times was 5.12 minutes, and an overall improvement in walking ability was estimated to be approximately 50% to 200%. Pain-free walking distance as well as maximum walking distance was also significantly improved. Although the benefits of unsupervised exercise are not as well established, it is obviously still strongly recommended.

Pharmacotherapy

Data from clinical trials do suggest presence of significant differences in claudication endpoints for some of the available agents. Nevertheless, pharmacotherapy in the treatment of IC has not gained a significant popularity in the United States. Its use here has been considerably lower when compared with European countries.

- Cilostazol is one of the newer and more commonly used pharmacologic agents. Its wide range of action, which encompasses antiplatelet, vasodilatory, and antithrombotic effects, is mediated mostly through inhibition of phosphodiesterase 3 activity. Money and colleagues[32] published results of a multicenter, randomized, double-blind, placebo-controlled trial where 239 patients with IC were randomly assigned to receive cilostazol or a placebo. At week 16, patients in the cilostazol group had a 96.4 m (47%) increase in absolute claudication distance compared with 31.4 m (12.9%) noted in the placebo group.
- Pentoxifylline is the most researched agent used in the treatment of IC. Currently it is considered a second-line therapy to cilostazol. Its main mechanism of action is improvement of blood flow by decreasing blood viscosity and improving erythrocyte flexibility. It has also been described to inhibit platelet aggregation. Its efficacy has been supported by clinical trials showing improvement in absolute as well as initial claudication distance.[33,34] Dawson and colleagues[35] in randomized, double-blind, placebo-controlled, multicenter trial compared the efficacy and safety of cilostazol and pentoxifylline. After 24 weeks of treatment, cilostazol was associated with a mean 54% increase in maximal walking distance, which was significantly more than 30% increase noted with pentoxifylline. In this study, the improvement with pentoxifylline was comparable to the placebo group.
- There are several other agents available that are either prescribed by physicians or self-administered by patients. They include substances like ethylenediaminetetraacetic acid, iloprost, ginkgo biloba, Vitamin E, and many others. In most cases, there are no data supporting use of those agents (L-arginine, ginkgo biloba) or its use is not indicated and may have harmful adverse effects (Chelation).

Overall, smoking cessation, exercise, and antiplatelet therapy are the cornerstones of treatment in patients with PAD. Although pharmacologic agents do show improvement in trials, the "real-life" clinical benefit may not be sufficient for some physicians and patients to justify its everyday use.

SURGICAL TREATMENT OF OCCLUSIVE AORTOILIAC DISEASE

Before prosthetic grafts for aortic bypasses became available, the first direct surgical reconstructions on the aorta were performed using thromboendarterectomy. This technique was first described by Dos Santos in 1947.[36] During the 1950s and 1960s, aortoiliac endarterectomy and its modifications became a standard in the treatment of AIOD. These long operations require substantial surgical skills and were later replaced by simpler and more convenient prosthetic bypass techniques. Over the last 30 years, aortofemoral bypass (AFB), iliofemoral bypass, and aortoiliac endarterectomy (AIE) have been the most widely used anatomic open surgical reconstructions. Although extra-anatomical bypass techniques were developed for patients at high risk or unsuitable for laparotomy, patency outcomes were less favorable and the treatment of choice in AIOD remained anatomic bypass procedures.

Throughout the 1980s, excellent long-term outcomes of AFB or AIE with patency rates of 80% and 90% defined surgery as a the gold standard therapy.[37] Chiu and colleagues[38] performed one of the largest meta-analysis of open surgical management of AIOD (**Table 1**). In their analysis, the observed 5-year primary patency rates for all most common surgical techniques were between

Table 1
Five-year patency rates, mortality, and morbidity for AFB, iliofemoral bypass, and AIE in patients with intermittent claudication and chronic lower extremity ischemia

Technique	Patency	IC	CLI	Mortality	Systemic Morbidity
AFB	86.3%	89.8%	79.8%	4.1%	16%
IFB	85.3%	86.7%	74.1%	2.7%	18.9%
AIE	88.3%	90.8%	81.7%	2.7%	12.5%

Abbreviations: CLI, chronic lower extremity ischemia; IFB, iliofemoral bypass.
Data from Chiu KW, Davies RS, Nightingale PG, et al. Review of direct anatomic open surgical management of atherosclerotic aorto-iliac occlusive disease. Eur J Vasc Endovasc Surg 2010;39(4):460–71.

85.3% and 88.3%. The 5-year patency rates were significantly higher in patients with IC when compared with surgeries on patients with chronic limb ischemia.

Inspite of good long-term outcomes, there has been a noticeable change over the past 15 years in patient population undergoing surgical reconstruction. It has been noticed that after year 2000, more procedures have been performed for chronic lower extremity ischemia rather than for claudication.[39] Furthermore, there has been a considerable shift in recent years in peripheral vascular surgeries toward increasingly complex procedures.[40] This finding seems to be related to change in patient selection for open reconstruction as a result of more widespread use of endovascular techniques. The shift away from open surgical techniques is driven also by considerable operative mortality and morbidity (see **Table 1**). Systemic or major morbidity rates are reported to occur in up to 10% of cases, with overall morbidity ranging between 11% and 32%.[41]

Another important factor when considering an intervention is the time of return to normal activities. This includes also sexual function, which is an important issue for many patients. All those considerations were a strong driving force, which led to development of new promising alternatives to open surgery. An example of such an advance is laparoscopic vascular surgery, which may be performed with or without robot assistance. This particular technique was developed as a minimally invasive option and resulted in a reduction in operative trauma and faster post-op ambulation.[42,43] Nonetheless, laparoscopic AIOD repair remains a challenging intervention from a technical standpoint. It is associated with a longer total operative time and longer aortic clamping times when compared with open repair.[44] Post-operative data suggest that the technical challenge of laparoscopic AIOD repair is not associated with worsening of the post-operative course.[44] Tiek and colleagues[45] reported a significantly faster post-operative recovery after laparoscopic surgery, earlier introduction of a fluid and solid diet, earlier mobilization, and overall shorter in-hospital stays. In their analysis, more than 50% of patients treated laparoscopically returned to normal activities at 2 weeks, whereas no patient had done so in the conventional open group. Moreover, the other advantage of laparoscopy is the lack of abdominal wall dehiscence, which happens in 10% to 15% of cases after open AFB.[44,46]

Hybrid procedures comprising both endovascular and surgical techniques are used particularly in challenging cases. Multilevel reconstructions using both techniques have been performed both simultaneously and in a staged fashion. In hybrid procedures, open access to femoral arteries is created with subsequent endovascular intervention performed on proximal as well as distal vessel. This approach can allow for the repair of occlusions from a single incision with outcomes and complications comparable to percutaneous interventions. Femoral endarterectomy also is a key step in complex hybrid repairs, which have been increasingly used for multilevel revascularization particularly in high-risk patients. Hybrid repairs currently comprise 15% of all revascularizations.[47]

ENDOVASCULAR TREATMENT OF AIOD

Endovascular treatment is an excellent treatment option for increasingly more types of AIOD. In addition to faster recovery time, it is associated with significantly lower morbidity and mortality when compared with standard surgical techniques. Endovascular therapy (EVT) for iliac artery lesions results in almost immediate improvement in quality of life approaching the level of age-matched controls.[48]

Perioperative Risk and Complications

Significantly lower mortality as well as faster recovery times are major factors facilitating ongoing expansion of indications to EVT. Thirty days mortality following EVT has been reported throughout the literature to range anywhere between 0% and 6.7%.[41] In addition, morbidity rates associated with percutaneous treatment are also lower when compared with surgical interventions. Most commonly reported complications associated with EVT are access site hematomas and episodes of distal embolization. Access site hematomas are reported to occur in 4% to 17% of cases, and the reported occurrence of pseudoaneurysms is less than 3%.[41] The rate of distal embolization and iliac or aortic vessel ruptures is estimated to be between 1% and 11% and 0.5% and 3%, respectively.[41] The rate of vessel wall dissections is estimated to be between 2% and 5%.[41] Higher complication rates are noted especially during complex procedures like reconstruction of the aortic bifurcation or interventions on the abdominal aorta. Increased complication rates during those procedures used to be related to factors like multiple access sites or lack of appropriate endovascular tools or techniques. However, as discussed later, introduction of new devices and techniques resulted in significant reduction in complications rates during those complex interventions. It is also important to remember that most complications occurring during percutaneous interventions can be relatively easily managed with endovascular approach or conservatively. Stent grafts covered with Dacron or polytetrafluoroethylene membranes allow to manage complications, such as arterial ruptures or tears with high success rates immediately after they occur.

Indications

In the recent years, the authors have witnessed significant technical advances in the field of endovascular interventions. Nevertheless, still the most substantial barrier obstructing widespread application of EVT in all aortoiliac lesions is the paucity of large randomized clinical trials. Endovascular approach for the treatment of the aortoiliac vessels in the United States has been officially recommended so far only for TASC lesions categorized in groups A and B.[20] There are several investigators questioning those restrictions and suggesting a need for significant expansion of indications to EVT. Just recently published 2014 guidelines developed by the Cardiovascular and Interventional Radiological Society of Europe officially expanded recommendations for endovascular interventions to lesions in TASC group C. Furthermore, recently published BRAVISSIMO questioned TASC guidelines recommending surgery as the treatment of choice for type D lesions.[20] BRAVISSIMO was a prospective, nonrandomized, multicenter trial designed to answer the question whether an endovascular treatment can be extended as the primary approach for aortoiliac lesions TASC C and D. Not surprisingly, the study confirmed the safety as well as effectiveness of modern EVT in those categories.[49] High technical success rates in treatment of TASC D lesions were also reported by other investigators.[50] Currently endovascular interventions on TASC C and D lesions are routinely performed in experienced high volume centers.

Long-Term Results

Long-term patency rates following endovascular treatment used to be inferior when compared with surgery. Becker and colleagues[51] in their work from 1989 after analysis of almost 2700 patients reported a 5-year patency rate of 72% for EVT. Almost 10 years after Becker, Rutherford reported a similar 5-year patency rate of 70%.[52] Murphy and colleagues[53] after an 8-year follow-up period reported a primary patency rate of 74%. Simons and colleagues[54] evaluated the outcomes of endovascular interventions for occlusive lesions localized to distal aorta. Reported primary clinical patency in this study was 68% at 3 years with primary hemodynamic patency reaching 83%. Increasing numbers of recent studies using modern percutaneous techniques report outcomes more comparable with open surgical procedures. Jongkind and colleagues[41] performed the largest analysis of literature regarding interventional treatment of aortoiliac disease. In their work, they included studies dating from 2000 to 2009 and found a 1-year primary patency rate between 70% and 97%. Interestingly, there were only 2 studies out of 19 analyzed, which reported patency rates of 70%. The remaining 16 studies reported a primary patency greater than 85% with most of them reporting a primary patency greater than 90%. Secondary 1-year patency ranged between 88% and 100%. Long-term (4 and 5 years) primary patency rates ranged from 60% to 86% and secondary patencies were between 80% and 98%.[41] Sixt and colleagues[50] reported the primary 1-year patency rate of 86% for the entire study cohort, which included TASC lesions A to D. Remarkably, reported patency for complex TASC D lesions in this study was also 85%. BRAVISSIMO reported even higher primary patency rates and at 12 months. The patency rates for the TASC A, B, C, and D lesions were 94.0%, 96.5%, 91.3%, and 90.2%, respectively. Kashyap and colleagues[55] conducted a retrospective study comparing an open repair against a percutaneous intervention in treatment of extensive AIOD. Although their reported limb-based primary patency rate at 3 years was greater for aortobifemoral bypass (93% vs 74%), the secondary patency (97% vs 95%), limb salvage (98% vs 98%), and long-term survival (80% vs 80%) were similar.

Revascularization Strategies in Endovascular Therapy

The choice of endovascular strategy is largely based on available access site, known biomechanical properties of iliac vessels, and complexity of the lesion.[56] Although the treatment of short iliac stenosis is a relatively simple procedure, a recanalization of complex aortoiliac occlusions can be a long and extremely challenging endeavor. Those procedures are commonly associated with increased procedure time, contrast load, exposure to radiation, and increased rates of periprocedural complications.[57,58] However, recent technological advances led to significant improvements in procedural times, success rates, and patient safety. At the present time, there are 2 major treatment pathways available when forming a revascularization strategy for patients with complex atherosclerotic lesions: classic percutaneous intraluminal angioplasty (PTA) or newer percutaneous intentional extraluminal revascularization (PIER).

Percutaneous intraluminal angioplasty

Successful revascularization of complex occlusive lesions with standard wires and balloons used to be achievable in less than the 60% of cases.[59] Although this tactic is still the most commonly used approach in EVT, the development of intraluminal crossing devices led to considerable improvement in success rates and reduction of perioperative complications. The Crosser (Bard Peripheral Vascular, Inc, Tempe, AZ, USA) is one of the most commonly used recanalization catheters designed to facilitate intraluminal angioplasty especially in long chronic total occlusions (CTOs). Crosser uses high-frequency vibrations to facilitate penetration of the occlusion, which appears to be particularly useful in long, calcified, and guidewire resistant CTOs. The PATRIOT trial (Peripheral Approach to Recanalization of Occluded Lesions) reported 84% successful crossing of guidewire resistant CTOs with Crosser and remarkable 0% rate of perforations.[60] The Crosser device is safe and shows excellent efficacy in facilitating guidewire distal lumen entry, especially for aortoiliac and tibial occlusions.[61] The Avinger Wildcat (Avinger, Redwood City, CA, USA) is another type of crossing catheter with demonstrated successful crossing rate of 89%.[62]

Percutaneous intentional extraluminal revascularization

PIER or Subintimal Angioplasty is a relatively new percutaneous technique implemented nowadays with increasing frequency. Subintimal entries during CTO procedures and inability to reenter the true lumen were major problems discouraging from percutaneous attempts in complex lesions. Development of true lumen reentry devices allowing for precise reintroduction of the guidewire to true lumen drastically changed the approach to treatment of CTOs. Currently there are 2 Food and Drug Administration (FDA)-approved reentry catheters: Outback LTD Re-Entry Catheter (Cordis, Johnson & Johnson company; Bridgewater, NJ, USA) and Pioneer Plus Catheter PPlus 120 (Medtronic CardioVascular; Santa Rosa, CA, USA).[63,64] Outback as well as Pioneer have been extensively used in infrainguinal lesions; however, their safety and efficacy in aortoiliac disease have also been confirmed.[65,66] Successful true lumen reentry rates have been estimated to reach 87% in femoropopliteal lesions and 91% in aortoiliac occlusions.[67] Furthermore, reentry times with reentry catheter manipulation require significantly less time (<10 minutes) and can be accomplished in less than 3 minutes.[66]

Balloon angioplasty in management of AIOD

Among all factors, which can negatively affect the patency rate after the intervention, the role of stent placement has been the mostly vastly discussed and investigated.[52] Improved results associated with stenting are commonly attributed to decreased elastic recoil, improved management of dissections as well as lower restenosis rates.[68] Rationale for a routine stent implantation was further supported by work of Bosch and Hunink. Their meta-analysis showed a significant 39% reduction of long-term failure after stent placement compared with PTA alone.[69] The benefits of routine stenting became questioned after the publication of the DUTCH trial. The Dutch Iliac Stent Trial Study was a multicenter, randomized trial evaluating a choice of stent versus PTA with provisional stenting.[70] Primary study as well as later published long-term outcomes surprisingly showed similar outcomes of provisional and primary stenting. There was no significant difference in 2-year reintervention rates, which were 7% for PTA and 4% for primary stenting. After a mean follow-up of 5.6 years, outcomes in both groups remained similar with primary patency rates of 82% and 80%.[71,72] Moreover, patients treated with PTA and selective stent placement in the iliac artery had a better outcome for symptomatic success.[72] When looking at the results of this study, it is important to remember a very high crossover rate reaching 43%. Nearly half of the patients randomized to balloon angioplasty received a stent due to suboptimal result during the primary procedure. Such high crossover rate makes the interpretation of study results somewhat difficult. Similarly to DUTCH trial, Piffaretti and colleagues[73] also did not find a significant difference in primary patency rates between PTA and stented lesions. Sixt and colleagues[50] on the other hand reported improved 1-year primary patency rate after stenting. Most recently published BRAVISSIMO also suggested primary stenting as the preferred treatment of patients with all types of aortoiliac lesions.[49] The 2013 ACC/AHA guidelines recommend stents as primary therapy in CIA and EIA lesions as class IB and IC indication, respectively.[23]

Stents in the management of AIOD

In contrast to coronary interventions, there are several different types of stents used in revascularization of aortoiliac lesions (**Table 2**). The differences among available stents are tremendous and include delivery systems, design, and used materials (see **Table 2**). The introduction of the first balloon expandable stent (BES) (Palmaz, Cordis Corporation, Bridgewater, NJ, USA) has been considered a breakthrough in the field of

Table 2
Examples of FDA-approved stents currently used in aortoiliac disease

Stent	Company	Trial	FDA Approval	Type
S.M.A.R.T Nitinol Stent System	Cordis Corporation	CRISP	August 12, 2003	Self-expandable Nitinol stent
The Express LD Iliac Stent	Boston Scientific Corporation	MELODIE	March 5, 2010	Balloon expandable Nitinol stent
Epic Vascular Self-Expanding Stent System	Boston Scientific Corporation	ORION	April 13, 2012	Self-expandable Nitinol stent
Omnilink Elite Vascular Balloon-Expandable Stent System	Abbott Vascular	MOBILITY	July 31, 2012	Balloon expandable Nitinol stent
Assurant Cobalt Iliac Balloon-Expandable Stent System	Medtronic Endovascular	ACTIVE	October, 2011	Balloon expandable Cobalt stent
E-LUMINEXX Vascular Stent	Bard Peripheral Vascular, Inc	A clinical evaluation of the Bard LUMINEXX Iliac Stent and Delivery System	December 4, 2008	Self-expanding Nitinol stent
GORE VIABAHN Endoprosthesis	W.L. Gore & Associates, Inc	GORE VIABAHN Endoprosthesis Feasibility Study	June 14, 2005	Self-expanding ePTFE covered/ also available with heparin bioactive surface
Zilver Vascular Stent	Cook, Incorporated	Clinical evaluation of the Zilver Vascular Stent for symptomatic iliac artery disease	June 26, 2006	Self-expanding Nitinol

percutaneous interventions. FDA approved Palmaz stents for iliac use in 1991. Wallstent (Boston Scientific, Natic, MA, USA) was the first self-expandable "closed-cell" stent (SES) approved for the treatment of iliac disease. In the last decade, however, those stents have been largely replaced by newer stents with "open-cell" structure. Nitinol-based stents are the most commonly used SESs available on the market today. Nitinol is a metal alloy of nickel and titanium and its popularity stems from unique combination of properties: biocompatibility, excellent shape memory, and high radial resistive force.[74] Open-cell structure used in new stents gives them high conformability along curvatures and allows for complete stent apposition throughout changing calibers of the vessel.

The common iliac artery is a straight and essentially immobile vessel, which is considered to be more amenable to stenting with BESs. The main advantage of BES is their substantial radial strength. Furthermore, the delivery system permits more accurate stent placement, which is of utmost importance particularly in the proximal segment of the CIA as well as bifurcations.[75,76] The external iliac artery is usually more tortuous and undergoes longitudinal stretching during hip movements. Because of those features, some investigators believe SESs to be more suitable for the management of lesions in this localization.[77] Provisional stenting with SESs has been preferred in EIAs mainly due to a lower risk of dissection and elastic recoil. Obviously, the final choice of BESs versus SESs is determined mainly by operator preference.

Despite relatively good results achieved with open-cell stents, the risk of restenosis particularly after treatment of complex lesions still remains substantial. Covering of the stent with fabric or graft material seemed to be a perfect solution to prevent neointimal proliferation in the healing artery. However, covering material does not protect from development of restenosis at the edges of the stent. Edge restenosis appears to be the primary pattern of restenosis associated with these devices. The Covered Versus Balloon Expandable Stent Trial (COBEST) compared Advanta Vascular V12 (Atrium Medical Corporation, Hudson, NH, USA) to bare-metal stents and revealed better outcomes with covered stents in TASC C and D lesions. Covered stents were associated with lower rates of restenosis and target vessel revascularization.[78] Additionally, covered stents are the first choice when it comes to treatment of iatrogenic vessel perforations, aneurysms, and possibly pseudoaneurysms. At present, GORE VIABAHN Endoprosthesis (Gore & Associates, Flagstaff, AZ, USA) is the only covered stent approved for iliac and superficial femoral artery use in the United States. The US equivalent of Advanta, the iCast stent (Atrium Medical Corporation) has not yet received FDA approval.

Introduction of drug-eluting stents and drug-coated balloons opened an exiting new article in EVT. Up to date trials evaluating those devices were focused primarily on infrainguinal disease.

SUMMARY

Over the last 40 years there has been amazing progress in understanding and managing atherosclerosis. Self-management strategies like smoking cessation and exercise as well as risk factor modification still play a pivotal role in the treatment. The continuous improvement in safety and long-term patency associated with EVT caused a significant shift from open surgical techniques toward percutaneous interventions. The latter, associated with significantly less morbidity and mortality, are inevitably the future of peripheral interventions. Unfortunately, the evidence base supporting decision making in the treatment of AIOD is still very limited. The ongoing research on recanalization techniques as well as on angiogenesis and pharmacotherapy is necessary to further advance the field and improve long-term outcomes.

REFERENCES

1. Jaff MR, Cahill KE, Yu AP, et al. Clinical outcomes and medical care costs among medicare beneficiaries receiving therapy for peripheral arterial disease. Ann Vasc Surg 2010;24(5):577–87.
2. Graham IM, Daly LE, Refsum HM, et al. Plasma homocysteine as a risk factor for vascular disease. The European Concerted Action Project. JAMA 1997;277(22):1775–81.
3. Selvin E, Erlinger TP. Prevalence of and risk factors for peripheral arterial disease in the United States: results from the National Health and Nutrition Examination Survey, 1999–2000. Circulation 2004; 110(6):738–43.
4. Ridker PM, Stampfer MJ, Rifai N. Novel risk factors for systemic atherosclerosis: a comparison of C-reactive protein, fibrinogen, homocysteine, lipoprotein(a), and standard cholesterol screening as predictors of peripheral arterial disease. JAMA 2001;285(19):2481–5.
5. Levy PJ. Epidemiology and pathophysiology of peripheral arterial disease. Clin Cornerstone 2002; 4(5):1–15.
6. Vogt MT, Wolfson SK, Kuller LH. Segmental arterial disease in the lower extremities: correlates of disease and relationship to mortality. J Clin Epidemiol 1993;46(11):1267–76.
7. Smith FB, Lee AJ, Fowkes FG, et al. Smoking, haemostatic factors and the severity of aorto-iliac and femoro-popliteal disease. Thromb Haemost 1996; 75(1):19–24.
8. Diehm N, Shang A, Silvestro A, et al. Association of cardiovascular risk factors with pattern of lower limb atherosclerosis in 2659 patients undergoing angioplasty. Eur J Vasc Endovasc Surg 2006; 31(1):59–63.
9. Coran AG, Warren R. Arteriographic changes in femoropopliteal arteriosclerosis obliterans. A five-year follow-up study. N Engl J Med 1966;274(12):643–7.
10. Aboyans V, Lacroix P, Criqui MH. Large and small vessels atherosclerosis: similarities and differences. Prog Cardiovasc Dis 2007;50(2):112–25.
11. Haltmayer M, Mueller T, Horvath W, et al. Impact of atherosclerotic risk factors on the anatomical distribution of peripheral arterial disease. Int Angiol 2001;20(3):200–7.
12. Lord JW Jr. Cigarette smoking and peripheral atherosclerotic occlusive disease. JAMA 1965; 191:249–51.
13. Strong JP, Richards ML. Cigarette smoking and atherosclerosis in autopsied men. Atherosclerosis 1976;23(3):451–76.
14. Selvin E, Marinopoulos S, Berkenblit G, et al. Meta-analysis: glycosylated hemoglobin and cardiovascular disease in diabetes mellitus. Ann Intern Med 2004;141(6):421–31.
15. van der Feen C, Neijens FS, Kanters SD, et al. Angiographic distribution of lower extremity atherosclerosis in patients with and without diabetes. Diabet Med 2002;19(5):366–70.
16. Murabito JM, Evans JC, Nieto K, et al. Prevalence and clinical correlates of peripheral arterial disease in the Framingham Offspring Study. Am Heart J 2002;143(6):961–5.

17. Hansen ME, Valentine RJ, McIntire DD, et al. Age-related differences in the distribution of peripheral atherosclerosis: when is atherosclerosis truly premature? Surgery 1995;118(5):834–9.
18. Vogelberg KH, Berchtold P, Berger H, et al. Primary hyperlipoproteinemias as risk factors in peripheral artery disease documented by arteriography. Atherosclerosis 1975;22(2):271–85.
19. Brewster DC. Clinical and anatomical considerations for surgery in aortoiliac disease and results of surgical treatment. Circulation 1991;83(2 Suppl):I42–52.
20. Norgren L, Hiatt WR, Dormandy JA, et al. Inter-Society Consensus for the management of peripheral arterial disease (TASC II). J Vasc Surg 2007; 45(Suppl S):S5–67.
21. Newman AB, Siscovick DS, Manolio TA, et al. Ankle-arm index as a marker of atherosclerosis in the cardiovascular health study. Cardiovascular Heart Study (CHS) Collaborative Research Group. Circulation 1993;88(3):837–45.
22. Aboyans V, Desormais I, Lacroix P, et al. The general prognosis of patients with peripheral arterial disease differs according to the disease localization. J Am Coll Cardiol 2010;55(9):898–903.
23. Anderson JL, Halperin JL, Albert NM, et al. Management of patients with peripheral artery disease (compilation of 2005 and 2011 ACCF/AHA guideline recommendations): a report of the American College of Cardiology Foundation/American Heart Association task force on practice guidelines. Circulation 2013;127(13):1425–43.
24. Antithrombotic Trialists' Collaboration. Collaborative meta-analysis of randomised trials of antiplatelet therapy for prevention of death, myocardial infarction, and stroke in high risk patients. BMJ 2002;324(7329):71–86.
25. Critical Leg Ischaemia Prevention Study Group, Catalano M, Born G, et al. Prevention of serious vascular events by aspirin amongst patients with peripheral arterial disease: randomized, double-blind trial. J Intern Med 2007;261(3):276–84.
26. Berger JS, Krantz MJ, Kittelson JM, et al. Aspirin for the prevention of cardiovascular events in patients with peripheral artery disease: a meta-analysis of randomized trials. JAMA 2009;301(18):1909–19.
27. Heart Protection Study Collaborative Group. MRC/BHF heart protection study of cholesterol lowering with simvastatin in 20,536 high-risk individuals: a randomised placebo-controlled trial. Lancet 2002; 360(9326):7–22.
28. Stone NJ, Robinson J, Lichtenstein AH, et al. 2013 ACC/AHA guideline on the treatment of blood cholesterol to reduce atherosclerotic cardiovascular risk in adults: a report of the American College of Cardiology/American Heart Association task force on practice guidelines. J Am Coll Cardiol 2014;63(25 Pt B):2889–934.
29. Hirsch AT, Haskal ZJ, Hertzer NR, et al. ACC/AHA 2005 practice guidelines for the management of patients with peripheral arterial disease (lower extremity, renal, mesenteric, and abdominal aortic): a collaborative report from the American Association for Vascular Surgery/Society for Vascular Surgery, Society for Cardiovascular Angiography and Interventions, Society for Vascular Medicine and Biology, Society of Interventional Radiology, and the ACC/AHA task force on practice guidelines (writing committee to develop guidelines for the management of patients with peripheral arterial disease): endorsed by the American Association of Cardiovascular and Pulmonary Rehabilitation; National Heart, Lung, and Blood Institute; Society for Vascular Nursing; TransAtlantic Inter-Society Consensus; and Vascular Disease Foundation. Circulation 2006;113(11):e463–654.
30. Fokkenrood HJ, Bendermacher BL, Lauret GJ, et al. Supervised exercise therapy versus non-supervised exercise therapy for intermittent claudication. Cochrane Database Syst Rev 2013;(8):CD005263.
31. Watson L, Ellis B, Leng GC. Exercise for intermittent claudication. Cochrane Database Syst Rev 2008;(4):CD000990.
32. Money SR, Herd JA, Isaacsohn JL, et al. Effect of cilostazol on walking distances in patients with intermittent claudication caused by peripheral vascular disease. J Vasc Surg 1998;27(2):267–74 [discussion: 274–5].
33. Ernst E, Kollar L, Resch KL. Does pentoxifylline prolong the walking distance in exercised claudicants? A placebo-controlled double-blind trial. Angiology 1992;43(2):121–5.
34. Porter JM, Cutler BS, Lee BY, et al. Pentoxifylline efficacy in the treatment of intermittent claudication: multicenter controlled double-blind trial with objective assessment of chronic occlusive arterial disease patients. Am Heart J 1982;104(1):66–72.
35. Dawson DL, Cutler BS, Hiatt WR, et al. A comparison of cilostazol and pentoxifylline for treating intermittent claudication. Am J Med 2000;109(7):523–30.
36. Dos Santos JC. Sur la desobstruction des thrombus arterielles anciennes. Mem Acad Chir (Paris) 1947;73:409.
37. Szilagyi DE, Elliott JP Jr, Smith RF, et al. A thirty-year survey of the reconstructive surgical treatment of aortoiliac occlusive disease. J Vasc Surg 1986; 3(3):421–36.
38. Chiu KW, Davies RS, Nightingale PG, et al. Review of direct anatomical open surgical management of atherosclerotic aorto-iliac occlusive disease. Eur J Vasc Endovasc Surg 2010;39(4):460–71.
39. Kakkos SK, Haurani MJ, Shepard AD, et al. Patterns and outcomes of aortofemoral bypass grafting in the era of endovascular interventions. Eur J Vasc Endovasc Surg 2011;42(5):658–66.

40. Back MR, Johnson BL, Shames ML, et al. Evolving complexity of open aortofemoral reconstruction done for occlusive disease in the endovascular era. Ann Vasc Surg 2003;17(6):596–603.
41. Jongkind V, Akkersdijk GJ, Yeung KK, et al. A systematic review of endovascular treatment of extensive aortoiliac occlusive disease. J Vasc Surg 2010;52(5):1376–83.
42. Nio D, Diks J, Bemelman WA, et al. Laparoscopic vascular surgery: a systematic review. Eur J Vasc Endovasc Surg 2007;33(3):263–71.
43. Diks J, Nio D, Jongkind V, et al. Robot-assisted laparoscopic surgery of the infrarenal aorta: the early learning curve. Surg Endosc 2007;21(10):1760–3.
44. Di Centa I, Coggia M, Cerceau P, et al. Total laparoscopic aortobifemoral bypass: short- and middle-term results. Ann Vasc Surg 2008;22(2):227–32.
45. Tiek J, Remy P, Sabbe T, et al. Laparoscopic versus open approach for aortobifemoral bypass for severe aorto-iliac occlusive disease–a multicentre randomised controlled trial. Eur J Vasc Endovasc Surg 2012;43(6):711–5.
46. Adye B, Luna G. Incidence of abdominal wall hernia in aortic surgery. Am J Surg 1998;175(5):400–2.
47. Dosluoglu HH, Lall P, Cherr GS, et al. Role of simple and complex hybrid revascularization procedures for symptomatic lower extremity occlusive disease. J Vasc Surg 2010;51(6):1425–35.e1.
48. Chetter IC, Spark JI, Kent PJ, et al. Percutaneous transluminal angioplasty for intermittent claudication: evidence on which to base the medicine. Eur J Vasc Endovasc Surg 1998;16(6):477–84.
49. Bosiers M, Deloose K, Callaert J, et al. BRAVISSIMO: 12-month results from a large scale prospective trial. J Cardiovasc Surg (Torino) 2013;54(2):235–53.
50. Sixt S, Alawied Ak, Rastan A, et al. Acute and long-term outcome of endovascular therapy for aortoiliac occlusive lesions stratified according to the TASC classification: a single-center experience. J Endovasc Ther 2008;15(4):408–16.
51. Becker GJ, Katzen BT, Dake MD. Noncoronary angioplasty. Radiology 1989;170(3 Pt 2):921–40.
52. Timaran CH, Stevens SL, Freeman MB, et al. External iliac and common iliac artery angioplasty and stenting in men and women. J Vasc Surg 2001;34(3):440–6.
53. Murphy TP, Ariaratnam NS, Carney WI Jr, et al. Aortoiliac insufficiency: long-term experience with stent placement for treatment. Radiology 2004;231(1):243–9.
54. Simons PC, Nawijn AA, Bruijninckx CM, et al. Long-term results of primary stent placement to treat infrarenal aortic stenosis. Eur J Vasc Endovasc Surg 2006;32(6):627–33.
55. Kashyap VS, Pavkov ML, Bena JF, et al. The management of severe aortoiliac occlusive disease: endovascular therapy rivals open reconstruction. J Vasc Surg 2008;48(6):1451–7, 1457.e1–3.
56. Dyet JF, Watts WG, Ettles DF, et al. Mechanical properties of metallic stents: how do these properties influence the choice of stent for specific lesions? Cardiovasc Intervent Radiol 2000;23(1):47–54.
57. Gandini R, Volpi T, Pipitone V, et al. Intraluminal recanalization of long infrainguinal chronic total occlusions using the Crosser system. J Endovasc Ther 2009;16(1):23–7.
58. Markose G, Miller FN, Bolia A. Subintimal angioplasty for femoro-popliteal occlusive disease. J Vasc Surg 2010;52(5):1410–6.
59. Bolia A, Miles KA, Brennan J, et al. Percutaneous transluminal angioplasty of occlusions of the femoral and popliteal arteries by subintimal dissection. Cardiovasc Intervent Radiol 1990;13(6):357–63.
60. Endovascular-Today. PATRIOT evaluates FlowCardia's Crosser to mediate CTO recanalization. 2009. Available at: http://www.evtoday.com/eNews/eNews102909.htm. Accessed July 20, 2014.
61. Staniloae CS, Mody KP, Yadav SS, et al. Endoluminal treatment of peripheral chronic total occlusions using the Crosser(R) recanalization catheter. J Invasive Cardiol 2011;23(9):359–62.
62. Pigott JP, Raja ML, Davis T. A multicenter experience evaluating chronic total occlusion crossing with the Wildcat catheter (the CONNECT study). J Vasc Surg 2012;56(6):1615–21.
63. Smith M, Pappy R, Hennebry TA. Re-entry devices in the treatment of peripheral chronic occlusions. Tex Heart Inst J 2011;38(4):392–7.
64. Shin SH, Baril D, Chaer R, et al. Limitations of the Outback LTD re-entry device in femoropopliteal chronic total occlusions. J Vasc Surg 2011;53(5):1260–4.
65. Varcoe RL, Nammuni I, Lennox AF, et al. Endovascular reconstruction of the occluded aortoiliac segment using "double-barrel" self-expanding stents and selective use of the Outback LTD catheter. J Endovasc Ther 2011;18(1):25–31.
66. Jacobs DL, Motaganahalli RL, Cox DE, et al. True lumen re-entry devices facilitate subintimal angioplasty and stenting of total chronic occlusions: initial report. J Vasc Surg 2006;43(6):1291–6.
67. Etezadi V, Benenati JF, Patel PJ, et al. The reentry catheter: a second chance for endoluminal reentry at difficult lower extremity subintimal arterial recanalizations. J Vasc Interv Radiol 2010;21(5):730–4.
68. Palmaz JC, Garcia OJ, Schatz RA, et al. Placement of balloon-expandable intraluminal stents in iliac arteries: first 171 procedures. Radiology 1990;174(3 Pt 2):969–75.
69. Bosch JL, Hunink MG. Meta-analysis of the results of percutaneous transluminal angioplasty and stent

placement for aortoiliac occlusive disease. Radiology 1997;204(1):87–96.
70. Tetteroo E, van der Graaf Y, Bosch JL, et al. Randomised comparison of primary stent placement versus primary angioplasty followed by selective stent placement in patients with iliac-artery occlusive disease. Dutch Iliac Stent Trial Study Group. Lancet 1998;351(9110):1153–9.
71. Klein WM, van der Graaf Y, Seegers J, et al. Long-term cardiovascular morbidity, mortality, and reintervention after endovascular treatment in patients with iliac artery disease: the Dutch Iliac Stent Trial Study. Radiology 2004;232(2):491–8.
72. Klein WM, van der Graaf Y, Seegers J, et al. Dutch iliac stent trial: long-term results in patients randomized for primary or selective stent placement. Radiology 2006;238(2):734–44.
73. Piffaretti G, Tozzi M, Lomazzi C, et al. Mid-term results of endovascular reconstruction for aorto-iliac obstructive disease. Int Angiol 2007;26(1):18–25.
74. Stoeckel D, Pelton A, Duerig T. Self-expanding nitinol stents: material and design considerations. Eur Radiol 2004;14(2):292–301.
75. Ichihashi S, Higashiura W, Itoh H, et al. Long-term outcomes for systematic primary stent placement in complex iliac artery occlusive disease classified according to Trans-Atlantic Inter-Society Consensus (TASC)-II. J Vasc Surg 2011;53(4):992–9.
76. Grenacher L, Rohde S, Ganger E, et al. In vitro comparison of self-expanding versus balloon-expandable stents in a human ex vivo model. Cardiovasc Intervent Radiol 2006;29(2):249–54.
77. Bekken JA, Fioole B. Regarding “A comparison of covered vs bare expandable stents for the treatment of aortoiliac occlusive disease”. J Vasc Surg 2012;55(5):1545–6 [author reply: 1546].
78. Mwipatayi BP, Thomas S, Wong J, et al. A comparison of covered vs bare expandable stents for the treatment of aortoiliac occlusive disease. J Vasc Surg 2011;54(6):1561–70.

Management of Aneurysmal Disease of the Aorta

Vishal Kapur, MD[a,*], William A. Gray, MD[b]

KEYWORDS

- Thoracic aortic aneurysm • Abdominal aortic aneurysm • Aortic dissection • TEVAR • EVAR

KEY POINTS

- Aneurysmal disease of the aorta is a degenerative disease of the wall of the aorta usually involving the elderly.
- Aneurysmal disease carries a high morbidity and mortality, especially when associated with complications, such as dissection and rupture.
- Early diagnosis and treatment forms the mainstay of management.
- Recent developments in both surgical and endovascular techniques have made a significant impact on the survival of these groups of patients.

INTRODUCTION

Aortic aneurysm (true aneurysm) is defined as a permanent increase in size of the vessel more than 50% of its normal diameter with the presence of all 3 layers of the arterial wall.[1] The normal size of the aorta ranges from 3 cm in the ascending part, 2.5 to 3.5 cm in arch segment, to 2 cm in the descending thoracic and abdominal part. Aortic aneurysms are classified based on their location into ascending aorta, arch, descending thoracic aortic aneurysm (TAA), thoracoabdominal aortic aneurysm (TAAA), and abdominal aortic aneurysm (AAA). In this article, the authors discuss in detail the management of descending thoracic/thoracoabdominal and AAA.

THORACIC AND THORACOABDOMINAL ANEURYSMAL DISEASE

The annual incidence of TAA and TAAA is 5.9 per 100,000 persons, with an increased predisposition to male sex (1.7 times) and increasing age.[2] In most cases, TAAs are asymptomatic; however, they can present as vague pain localized to the chest, back, flank, or abdomen; hoarseness of voice; chronic cough and pulmonary symptoms; dysphagia; hemoptysis; and hematemesis. In rare cases, paraplegia and distal atheroembolism can be the presenting signs and symptoms of the TAA/TAAA. Factors predisposing to aneurysm formation are described in **Box 1**.

MANAGEMENT GOALS

The main principle in the management of TAA is the prevention of rupture and associated catastrophic complications. Crawford and DeNatale[3] noted that those in whom TAA were left untreated had a survival rate of only 24% at the end of 2 years. Dapunt and coworkers[4] documented that TAAAs greater than 8 cm have an 80% risk for rupture within 1 year of diagnosis. The size of the aneurysm is the single biggest predictor of

The authors have nothing to disclose.

[a] Department of Medicine, Icahn School of Medicine, Mount Sinai Medical Center, 1 Gustave L. Levy Place, New York, NY 10029, USA; [b] Department of Medicine, Columbia University Medical Center, NY Presbyterian Hospital, 161 Fort Washington Avenue, New York, NY 10032, USA
* Corresponding author.
E-mail address: vishal.kapur@mountsinai.org

Intervent Cardiol Clin 3 (2014) 545–555
http://dx.doi.org/10.1016/j.iccl.2014.06.003
2211-7458/14/$ – see front matter

Box 1
Risk factors associated with aneurysm formation

1. Older age
2. Male sex
3. White race
4. Positive family history
5. Smoking
6. Hypertension
7. Hypercholesterolemia
8. Coronary artery disease
9. Peripheral vascular disease

rupture. The average expansion rate of a TAAA is approximately 0.10 to 0.42 cm/y.[5] In order to treat the aneurysm, it is essential to determine the underlying cause, most commonly being atherosclerotic degenerative disease (**Box 2**).

The management strategy includes nonoperative (medical) and operative (surgical/endovascular) options. The management of TAA is mainly governed by the size and the presentation of the aneurysm.

EVALUATION

Diagnosis of TAA/TAAA is mainly supported by the radiological assessment of the thorax. Various imaging modalities that help in the diagnosis of TAA/TAAA are described in **Table 1**.

Table 1
Radiological imaging in diagnosis of TAA

Modality	Characteristics
Chest radiograph	Low sensitivity and specificity for the diagnosis of TAA findings • Enlarged thoracic aorta with calcified aortic wall • Widened mediastinum • Enlargement of the aortic knob • Tracheal deviation may suggest aneurysmal changes
CT scan	• Gold standard • Comprehensive assessment of the aneurysm including the size, side branch assessment, patency of intercostal vessels, and presence of thrombus and dissection • Caution in patients with chronic renal insufficiency and allergy to iodinated contrast
MRI scan	• Alternative imaging technique to CT scan • Caution noted in patients with renal insufficiency and gadolinium use because of a high risk of NSF
Arteriography	• Mainly used intraprocedurally during endovascular repair for final evaluation and confirmation of the size and placement of the stent graft

Abbreviations: CT, computed tomography; MRI, magnetic resonance imaging; NSF, nephrogenic systemic fibrosis.

MEDICAL MANAGEMENT

This form of treatment strategy lays emphasis on blood pressure (BP) control, smoking cessation, and serial monitoring of the aneurysm size.

Antihypertensive Medications

Two classes of antihypertensives have been studied extensively for BP control: beta-blockers and angiotensin converting enzyme inhibitors (ACEi). Wheat and colleagues[6] noted a decrease in progression of the aneurysm by decreasing the force on the wall achieved by strict BP control. In clinical studies, Shores and colleagues[7] showed that with the use of propranolol there was a significant reduction in growth of the aortic root and mortality in patients with Marfan syndrome. However, there is still a lack of substantial data suggestive of direct effect of beta-blocker on TAA progression. Beta-blocker use in vascular surgery is known to have perioperative mortality benefits.

Box 2
Causes of TAA/TAAA

1. Degeneration
2. Dissection
3. Connective tissue disorders (Marfan syndrome, Ehlers-Danlos syndrome)
4. Infection (syphilis, tuberculosis, mycotic)
5. Inflammation (aortitis): Takayasu, giant cell arteritis
6. Trauma

Statin Therapy

The pleotropic properties of statins have a beneficial effect on the vascular biology and aneurysmal disease process. The role of statin in TAA comes from a study that suggested that statins might have inhibitory effects on the formation of TAAAs via the suppression of nicotinamide adenine dinucleotide/nicotinamide adenine dinucleotide phosphate oxidase.[8] However, there is a lack of convincing data of benefit in humans.

Smoking Cessation

It has been proposed that smokers have a higher proteolytic enzymatic activity, which results in degenerative changes in the medial wall of the aorta leading to TAA formation. Hence, smoking cessation serves as an important adjuvant therapy in the management of patients with TAA.

OPERATIVE MANAGEMENT

The indication to treat a thoracic aneurysm depends on the size, rate of growth, location, symptoms, and general medical condition of patients. Based on the available data, it is recommended that TAA repair should be considered before rupture when aneurysms are 5 cm or larger and in patients with symptomatic aneurysms. In general, patients who have significant comorbid conditions like old age, severe cardiovascular disease, and pulmonary or renal dysfunction are not considered good surgical candidates and may opt for endovascular repair.

Graft placement under direct surgical approach is the treatment of choice in patients eligible for surgery. The main goal of surgery is successful placement of a graft with reconstruction of the visceral vessels in case of anticipated coverage by the graft itself.

ENDOVASCULAR INTERVENTION

Initial work with endovascular repair was demonstrated in the 1990s, with Volodos and colleagues[9] credited with the placement of the first thoracic aortic endograft. With the advancements in technology, there has been an increase in the availability and use of stent grafts in the market with Food and Drug Administration–approved devices available for the treatment of TAAs (**Table 2**).

Most of the data regarding endovascular repair of TAA/TAAA are essentially based on observational studies and suggest that thoracic endovascular repair (TEVAR) of TAAs is a safe alternative to open surgery and is associated with lower mortality and morbidity.[10] **Table 3** however, long-term results are not yet available to substantiate the findings.

As a prerequisite to the success of TEVAR, the proximal and distal neck diameters should not exceed the largest diameter of the graft available, for a leak-proof seal. Also, the proximal and distal necks should be at least 20 mm long for an adequate landing zone. Impingement of the major arterial branches that might be occluded for adequate sealing have to be carefully assessed for risks associated with occlusion, with an option of surgical bypass or debranching to maintain perfusion while extending the sealing zone. Another anatomic limitation for this therapy relates to vascular access: The femoral and iliac arteries have to be wide enough to accommodate the large sheaths necessary to deploy the stent grafts. In case any of these anatomic criteria is not met, an open approach is preferred to an endovascular approach.

COMPLICATIONS OF ENDOVASCULAR TECHNIQUE

As with any procedure, there are risks and complications associated with endovascular therapy that need to be assessed and addressed. With TEVAR use, there is considerably less known major side effects compared with open surgical intervention as shown in the TAG Study[11] and VALOR (Evaluation of the Medtronic Vascular Talent Thoracic Stent Graft System for the Treatment of Thoracic Aortic Aneurysms) Medical studies.[12]

Table 2
Endografts available for TAA repair

Product Name	Company Name	Stent Material	Graft Material	Expansion
Relay Thoracic	Boston Scientific (Marlborough, MA)	Nitinol	Woven polyester with PTFE sutures	Self-expanding
TX	Cook Medical (Bloomington, IN)	Stainless steel	Woven polyester	Self-expanding
Gore TAG	Gore & Associates (Newark, DE)	Nitinol	ePTFE	Self-expanding
Valiant Thoracic	Medtronic Inc (Minneapolis, MN)	Nitinol	Woven polyester	Self-expanding

Abbreviations: ePTFE, expanded PTFE; PTFE, polytetrafluoroethylene.

Table 3
TAA trials

Trial	Population	Results
Gore TAG Trial	140 Patients with Gore TAG device compared with 94 patients in the open surgical arm	• There was significantly reduced perioperative mortality (2.4% vs 11.7%, *P*<.001) in the endovascular arm. • Perioperative complication rates and intensive care unit and hospital length of stay also significantly reduced in the TEVAR group. • At 2 y, there was no difference in overall mortality.
Cook TX2 Trial	160 Patients undergoing TEVAR with the Zenith TX2 Endovascular Graft with 70 patients undergoing open TAA repair	• The 30-day survival rate was better for the TEVAR group than for the open group (98.1% vs 94.3%, *P*<.01). • The TEVAR group also had fewer cardiovascular, pulmonary, and vascular adverse events, although neurologic events were not significantly different.
Medtronic VALOR Trial	195 Patients with TEVAR vs 189 open surgical repair	• The 30-day perioperative mortality rate in the TEVAR group was 2.1%. • Major adverse advents occurred in 41% of the stent-graft group, including paraplegia in 1.5%, paraparesis in 7.2%, and stroke in 3.6%. • At 12 mo, the TEVAR group had an all-cause mortality rate of 16.1% and an aneurysm-related mortality rate of 3.1%.

Abbreviation: TEVAR, thoracic endovascular repair.

Vascular Complications

These complications are mainly attributed to the large size of the sheath for the deployment of the device. In the presence of tortuous, calcified, and small-sized iliac arteries, the incidence of vascular complications increases. Use of arterial conduits can help bypass the hostile arterial anatomy and provide direct access thereby lowering the access site complication rates.

Neurologic Complications

This subset of complications are mainly caused because of embolization during placement of the graft leading to stroke or occlusion of the spinal arteries leading to spinal ischemia. There is a higher chance of neurologic involvement when the graft involves covering the hypogastric artery, left subclavian artery, extensive thoracic aortic coverage.[3,13] Associated comorbid conditions such as renal insufficiency[3] and intraoperative hypotension (systolic blood pressure <80 mm Hg) also puts a patient at high risk of neurological complications.[14] Procedural techniques such as minimal manipulations, knowledge of important vascular anatomy and optimization of graft location can help minimize the risk of stroke during TEAVR.

Endoleaks

These are well-documented complications of TEVAR. The prevalence of complications are noted to vary from 26.0% in the VALOR Trial[14] to 3.6% in Gore TAG Trial.[12] The incidence is reported to be decreasing with advent of second-generation devices.

ABDOMINAL AORTIC ANEURYSM

AAA is the most common form of aortic aneurysm, occurring in 3% to 10% of people older than 50 years. Most of the AAAs are located infrarenal, with approximately 25% involving the iliac arteries.[15] AAA rupture is a major catastrophic complication of the AAA disease with an overall mortality of 90% which needs prompt diagnosis and attention.[16] In the United States, AAA rupture is the 15th leading cause of death overall and the 10th leading cause of death in men older than 55 years.[17]

Most of the AAAs are asymptomatic; however, in some cases, it can present as satiety, nausea or vomiting, urinary symptoms from compression of urinary bladder, or venous thrombosis from iliocaval venous compression. AAA can also present with vague chronic back pain or abdominal pain.

EVALUATION

AAA is primarily a radiological diagnosis, as physical examination has a variable sensitivity and specificity and depends largely on the AAA size, presence of obesity, and the examinee's skills. As the AAA size increases, the sensitivity of detecting AAA increases, with a diagnosis being made in 29% of AAAs with a size between 3.0 and 3.9 cm, 50% between 4.0 and 4.9 cm, and 75% in AAAs greater than 5.0 cm.[18] Radiological examination is the mainstay of diagnosis of AAA (**Table 4**). Screening for AAA is based on the US Preventive Task Force's guidelines (**Box 3**).[19]

MANAGEMENT

The management of AAA is a complex decision involving a comprehensive assessment of patients and the disease process and includes multiple factors such as the size of the AAA, patient presentation, the rate of growth, and the comorbid conditions. The critical driving force in the decision making for the treatment of AAA is the risk of rupture. An expansion of 0.5 cm in 6 months or 1 cm over 12 months is defined as rapid enlargement and indicates that the aneurysm is unstable and should be repaired.

Szilagyi and colleagues[20] first established that aneurysm size is the best determinant of rupture risk in 1966. In a study by Darling and colleagues,[21] it was noted that the probability of rupture was increased with an increase in size: less than 4 cm, 10%; 4 to 7 cm, 25%; 7 to 10 cm, 46%; and greater than 10 cm, 61%.

MEDICAL MANAGEMENT

Medical management plays a crucial role in patients with AAAs, especially patients who do not meet the criteria for intervention. The main focus of management is to reduce the rate of expansion of the AAA and treat the comorbid conditions, thereby reducing the cardiovascular complications associated with the disease.

Table 4
Radiological imaging in diagnosis of AAA

Modality	Characteristics
Abdominal radiograph	• Less sensitive and specific • Calcifications suggest presence of aneurysm/gives gross estimate of size of aneurysm
Ultrasound	• Least expensive, abundantly used, noninvasive imaging modality • Limitation of view in suprarenal segment and obese patients • Limited to diagnose rupture
CT scan	• Gold standard • Assessment of the size, orientation, diameter, proximal and distal extent, adjacent structures like renal artery position and involvement, ectopic kidneys, duplicate vena cava • Operative planning for endovascular/surgical repair
MRI scan	• Alternative to CT scan
Aortography	• Mainly used intraprocedural during endovascular repair for final evaluation and confirmation of the size and placement of the stent graft

Abbreviations: CT, computed tomography; MRI, magnetic resonance imaging.

Smoking Cessation

This risk factor is the single most modifiable risk factor in the medical management of patients with AAA disease. Lederle and colleagues[22] determined that smokers have a 3 to 6 times higher incidence of

Box 3
US Preventive Task Force's recommendations for screening of AAA

- Recommends one-time screening for AAA by ultrasound in men aged 65–75 years who have ever smoked (grade B recommendation)
- No recommendations for or against screening in men aged 65 to 75 years who have never smoked (grade C recommendation)
- Recommends against routine screening for AAA in women (grade D recommendation)

Data from U.S. Preventive Services Task Force. Screening for abdominal aortic aneurysm: recommendation statement. Ann Intern Med 2005;142(3):198–202.

aortic aneurysm–related events as compared with nonsmokers. Hence, smoking cessation forms a cornerstone of medical treatment.

Medications

Various medications have been used in the management of AAA like beta-blockers, ACEi, statins, and even doxycycline.

Beta-blockers

Certain animal models have demonstrated a decrease in the rate of progression of AAA with the use of beta-blocker therapy. However, a randomized trial by Wilmink and Quick[23] did not show any beneficial effect of the use of propranolol in patients with AAA. Hence, the use of beta-blocker therapy solely for the purpose of reducing AAA expansion is still controversial. However, the use of beta-blocker therapy has been advocated as an adjuvant therapy because of its beneficial perioperative and long-term mortality benefits in patients undergoing vascular surgery. ACEi are known to provide similar antihypertensive benefits.

Statins

Statins are thought to decrease the matrix metallopeptidase 9 (MMP-9) levels[24] within the vascular wall, thereby reducing the expansion rate; however, there have been no randomized trials to support this hypothesis.

Doxycycline

Mosorin and colleagues[25] have shown that with the use of a 3-month regimen of 150 mg daily, there was a reduction in the expansion rate by almost 50% at 18 months when compared with a placebo group. It has been postulated that the suppression of expression of MMP and decrease in MMP-9 levels in the aneurysmal wall might have some beneficial effect in reducing the rate of progression. Because of a lack of large randomized trials, the use is based on physician decision making.

OPERATIVE MANAGEMENT

Operative intervention (endovascular vs open surgical) is the treatment of choice for patients with asymptomatic AAAs greater than 5.5 cm, a rate of increase greater than 0.5 to 1 cm/y, or symptomatic patients. In rare situations, for example, very-high-risk patients or patients with a short life expectancy, patients are managed medically.

The factors that determine the mode of surgical intervention include high-risk patients (defined as diameter >6 cm, rate of increase >0.6 cm/y, elevated wall tension [>40 N/cm^2]), female sex, current smokers, severe chronic obstructive pulmonary disease on steroids, coronary artery disease (CAD), uncontrolled hypertension and significant family history, operative mortality, and patient preferences.

ENDOVASCULAR THERAPY

Parodi[26] first described endovascular aneurysm repair (EVAR) of AAAs in 1991. Since then, there have been significant advancements in stent graft material, deliverability, durability, and safety, making EVAR a viable alternative to open surgical repair. Certain anatomic considerations have proven to be ideal for EVAR therapy. These considerations include neck length greater than 15 mm, neck diameter less than 30 mm, neck angulation less than 60°, common iliac artery diameter less than 22 mm, and common iliac artery length greater than 35 mm. Careful assessment by using an imaging modality like a computed tomography (CT) scan helps define the aneurysmal anatomy and plan of care.

There are various devices on the market now that are available for endovascular repair of AAAs (**Table 5**).

COMPARISON BETWEEN ENDOVASCULAR (EVAR) AND OPEN SURGERY

With the advances in technology and the preference for minimally invasive treatment strategies, EVAR has been gaining popularity and precision in the treatment of AAA. There have been randomized trials and registry data to establish EVAR as an excellent alternative to a definitive surgical option. The 4 trials of note are EVAR-1 (Endovascular Aneurysm Repair), DREAM (Dutch Randomized Endovascular Aneurysm Management) Trial, ACE (Anevrysme de l'aorte abdominale: Chirurgie versus Endoprothese), and OVER (Open versus Endovascular Repair) trial.

EVAR-1

EVAR-1 is one of the earliest trials that randomized 1082 patients to open repair (n = 543) versus EVAR (n = 543). Four years after randomization, the all-cause mortality was similar in the two groups (28%; hazard ratio [HR]: 0.90, *P* = .46). There was a persistent reduction in aneurysm-related deaths in the EVAR group (4% vs 7%; HR: 0.55, *P* = .04). The proportion of patients with postoperative complications within 4 years of randomization was 41% in the EVAR group and 9% in the open-repair group (*P*<.0001).[27]

DREAM Trial

A total of 351 patients with an AAA of at least 5 cm in diameter were randomized to either endovascular

Table 5
Endografts available for abdominal aneurysmal repair

Product Name	Company Name	Stent Material	Graft Material	Fixation Location	Stent Expansion
Zenith Flex/Fenestrated	Cook Medical (Bloomington, IN)	Stainless steel and nitinol	Woven polyester	Suprarenal	Self-expanding
AFX Endovascular/IntuiTrak	Endologix (Irvine, CA)	Cobalt chromium	ePTFE	At the bifurcation of aorta, infrarenal/suprarenal for seal	Self-expanding
Gore Excluder	Gore & Associates (Newark, DE)	Nitinol	ePTFE	Suprarenal	Self-expanding
Aorfix	Lombard Medical (Irvine, CA)	Nitinol	Polyester	Infrarenal/transrenal	Self-expanding
Endurant II System	Medtronic Inc (Minneapolis, MN)	Nitinol	Woven polyester	Suprarenal	Self-expanding
Ovation Prime	TriVascular (Santa Rosa, CA)	Nitinol	PTFE	Suprarenal	Self-expanding

Abbreviations: ePTFE, expanded PTFE; PTFE, polytetrafluoroethylene.

repair or open surgical repair. At the 6-year follow-up, 69.9% of the open-repair patients were still alive compared with 68.9% of the EVAR group ($P = .97$). The reintervention rate was higher in patients in the EVAR group as compared with the open surgical arm (29.6% vs 18.1%, $P = .03$). This study showed comparable long-term benefits.[28]

ACE Trial

Anevrysme de l'aorte abdominale: Chirurgie versus Endoprothese was a randomized controlled trial comparing EVAR versus open surgery for AAA in low- to moderate-risk patients. Two hundred ninety-nine patients were randomized to EVAR versus open surgery. After a median follow-up of 3 years, there was no significant difference in death (8.0% open repair vs 11.3% EVAR, P = NS), major adverse cardiac event (MACE) (4.0% open repair vs 6.7% EVAR, P = NS) between the two groups. However, there was an increased rate of reintervention in the EVAR group (2.7% open repair vs 16.0% EVAR, $P<.001$).[29]

OVER Trial

Eight hundred eighty-one patients with asymptomatic AAA who were candidates for both procedures to either endovascular repair (444) or open repair (437) and followed them for up to 9 years (mean, 5.2 years). One hundred forty-six deaths occurred in each group (HR: 0.97, $P = .81$), with a decrease in perioperative mortality with EVAR until 3 years (HR = 0.72, $P = .05$) but not thereafter. The investigators concluded that perioperative survival in the EVAR group persisted for years, and increased survival was noted only in younger individuals.[30]

COMPLICATIONS OF ENDOVASCULAR ANEURYSM REPAIR

Endoleaks

Endoleaks (**Fig. 1**) are the most commonly noted complications encountered with the EVAR procedure. The management of the endoleaks is based on the classification of White and colleagues[31] (**Table 6**).

Graft Migration

Migration is a slow process caused by unstable proximal end attachment leading to distal/caudal migration of the stent graft. The incidence of migration has significantly reduced with the advent of barbed suprarenal fixation devices, which provide better anchorage and stability to the structure. Treatment options include endovascular placement of extra cuff on the proximal edge for better apposition of the edges and to prevent/treat endoleak.

Graft Occlusion

This complication is a rare known complication of endovascular management of AAA. Angulation, kinking, or poor outflow predisposes to the development of thrombus. Treatment of graft occlusion includes the removal of thrombus using thrombectomy devices and treatment of the underlying cause.

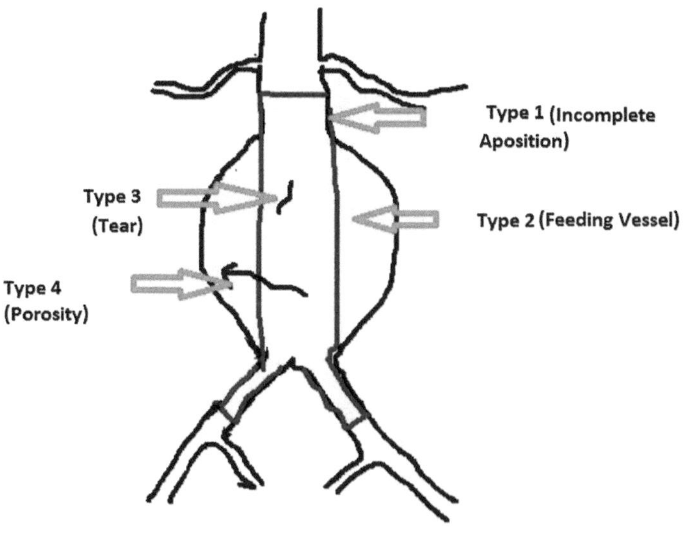

Fig. 1. Abdominal aneurysm endoleak classification, based on the classification of White and colleagues. (*Data from* White GH, May J, Waugh RC, et al. Type III and type IV endoleak: toward a complete definition of blood flow in the sac after endoluminal AAA repair. J Endovasc Surg 1998;5(4):305–9.)

Table 6
Endoleaks

Type	Characteristics	Treatment
Type 1	• At the ends of the graft because of incomplete apposition of the stent graft to the aortic wall, increase in the size of the aneurysmal neck or migration of the stent graft system • Type IA: proximal site • Type IB: distal site	• Balloon dilation • Additional stent placement • Coil embolization of perigraft space • Open surgical repair
Type 2	• Most common type • Because of the presence of a feeding vessel to the aneurysmal sac, most commonly the lumbar artery	• Monitor with serial CT scans • Embolization of the feeding vessel • Obliteration of the sac with a thrombogenic material • Open surgical ligation
Type 3	• Tear in the graft material or • Graft limb dislocation	• Extra limb to cover the tear and/or limb dislocation
Type 4 (rare)	• Graft porosity	• Additional stent graft placement

Endoleak types based on the classification of White and colleagues.[31]

Rupture of Vessels

This complication is the most feared complication of EVAR, with iliac and suprarenal aorta being the most common sites. Iliac artery rupture is caused by forceful delivery through a tortuous calcified iliac artery, whereas suprarenal aortic rupture is caused by an angulated neck and advancement of the system without a wire. Diagnosis is usually made clinically and confirmed by radiology, and treatment includes balloon tamponade and placement of a stent graft to cover the rupture site.

Side Branch Occlusion

Covering of the stent graft material causes occlusion of the side branches, such as renal and internal iliacs. The treatment options include stenting the renal artery above the proximal edge of the stent graft or puncturing through the graft material. With unilateral occlusion of the internal iliac artery, patients usually tolerate well, with only 15% developing buttock ischemia. Bilateral occlusion can lead to bowel and pelvic ischemia.

Stent Graft Infection

It has very low incidence of occurrence (0.43%) and usually occurs because of hematogenous spread from a distant site or after reintervention of the graft caused by endoleak repairs. Treatment is directed at the use of intravenous antibiotics and, in rare cases, surgical removal of the graft.

AORTIC DISSECTION

Aortic dissection is a potential catastrophic event of the aorta characterized by separation of the layers of the aorta through a tear in the intima. This tear results in the formation of a true and false lumen separated by an intimal flap. Blood can flow in either direction and in between the two lumens via fenestrations. Aortic dissection is classified by the site of origin (**Box 4**). The risk factors associated with this disease process include the presence of CAD, uncontrolled hypertension, coarctation of aorta, chromosomal abnormalities (Turner and Noonan syndrome), hereditary

Box 4
Classification of aortic dissection

1. DeBakey Classification

Type 1	Originates in the ascending aorta and extends into the descending aorta or abdominal aorta
Type 2	Originates and confined to the ascending aorta
Type 3A	Originates and confined to the descending aorta
Type 3B	Originates in the descending and extends to the abdominal aorta

2. Stanford Classification

Type A	Originates in the ascending aorta
Type B	Originates in the descending aorta after the origin of the left subclavian artery

disorders (Marfan syndrome and Ehlers-Danlos syndrome), pregnancy, and cocaine abuse. The most common symptom of acute aortic dissection is abrupt onset of pain located in the back, abdomen, or chest. Other symptoms suggestive of aortic dissection include syncope caused by cardiac tamponade or involvement of the brachiocephalic vessels. End-organ damage caused by malperfusion can present as stroke, hypotension, renal failure, or limb ischemia. Clinical suspicion should be high on the differential diagnosis to initiate the appropriate workup, including emergent radiological assessment. CT angiography is usually considered the gold standard test; however, the use of magnetic resonance angiography aortography, and transesophageal echocardiography can also provide valuable information. Optimal treatment of acute dissection is predicated on timely diagnosis and emergent intervention both medically and surgically. Stanford type A dissection warrants emergent surgical intervention with the aim of repair of the lesion and adequate end-organ perfusion, as the mortality can approach 1% per hour. Type B lesions are managed medically with admission to an intensive care unit for close monitoring and strict control of blood pressure. The primary late complication of survivors of aortic dissection is aneurysmal dilatation of the outer wall of the false lumen, which is treated as per standard protocol of any aneurysm in the aorta.

SUMMARY

Even though the incidence of aneurysmal disease of the aorta is well less than that of cardiovascular disease and cancer, the morbidity and mortality associated with the aneurysm is extremely high. With the improvements in endovascular techniques and rapid advancement in technology, the minimally invasive strategy has become a viable treatment of choice. However, there still remains much to be done in this field, from diagnosis to treatment and prevention of complications.

REFERENCES

1. Johnston KW, Rutherford RB, Tilson MD. Suggested standards for reporting on arterial aneurysms. Subcommittee on Reporting Standards for Arterial Aneurysms, Ad Hoc Committee on Reporting Standards, Society for Vascular Surgery and North American Chapter, International Society for Cardiovascular Surgery. J Vasc Surg 1991;13(3):452–8.
2. Bickerstaff LK, Pairolero PC, Hollier LH. Thoracic aortic aneurysms: a population-based study. Surgery 1982;92(6):1103–8.
3. Crawford ES, DeNatale RW. Thoracoabdominal aortic aneurysm: observations regarding the natural course of the disease. J Vasc Surg 1986;3(4): 578–82.
4. Dapunt OE. The natural history of thoracic aortic aneurysms. J Thorac Cardiovasc Surg 1994;107(5): 1323–32 [discussion: 1332–3].
5. Davies RR. Yearly rupture or dissection rates for thoracic aortic aneurysms: simple prediction based on size. Ann Thorac Surg 2002;73(1):17–27 [discussion: 27–8].
6. Wheat MW Jr, Palmer RF. Dissecting aneurysms of the aorta: present status of drug versus surgical therapy. Prog Cardiovasc Dis 1968;11(3):198–210.
7. Shores J. Progression of aortic dilatation and the benefit of long-term beta-adrenergic blockade in Marfan's syndrome. N Engl J Med 1994;330(19): 1335–41.
8. Ejiri J. Oxidative stress in the pathogenesis of thoracic aortic aneurysm: protective role of statin and angiotensin II type 1 receptor blocker. Cardiovasc Res 2003;59(4):988–96.
9. Volodos NL. Clinical experience of the use of self-fixing synthetic prostheses for remote endoprosthetics of the thoracic and the abdominal aorta and iliac arteries through the femoral artery and as intraoperative endoprosthesis for aorta reconstruction. Vasa Suppl 1991;33:93–5.
10. Heijmen RH. Endovascular stent-grafting for descending thoracic aortic aneurysms. Eur J Cardiothorac Surg 2002;21(1):5–9.
11. Makaroun MS. Endovascular treatment of thoracic aortic aneurysms: results of the phase II multicenter trial of the GORE TAG thoracic endoprosthesis. J Vasc Surg 2005;41(1):1–9.
12. Fairman RM. Pivotal results of the Medtronic Vascular Talent Thoracic Stent Graft System: the VALOR trial. J Vasc Surg 2008;48(3):546–54.
13. Kato N. Traumatic thoracic aortic aneurysm: treatment with endovascular stent-grafts. Radiology 1997;205(3):657–62.
14. Dake MD. The "first generation" of endovascular stent-grafts for patients with aneurysms of the descending thoracic aorta. J Thorac Cardiovasc Surg 1998;116(5):689–703 [discussion: 703–4].
15. Olsen PS. Surgery for abdominal aortic aneurysms. A survey of 656 patients. J Cardiovasc Surg (Torino) 1991;32(5):636–42.
16. Assar AN, Zarins CK. Ruptured abdominal aortic aneurysm: a surgical emergency with many clinical presentations. Postgrad Med J 2009;85: 268–73.
17. Heron M, Tejada-Vera B. Deaths: leading causes for 2005. Natl Vital Stat Rep 2009;58(8):1–97.
18. Lederle FA, Simel DL. The rational clinical examination. Does this patient have abdominal aortic aneurysm? JAMA 1999;281(1):77–82.

19. U.S. Preventive Services Task Force. Screening for abdominal aortic aneurysm: recommendation statement. Ann Intern Med 2005;142(3):198–202.
20. Szilagyi DE. Contribution of abdominal aortic aneurysmectomy to prolongation of life. Ann Surg 1966; 164(4):678–99.
21. Darling RC 3rd. Are familial abdominal aortic aneurysms different? J Vasc Surg 1989;10(1):39–43.
22. Lederle FA. Prevalence and associations of abdominal aortic aneurysm detected through screening. Aneurysm Detection and Management (ADAM) Veterans Affairs Cooperative Study Group. Ann Intern Med 1997;126(6):441–9.
23. Wilmink AB, Quick CR. Epidemiology and potential for prevention of abdominal aortic aneurysm. Br J Surg 1998;85(2):155–62.
24. Evans J. Simvastatin attenuates the activity of matrix metalloprotease-9 in aneurysmal aortic tissue. Eur J Vasc Endovasc Surg 2007;34(3):302–3.
25. Mosorin M. Use of doxycycline to decrease the growth rate of abdominal aortic aneurysms: a randomized, double-blind, placebo-controlled pilot study. J Vasc Surg 2001;34(4):606–10.
26. Parodi JC, Palmaz JC, Barone HD. Transfemoral intraluminal graft implantation for abdominal aortic aneurysms. Ann Vasc Surg 1991;5(6):491–9.
27. Greenhalgh RM. Comparison of endovascular aneurysm repair with open repair in patients with abdominal aortic aneurysm (EVAR trial 1), 30-day operative mortality results: randomised controlled trial. Lancet 2004;364(9437):843–8.
28. Blankensteijn JD. Two-year outcomes after conventional or endovascular repair of abdominal aortic aneurysms. N Engl J Med 2005;352(23): 2398–405.
29. Becquemin JP. The ACE trial: a randomized comparison of open versus endovascular repair in good risk patients with abdominal aortic aneurysm. J Vasc Surg 2009;50(1):222–4 [discussion: 224].
30. Lederle FA. Long-term comparison of endovascular and open repair of abdominal aortic aneurysm. N Engl J Med 2012;367(21):1988–97.
31. White GH, May J, Waugh RC, et al. Type III and type IV endoleak: toward a complete definition of blood flow in the sac after endoluminal AAA repair. J Endovasc Surg 1998;5(4):305–9.

Acute Limb Ischemia

Bhaskar Purushottam, MD, Karthik Gujja, MD, MPH, Adrian Zalewski, BSc, Prakash Krishnan, MD*

KEYWORDS

- Acute limb ischemia • Aspiration devices • Catheter directed thrombolysis
- Percutaneous mechanical thrombectomy • Severe limb ischemia • Thromboembolectomy

KEY POINTS

- Acute limb ischemia is a vascular event presenting with sudden decrease in limb perfusion (of <14 days' duration) that threatens limb viability.
- Acute thrombosis of the native artery or graft makes up the bulk of etiopathogenesis.
- Prompt revascularization is the cornerstone of management of acute limb ischemia as long as the limb has not undergone irreversible tissue and nerve damage.
- Amputation is performed in patients with irreversible tissue and nerve damage.

INTRODUCTION AND EPIDEMIOLOGY

Acute limb ischemia (ALI) is considered a vascular emergency. It comprises 10% to 16% of the vascular workload.[1] Despite several advances in the management of peripheral arterial disease (PAD), the morbidity and mortality associated with ALI is high when compared with the other clinical syndromes of PAD. ALI is a clinical syndrome of less than 14 days' presentation, which is defined as a sudden decrease in limb perfusion in which the limb viability is threatened.[2] The term "acute ischemia" does not imply severe ischemia, but that the survival of the limb is in immediate jeopardy.[3,4] There are approximately 13 to 17 cases per 100,000 persons per year.[5,6] Earnshaw[7] reports that a vascular unit serving a community of half a million people can expect to treat at least 75 cases of ALI in a year. The incidence is higher in regions with an older patient population with multiple medical comorbidities, especially with congestive heart failure and atrial fibrillation. It is also high among the PAD subpopulation that undergo endovascular and surgical procedures. Upper extremity ALI is uncommon because of the extensive collateral network and the infrequency of atherosclerosis and accounts for only 17% of all the ALI cases.[8] The annual incidence of upper-extremity ALI is reported at 1.2 to 3.5 cases per 100,000 persons per year.[9] Men and women are equally affected. Patients tend to be middle aged and older.

ETIOLOGY

The different causes leading to ALI can be broadly categorized into 3 mechanistic categories, which include embolism, thrombosis, and other causes (as listed in **Table 1**). The approach to the etiopathogenesis of ALI also can be segregated as upper-extremity and lower-extremity ALI. In lower-extremity ALI, the proportion of cases from in situ thrombosis is on the rise and that of embolism has been on the decline in the past few decades. This trend is a consequence of the increasing number of endovascular and surgical procedures performed and the effective management of atrial fibrillation and congestive cardiac failure. Klonaris and colleagues[10] found that 50% of ALI cases were due to in situ thrombosis, 40% were embolic in origin, and 10% were from other miscellaneous causes. When looking at the North

The authors have nothing to disclose.
Zena and Michael A. Weiner Cardiovascular Institute, Mount Sinai School of Medicine, One Gustave Levy L. Place, New York, NY 10029, USA
* Corresponding author. One Gustave L. Levy Place, Box 1030, New York, NY 10029.
E-mail address: prakash.krishnan@mountsinai.org

Intervent Cardiol Clin 3 (2014) 557–572
http://dx.doi.org/10.1016/j.iccl.2014.07.004
2211-7458/14/$ – see front matter

Table 1
Causes of acute limb ischemia

Embolic (40%)	Thrombotic (50%)	Other Etiologies (10%)	Upper Extremity Etiologies
I. Cardiac Source (80%) a. Atrial fibrillation b. Left ventricular thrombus c. Left atrial myxoma or other cardiac tumors d. Valvular heart disease i. Infective endocarditis ii. Prosthetic valve thrombosis iii. Rheumatic valve disease e. Paradoxic embolism via patent foramen ovale *II. Vascular tree source* a. Aneurysms (aortic, iliac, popliteal) b. Atherosclerotic plaque *III. Procedure related* a. Coronary artery bypass b. Endovascular procedures *IV. Other* a. Air b. Amniotic fluid c. Tumor d. Fat e. Intra-arterial drug injection	*I. Underlying PAD related* a. De novo plaque rupture (30%) b. Stent and graft thrombosis (70%) c. Thrombosed aneurysm d. Severe hypoperfusion from cardiogenic shock *II. Absence of underlying PAD* a. Arteritis with thrombosis i. Giant cell arteritis ii. Thromboangiitis obliterans b. Catheter associated c. Hypercoagulable i. Antiphospholipid antibody syndrome ii. Malignancy iii. Hyperviscosity syndromes d. Popliteal adventitial cyst e. Popliteal entrapment f. Vasospasm g. Ergotism h. Cocaine i. Vasopressor	a. Arterial trauma b. Aortic or arterial dissection c. HIV arteriopathy d. Compartment syndrome e. Phlegmasia cerulean dolens (treat the underlying venous thrombosis) f. External compression	a. Embolism (>75%); most (>70%) are cardioembolic b. Thrombosis c. Trauma d. Dissecting aneurysm e. Small vessel disease f. Radiation fibrosis g. Hypercoagulable states h. Inflammatory vasculitides i. Arterial catheterization j. Thoracic outlet obstruction

Data from Refs.[2,3,7,8,84]

American and European database from the TOPAS trial,[11] among the 542 patients with ALI, 85% of the patients had an in situ thrombosis as the etiology. The most common source for embolic etiology is cardiac. As much as 80% to 90%[12,13] of arterial emboli originate from the heart, and 60% to 70% of these patients have underlying myocardial disease.[14,15] It is estimated that patients with chronic atrial fibrillation who are not on anticoagulation have a 3% to 6% annual risk of thromboembolic complications.[16] Most upper-extremity ALIs have a cardioembolic source.[17] Atrial fibrillation and left ventricular thrombus in patients with severe left ventricular systolic dysfunction are the most common causes of cardiac emboli. The upper-extremity arterial tree is relatively spared from atherosclerotic disease, when compared with lower extremities. Therefore, in situ thrombosis is a rare phenomenon in the upper extremity. Finally, blue toe syndrome is a manifestation of atheroembolism and presents as digital ischemia rather than as ALI.

PATHOPHYSIOLOGY

ALI triggers a cascade of events resulting in irreversible muscle damage in about 6 hours (in patients without a good collateral system and those who do not have a preconditioned limb). With ALI, there is a significant loss of ATP reserves and also the capacity to generate ATP with resultant accumulation of lactate. Malfunction of the sodium-potassium ATPase pump results in the leakage of intracellular calcium. Persistent elevated levels of calcium trigger a whole host of calcium-activated enzymes, which results in necrosis. Thus, with the loss of cell membrane and mitochondrial integrity, the irreversible process of cell death is heralded. A key concept in patients with ALI is the phenomenon of reperfusion injury. Reperfusion injury refers to the damage caused to the ischemic tissue when blood supply is restored after a period of ischemia. Reperfusion injury is mediated through the induction of oxidative stress, which causes aggravation of inflammatory changes. With reperfusion, the oxygen supply is restored to the ischemic tissues that results in activation of xanthine dehydrogenase. This leads to the conversion of large amounts of hypoxanthine to xanthine, which results in the generation of toxic-inflammatory reactive oxygen radicals. These reactive oxygen species then trigger a chain of inflammatory events, which are mediated by a complex cascade of cytokines, neutrophils, and other inflammatory cells. The clinical presentation of reperfusion injury ranges from a local phenomenon of compartment syndrome to a systemic inflammatory state with toxemia and multiorgan failure.

CLINICAL PRESENTATION

The classic presentation of ALI consists of the 6 Ps: pulselessness, pallor, pain, poikilothermia, paralysis, and paresthesia. The most common manifestation of ischemia is pain, which is directly proportionate to the severity of ischemia.[18] The order of symptom presentation would be pain, followed by pallor (an early finding caused by vasospasm of the arteries), mottling of the skin (caused by stagnation of microvascular circulation, which blanches initially on pressure), paresthesia, numbness (replaces pain), nonblanching fixed mottled skin, and paralysis.[8] The final 2 features reflect irreversible ischemic injury. Other signs indicative of this irreversible process are stiffness of the extremity, firm muscle compartments on palpation, and anesthesia.

The anterior compartment of the lower extremity is most sensitive to ischemia-induced neurologic impairment. Thus, numbness and tingling in the toes or the first web space are the initial neurological symptoms, which then progresses more cranially. Pain on passive dorsiflexion is an indicator of advanced ischemia and also heralds the onset on compartment syndrome. Physical examination can help decipher the level of occlusion (detecting a temperature gradient, pallor, and loss of pulses, which are usually a level below the occluded segment), potential sources of embolism (irregular rhythm of atrial fibrillation, pulsus alternans of cardiogenic shock with potential left ventricular thrombus, dermatologic findings and torrential mitral or aortic regurgitation in a patient with fulminant infective endocarditis, mitral stenosis murmur with a "plop" suggestive of an obstructing left atrial myxoma, or loss of the artificial crisp click of a mechanical heart valve, which suggests prosthetic valve thrombosis), stigmata of chronic PAD in the contralateral limb (suggestive of potential in situ thrombosis, especially if the patient has undergone an interventional procedure on the limb of interest), severity of ischemia, and the extent of neurologic impairment. Palpation of the pulse is an unreliable physical sign, with a false positivity of 14% among nonspecialists.[19] ALI should be considered in every individual who presents with sudden onset of leg pain, irrespective of the presence or absence of risk factors.

DIAGNOSTIC STUDIES

A thorough evaluation of the concerned circulation system with ankle-brachial index, pulse volume recording and arterial Doppler is strongly recommended. The 3 findings that identify a threatened limb are the presence of rest pain, sensory loss, and muscle weakness. Based on these findings and arterio-venous Doppler signals, ALI is categorized by the Rutherford classification (**Table 2**). The decision to perform diagnostic imaging depends on the Rutherford classification of the ALI. Category IIb (immediately threatened limb) should proceed to revascularization without any delay. It is in patients with category I (viable limb) ALI that noninvasive imaging can be performed to delineate the site of occlusion and to help in planning the appropriate interventional strategy. The intermediate group, category IIa (marginally threatened) represents the challenging group. The decision to perform imaging studies should be individualized. Factors that should be taken into account are complex underlying anatomy, determining the best site of access, recent interventional procedures, and anticipate any difficulties in reaching the site of occlusion or to rule out any severe inflow or suprainguinal disease. The choice of imaging study to further determine the nature and extent of the occlusion should be individualized. Magnetic resonance imaging of the arterial tree is laborious and time-consuming. On the other hand, computed tomographic arteriography has its ease of application in an emergency setting at the cost of iodinated contrast media and radiation exposure. Duplex ultrasonography overcomes these two drawbacks, but lacks the detail provided by the former two imaging modalities and is very operator dependent. These imaging modalities have sensitivities and specificities in the 90% range, when evaluating chronic PAD.[20–22] The following studies should be obtained in all patients with ALI: electrocardiogram, standard chemistry, complete blood count, prothrombin time, partial thromboplastin time, and creatine phosphokinase levels.[2] In certain scenarios, a 2-dimensional transthoracic or transesophageal echocardiography should be considered. Diagnostic studies should not delay or interrupt treatment.

PROGNOSIS

Approximately 10% to 15% of patients undergo amputation during the hospitalization, despite urgent revascularization.[23,24] Amputation-free survival is adversely affected by delay in diagnosis, diabetes, non-White race, older age, congestive heart failure, malignancy, and low body weight. Systemic atherosclerosis has a favorable impact on amputation-free survival.[14,25,26] This is because of the phenomenon of preconditioning and the development of collateral bypasses, which allows the limb an additional 6 hours before its viability is threatened. The major modifiable factor, which is responsible for adverse outcomes, is delay in recognition and treatment. The 30-day mortality rates are approximately 42% in patients older than 75 years.[27]

MANAGEMENT

The key factors in the management of ALI are early diagnosis and urgent revascularization. We divide

Table 2
Rutherford classification of acute limb ischemia

Rutherford Class	Prognosis	Sensory Examination	Motor Examination	Arterial Doppler Signal	Venous Doppler Signal	Skin Examination
Class I: Viable/ Not threatened	Threatened	Normal	Normal	Audible	Audible	Normal capillary return
Class IIa: Marginally threatened	Salvageable with prompt therapy	Minimal (toes are involved)	Normal	Often audible	Audible	Decreased capillary return
Class IIb: Immediately threatened	Salvageable if treated immediately	Mild sensory loss (more than toes) and rest pain	Normal	Usually inaudible	Audible	Pallor
Class III: Irreversible	Irreversible tissue and nerve damage	Profound sensory loss	Paralysis and rigor	Inaudible	Inaudible	No capillary return, skin marbling

Adapted from Rutherford RB, Baker JD, Ernst C, et al. Recommended standards for reports dealing with lower extremity ischemia: revised version. J Vasc Surg 1997;26:517–38.

the management section into medical, endovascular, and surgical treatment.

Medical Treatment

The basics of medical treatment are as follows:

- Managing the patient in a critical care setting with continuous cardiac monitoring
- A multidisciplinary team approach
- Fluid resuscitation
- Correction of metabolic and electrolyte abnormalities
- Analgesia, antiplatelet and antithrombin therapy

The TASC II (Trans-Atlantic Inter-Society Consensus Document on Management of Peripheral Arterial Disease) guidelines recommend the initiation of intravenous heparin unless a specific contraindication exists.[2] However, in patients in whom thromboembolism is responsible for the ALI and the decision has been made to perform emergent surgical embolectomy, anticoagulation may be deferred to accommodate regional anesthesia. The recommended doses are in the range of 100 to 150 units/kg with a goal-activated partial thromboplastin time (APTT) that is 2.0-fold to 2.5-fold above the baseline. Patients with heparin-induced thrombocytopenia should be managed with intravenous direct thrombin inhibitors (argatroban or lepirudin). Bivalirudin can also be considered. Currently, there are no specific recommendations on the use of antiplatelet therapy in ALI. It is important to remember that ALI is a clinical syndrome with several etiologies. Given the increasing incidence of in situ thrombosis in patients with PAD (especially those who have undergone interventions) and also the high burden of cardiovascular morbidity, aspirin 75 to 325 mg should be considered.[2,28] We recommend all patients with ALI to be started with 325 mg aspirin. Clopidogrel can be considered as an alternative choice.[29] There are no definitive data (ie, randomized trials) on the use of dual antiplatelet therapy in ALI. Patients who present with irreversible tissue injury are at an increased risk of rhabdomyolysis. Alkalinization of the urine may benefit these patients with regard to acute kidney injury. Patients who present with serious systemic illness, such as cardiogenic shock with a left ventricular thrombus, aortic dissection, or infective endocarditis with severe native/prosthetic valvular incompetence; the focus should be on resuscitating the patient and stabilizing the cardiovascular status.

Endovascular Management

The main principles of endovascular therapy are immediate restoration of arterial flow, followed by definitive management of the underlying lesion. Endovascular strategy consists of 2 predominant modalities: catheter-directed thrombolysis (CDT) and percutaneous mechanical thrombectomy (PMT). The first step in endovascular therapy is planning the appropriate access. This is determined by the clinical examination, information obtained from noninvasive imaging, and the location of the arterial occlusion. Contralateral common femoral arterial (CFA) access is recommended for arterial occlusions at the CFA level. If the contralateral ilio-femoral system is not favorable, then brachial arterial access can be considered. For mid and distal superficial femoral arterial occlusion, ipsilateral antegrade or contralateral CFA access can be considered. For infrapopliteal occlusions, antegrade CFA is strongly recommended. For occluded femoral-popliteal grafts, contralateral CFA access would be advisable. Finally, for occluded aorto-femoral grafts, brachial access can be considered. Unfortunately, at this stage, the equipment is not built for radial access. **Table 3** lists the standard equipment used in endovascular management of ALI.

CDT

Dotter and colleagues[30] pioneered catheter-directed thrombolysis in 1974. All the thrombolytics (**Table 4**) work by converting plasminogen to plasmin, which then degrades fibrin. Thus, they act by enhancing the intrinsic fibrinolytic system. CDT is far more superior and safer than intravenous thrombolytics.[31] Procedural or technical success is defined as complete or near complete (>80%) dissolution of thrombus, restoration of antegrade flow, and the absence of the need for open surgical intervention.[32,33] The most powerful predictor of procedural success is the ability to position the infusion catheter within the thrombus.[34] Clinical success is defined as resolution of the acute ischemic symptoms or reduction of the level of the surgical procedure or amputation.[32] CDT achieves a satisfactory clinical result in 75% to 92% of ALI patients (including native, stent and graft cases).[11,24,25,35] After obtaining arterial access, diagnostic angiograms of the concerned limb of concern are obtained using a sidehole catheter. Once the arteriographic diagnosis is confirmed, a long sheath is exchanged for the short 5-Fr sheath (which was initially placed) and positioned proximal to the arterial occlusion. The thrombotic segment is crossed with a sturdy guidewire or exchanged for one after crossing the lesion. The infusion catheter is then advanced into the thrombotic segment over the sturdy wire. The infusion catheter should atleast be 5 cm longer than the length of the occlusion. An infusion wire is needed

Table 3
Standard equipment used in endovascular management of ALI

Devices	Details	Purpose
Sheaths	5 Fr and 6 Fr, 11- and 23-cm sheaths 5–7 Fr, 45–55-cm length, 0.018–0.038-inch guidewire compatible	Diagnostic angiogram For delivery of the ALI interventional devices
Guidewires	0.035 inch, 0.018 inch, or 0.014 inch	Cross the occluded segment
Catheters	4 or 5 Fr straight glide (65 and 120 cm) 0.014, 0.018, and 0.035 inch Quickcross (135 and 150 cm) Dedicated aspiration catheter, 6- or 7-Fr multipurpose guide Fountain, EKOS, Cragg-McNamara, MicroMewi, and Unifuse* Tuohy-Borst connector	Support and exchange catheters Mechanically aspirate the thrombus For CDT For the infusion wire
Rheolytic thrombectomy	AngioJet system (4–6 Fr, 0.014–0.035-inch guidewire)	PMT
Balloons	Range of lengths and diameters: 2.0-mm diameter for below the knee to 5.0 mm for suprainguinal lesions Over the wire and Rx systems	Treat the underlying lesion

Abbreviations: ALI, acute limb ischemia; CDT, catheter-directed thrombolysis; PMT, percutaneous mechanical thrombectomy.

* Fountain catheter (Merit Medical, South Jordan, UT); EKOS (EKOS Corporation, Bothell, WA); Cragg-McNamara catheter (Coviden, Plymouth, MN); MicroMewi catheter (Coviden, Plymouth, MN); UniFuse catheter (AngioDynamics, Latham, NY).

Adapted from Hynes BG, Margey RJ, Ruggiero N II, et al. Endovascular management of acute limb ischemia. Ann Vasc Surg 2012;26:110–24.

when the occlusion is multisegmental or when the occlusion length is longer than the infusion length of the catheter. Therefore, a Tuohy-Borst connector needs to be applied to the end of the infusion catheter through which the infusion wire can be inserted. The tissue plasminogen activator (t-PA) is then infused through the infusion catheter and unfractionated heparin is administered via the side arm of the long delivery sheath. All patients must receive unfractionated heparin via the side arm of the long delivery sheath to maintain an APTT of 45 to 50 seconds. Depending on the level of arterial occlusion, thrombus burden, bleeding risk, availability of equipment, operator experience, and comfort, CDT can be combined with PMT. The commonly used infusion catheters are Cragg-McNamara, MicroMewi, Fountain, Unifuse, and EkoSonic Endovascular System (EKOS). The commonly used infusion protocol consists of administering 1 mg/h of t-PA divided between the infusion catheter and the wire. The most common practice would be to cross the entire occluded segment, infuse recombinant t-PA at a rate of 0.5 to 1 mg/h for a minimum of 12 hours through an infusion catheter with multiple side holes. Concomitant unfractionated heparin is delivered through the side arm of the arterial access sheath at 500 to 800 units per hour (the dose can be weight based) to lower the risk of catheter-induced thrombosis.[36] Traditionally, thrombolytic infusion is not continued beyond 48 hours.[37,38] Guidelines[39] by the working party advocate regular measurement of hemoglobin and hematocrit levels. After the infusion period, the patient is brought back to the angiography suite and the vasculature is revisited and the next definitive intervention is planned. "Power pulse-spray" method consists of forced periodic lytic infusion, wherein the thrombolytic agent is forced under high pressure into the thrombus. Currently, there is no convincing evidence to show that one recombinant t-PA is better than the other in efficacy or safety. Distal embolization presents as worsening distal ischemia. It is managed with continued thrombolytic infusion and frequent monitoring. If this fails, then a relook angiography is performed with adjuvant PMT. Contraindications to the use of thrombolytics are listed in **Box 1**.

Complications of CDT The risk of major bleeding is 5.1%, minor bleeding is 15.0%,[39] and intracranial hemorrhage is 1.2% to 3.0%.[40] Bleeding occurs most commonly at the catheter-insertion site. Intensity and duration of thrombolysis, hypertension, octogenarians, and low platelet count have been associated with increased bleeding. In a bid to reduce the hemorrhagic complications of

Table 4
Commonly used thrombolytic agents in catheter-directed thrombolysis

Drug	Dose Range	Success	One-Year Amputation-Free Survival	Complication
Urokinase	240,000 IU/h for 4 h, then 120,000 IU/h	64%–79%	65%–75%	0%–17% ICH: 0%–2.1%
Alteplase (rt PA)	0.25–2.5 mg/h or Three 5-mg doses at 5–10-min intervals, then 0.05 mg/kg/h (intrathrombus lacing) or 0.5–1 mg/cm occlusion length with pulse spray delivery 0.2–0.5 units/h	84%–89%	94.3% at 6 mo	6%–19.2% ICH: 1%–4%
Reteplase (r-PA)	0.2–0.5 units/h	96.2% (>50% thrombus resolution)	69.7%	4.9% major complications No ICH in 81 cases
Tenecteplase (TNK-rtPA)	0.25–1 mg/h Low-dose regimen: 0.125 mg/h		5.4%–13.3% 2.9%	

Abbreviations: ICH, intra cranial hemorrhage.
Adapted from Hynes BG, Margey RJ, Ruggiero N II, et al. Endovascular management of acute limb ischemia. Ann Vasc Surg 2012;26:110–24.

Box 1
Contraindications to thrombolysis

Absolute contraindications

Established cerebrovascular event (excluding transient ischemic attack) within previous 2 months

Active bleeding diathesis

Recent gastrointestinal bleeding (within previous 10 days)

Neurosurgery (intracranial, spinal) within previous 3 months

Intracranial trauma within previous 3 months

Relative contraindications

Cardiopulmonary resuscitation within previous 10 days

Major nonvascular surgery or trauma within previous 10 days

Uncontrolled hypertension (systolic >180 mm Hg or diastolic >110 mm Hg)

Puncture of noncompressible vessel

Intracranial tumor

Recent eye surgery

Recent internal or noncompressible hemorrhage

Life expectancy less than 1 year

Minor contraindications

Hepatic failure, particularly those with coagulopathy

Bacterial endocarditis

Pregnancy and immediate postpartum

Active diabetic proliferative retinopathy

Adapted from Norgren L, Hiatt WR, Dormandy JA, et al. Inter-society consensus for the management of peripheral arterial disease (TASC II). J Vasc Surg 2007;45 Suppl S:S5–67.

the thrombolytic, multiple infusion protocols have been proposed without much success. Unfortunately, acute compartment syndrome is high at 20%.[41] Ischemic reperfusion injury is considered the culprit pathophysiological mechanism for acute limb compartment syndrome. Mortality rates associated with acute limb compartment syndrome range from 8% to 40%.[1] If the reperfusion is performed within 12 hours, mortality and limb salvage rates are 12% and 93%, respectively. However, if performed after more than 12 hours, the mortality and limb salvage rates are 31% and 78%, respectively.[12] As the intracompartmental pressure increases, arterial perfusion is finally impaired.[42] This is a surgical emergency warranting an emergent or salvage fasciotomy. The clinical features of compartment syndrome consist of rapidly progressive pain not relieved with narcotics, which appears out of proportion to the clinical situation. The characteristic finding of excruciating pain on passive stretching of the muscle (of the involved compartment) along with paresthesias and a pale and swollen limb nails the diagnosis.

PMT

PMT devices came into the market as a supplement to CDT to reduce thrombolytic infusion times, doses (with the aim to reduce hemorrhagic complications), reduce the delay in reperfusion, better penetration of the thrombolytic, debulk large thrombi burden, and in distal embolization failing continued CDT therapy. In this section, we briefly discuss the different devices. A summary of currently used PMT devices is listed in **Table 5**.

Aspiration devices Aspiration devices are the simplest forms of mechanical thrombectomy catheters. They work on the simple principle of aspirating the thrombus.[43,44] They are usually used in vessel sizes of 3 to 4 mm in diameter. They are not very effective in cases with large thrombus burden. These catheters are best used as pretreatment devices before the larger thrombectomy are used. When used along with CDT, the success rates can be high as 90%, with a limb salvage rate of 86% at 4 years.[45]

Hydrodynamic aspiration devices These thrombectomy devices use the principle of high-speed saline jets, which not only lyse the thrombus, but also the Venturi-Bernoulli effect created by the high-speed saline jets results in aspiration of the thrombus. There are mainly 2 kinds of such devices. The first is the AngioJet Xpeedior rheolytic thrombectomy catheter (Medrad Interventional/Possis, Warrendale, PA) is the most commonly used mechanical thrombectomy catheter. The system consists of a drive unit that monitors the performance of the system, a pump set that delivers and collects equal volumes of fluid, and the catheter. The drive unit and the pump set are housed in a console. This console can accommodate the 7 different kinds of catheters. The Xpeedior, DVX, and AVX catheters are used specifically for the peripheral vasculature. These catheters are identical except for their length. In smaller popliteal and infrapopliteal vessels, the XVG and XMI catheters can be used. The other alternatives would be the monorail catheters used in the coronaries and the saphenous vein grafts (Spiroflex and Spiroflex VG [Medrad Interventional/Possin, Warrendale, PA]). All the

Table 5
Summary of currently used PMT devices

Device	System	Details
Aspiration Catheter		
Export Catheter (Medtronic Inc, Minneapolis, MN)	6 or 7 Fr; maximum tip diameter 1.73–1.98 mm	Aspirates the thrombus
Pronto LP, V3, and .035 Extraction Catheter (Vascular Solutions Inc, Minneapolis, MN)	6 Fr; maximum tip diameter 1.34–3.25 mm	Aspirates the thrombus
Hydrodynamic Aspiration Devices		
AngioJet (Possis Medical, Inc, Minneapolis, MN/Medrad Interventional)	4 to 6 Fr; 0.014–0.035-inch guidewire	High-velocity saline solution jets enclosed in catheter use the Bernoulli principle for capture, microfragmentation, and removal
Hydrolyzer system (Cordis, Miami, FL)	6 Fr; 0.018 inch-guidewire, working length of 65 and 100 cm	Predominantly used in hemodialysis fistulas and acute arterial occlusion below the inguinal ligament (native arteries or synthetic grafts). Same principle as AngioJet
Fragmentation devices		
Helix (Microvena, White Bear Lake, MN)	7 Fr; 0.018 inch; working length of 75 and 120 cm	Mechanically fragmenting the thrombus and dispersing it. Please note that there is no aspiration. The theory is that the thrombus is broken down into microscopic fragments, which do not cause any clinically significant distal embolization
Ultrasound-induced thrombolysis		
EkoSonic Endovascular System with Rapid Pulse Modulation (Ekos Corporation, Bothell, WA)	5.2 Fr; 0.014–0.035-inch guidewire, catheter treatment length: 6–50 cm	Allows delivery of thrombolytics and ultrasonic energy to loosen and thin clot's fibrin to enhance lysis; also creates ultrasonic pressure waves to maintain lytics at clot site
Miscellaneous group		
X-Sizer system	6 and 7 Fr; 0.014 inch; working length of 135 cm	The stainless steel cutter (which rotates at 2100 rpm) at the catheter tip fragments the thrombus and aspirates it through a vacuum port
Trellis-8 and -6 infusion system (Covidien, Manchester, MA)	6 to 8 Fr, 0.035 inch guidewire	Isolated thrombolysis through lytic infusion between 2 occlusion balloons, oscillation of dispersion wire increases surface area to promote lysis, aspiration of lysate and remaining thrombolytic agent before removal

Data from Hynes BG, Margey RJ, Ruggiero N II, et al. Endovascular management of acute limb ischemia. Ann Vasc Surg 2012;26:110–24; and Hynes BG, Margey RJ, Rosenfield K, et al. Acute limb ischemia: overview, thrombolysis, and mechanical thrombectomy. In: Casserly IP, Sachar R, Yadav JS, editors. Practical peripheral vascular intervention. 2nd edition. Philadelphia: Lippincott Williams & Wilkins; 2011.

catheters have the same hydrodynamic principle. The fluid jet that emits the catheter is oriented toward the proximal portion of the catheter (essentially, the jet that is emitted, curls back to head into the proximal end of the catheter). Overall procedural success rate with AngioJet was in the range 56% to 95%, distal embolization rates of 9.5% and amputation-free survival rates approach 75% at 2 years. The limb salvage rates were as high as 95% when used without concomitant thrombolytics.[46,47] The second device is a hydrolyzer system, which is used predominantly in hemodialysis fistulas and acute arterial occlusion below the inguinal ligament (native arteries or synthetic grafts). The principle is the same as the AngioJet. Two studies[48,49] reported a success rate of 82% and 83%. The success rate was higher for grafts (88%) compared with native vessels (73%). Complications from these devices arise as they are bulky, emit high-speed jets, and are able to create a suction of 760 mm Hg; hence, they have the potential to cause embolization,[50] endothelial and vessel trauma,[51] and hemolysis. Some physicians use a distal-emboli protection device to reduce the amount of distal embolization.[52]

Rotational or fragmentation devices The HELIX Clot Buster Thrombectomy Device (formerly known as Amplatz Thrombectomy Device) (Microvena, White Bear Lake, MN) is the only device in this group. They work on the principle of mechanically fragmenting the thrombus and dispersing it. Please note that there is no aspiration. The theory is that the thrombus is broken down into microscopic fragments, which do not cause any clinically significant distal embolization. It is important to avoid any form of contact between the vessel wall and the device tip. Rilinger and colleagues[53] have the largest experience with this device. As a stand-alone therapy, complete thrombus removal is appreciated in 75% of the patients. Unfortunately, 7.5% of the patients could not have their device removed percutaneously.

Ultrasound-induced thrombolysis Ultrasound energy can cause thrombolysis as well as facilitate t-PA–induced thrombolysis through acoustic streaming and cavitation.[54–56] A high energy of ultrasound can fragment the thrombus.[57,58] However, a low energy of ultrasound accelerates enzymatic thrombolysis by exposing more fibrin-binding sites and increasing the penetration of thrombolytics.[59,60] The EKOS consists of a reusable control unit and an infusion catheter. The catheter delivers a frequency of 2.2 MHz at a power of 0.45 W. Motarjeme[61] reports a 100% procedural success rate with complete thrombus lysis in 96% of cases after a mean treatment of 16.4 hours. This resulted in a reduction in the lytic dose and therefore a reduction in bleeding complications. A few smaller studies have shown similar results.[62,63] The Dutch randomized trial[64] comparing standard catheter-directed thrombolysis versus ultrasound-accelerated thrombolysis for thromboembolic infrainguinal disease reported positive outcomes with a technical success rate of 80%, reduction in treatment time, and similar rates in serious adverse events.[65] This study has not been published yet. There are plans to start the DUET II nonrandomized study, which will use lower lytic doses. Some of the drawbacks of this system are the technical difficulty in positioning the catheter, distal embolization rate of 5% and possible vessel trauma.

Miscellaneous group (fragments and aspirates) The X-sizer catheter [EndiCOR Medical Inc, San Clemente, CA] works by fragmenting the thrombus and then aspirating it.[66,67] It is approved by the Food and Drug Administration (FDA) for removal of thrombus from synthetic hemodialysis grafts. The Trellis Thrombectomy system (Covidien, Manchester, MA) causes mechanical lysis of the clot and pharmacologic fibrinolysis of thrombus in the arterial circulation. Currently, the FDA has approved it only for the delivery of thrombolytic agent. This device has been used more so in venous thrombosis. The Rotarex device [Straub Medical AG, Wangs, Switzerland] is an over-the-wire catheter, which has a spiral at the end of the catheter that rotates at 40,000 rpm and aspirates particles at 180 mL/min.[68]

Surgical Management

The landmark study in the management of ALI was done by Fogarty and colleagues.[69] A balloon-tipped embolectomy catheter is advanced into the vessel from the proximal end into the occluded distal segment. The balloon is inflated distally, beyond the site of occlusion, and pulled back. Thus, the thrombus is removed en bloc. It is recommended to perform intraoperative angiography after every embolectomy to ensure removal of the complete thrombus and also to ensure that there has been no damage. As mentioned earlier, with the rise of in situ thrombosis, these patients with underlying PAD will need some form of definitive procedure after the embolectomy. Amputation is considered promptly in a nonviable limb. The level of amputation is determined based on the clinical findings, noninvasive techniques, and the viability of tissues at the time of surgery.

Comparison of Endovascular Versus Surgical Management Strategies

The 3 randomized prospective clinical trials that were instrumental in bringing CDT as a potential first-line therapy for ALI in category I, IIa, and possibly IIb patients was the Rochester, STILE and TOPAS trials. The Rochester trial[70] randomized patients with limb-threatening ischemia (embolic and thrombotic) of less than 7 days' duration to CDT (57 patients) and surgical therapy (57 patients). Cumulative limb-salvage rate was similar in the 2 treatment groups; however, the cumulative survival rate was significantly improved in patients who received CDT. The Surgery versus Thrombolysis for Ischemia of the Lower Extremity (STILE) trial[71] is a randomized prospective study that assigned patients with symptoms of worsening limb ischemia within the last 6 months to 3 treatment groups: surgery (n = 144), CDT with recombinant t-PA (n = 137), and CDT with urokinase (n = 112). Patients with acute embolic occlusion were excluded. Thirty-day outcomes, which consisted of a combined end point of death, major amputation, and recurrent ischemia, was better with surgery. The differences in the composite end point were the result of increased morbidity in the CDT arm (21% vs 16%) because of hemorrhagic, vascular access complications and recurrent ischemia. A post hoc analysis in the patient population whose symptom duration was 0 to 14 days (as per the ALI definition) found that the patients in the CDT arm had a lower amputation rate, shorter hospital stay, and lower rate of death and amputation at 6 months compared with the surgical arm. The STILE trial confirmed the Rochester study results of CDT being a potential first-line therapy for ALI. However, it also established that CDT was not effective in most cases of chronic limb ischemia. The TOPAS trial[11] is a randomized, multicenter trial that they compared vascular surgery (thrombectomy or bypass surgery) with CDT in thrombotic or embolic ALI (symptom duration of <14 days). Amputation-free survival rates were similar between the 2 groups at 6 months and 1 year. The CDT group had an increased rate of major hemorrhage and intracranial hemorrhage when compared with the surgical group. In a meta-analysis[72] of 5 randomized trials[11,70,71,73,74] consisting of 1283 participants, there was no significant difference in limb salvage or death at 30 days, 6 months, or 1 year between initial surgery and initial thrombolysis. Thrombolysis participants had significantly more stroke, major hemorrhage, and distal embolization when compared with surgery participants.

Hybrid Procedures

Several clinical and experimental studies have demonstrated that embolectomy results in incomplete removal of thrombus in most patients.[75] Thus, an endovascular intervention usually follows a surgical thromboembolectomy in patients with ALI from in situ thrombosis. The decision to perform complete revascularization after thromboembolectomy is based on outflow from the distal vessel, Doppler signals at the ankle, availability and familiarity of endovascular equipment in an operating room (which can also behave as hybrid operating room), and operator experience or availability of endovascular interventionalist. Setacci and colleagues[76] found that the patients who underwent the hybrid procedure had better primary patency and lower reintervention rates at 3 months, with similar mortality rates when compared with surgery.

Long-Term Anticoagulation and Antiplatelet Management

Anticoagulation is continued after the thrombolysis or surgical hemostasis has been achieved. Unfractionated heparin or low molecular weight heparin can be used. Further long-term antithrombotic therapy depends on the cause of ischemia. Patients with underlying thrombophilia and cardiac source of emboli should be on long-term anticoagulation. Long-term antiplatelet therapy is considered in patients with underlying PAD and those with an arterial aneurysm.

Management of Upper-Extremity Ischemia

Most of the data on the management of upper-extremity ischemia is from surgical experience. Medical treatment can be extrapolated from what we do for the lower-extremity ischemia. Surgical embolectomy has a more favorable[77,78] outcome (overall success rate of 85%–90%) in the treatment of upper-extremity ALI than lower-extremity ALI. In a series of 251 patients with upper-extremity ALI treated with surgical embolectomy, the amputation rate was 2% and mortality rate was 5.6%.[79] In the current clinical practice era, upper-extremity ALI is managed most commonly by surgery (86%), followed by conservative management (11%) and endovascular approaches (3%).[80] Until we have more robust randomized data, surgery will be the probable best treatment choice in a patient who has upper-extremity ALI, in the absence of significant medical comorbidities and acceptable surgical risk.

RECOMMENDATIONS AND GUIDELINES

Once again, we reiterate and reemphasize that early diagnosis and prompt initiation of treatment is the cornerstone to ALI management. Once the diagnosis has been made, the patient needs to be stratified into the appropriate category based on the Rutherford classification. Our recommended management algorithm is illustrated in **Fig. 1**.

For patients with category I, after the initiation of medical treatment, a decision should be made as to whether the patient will benefit from revascularization and if so what would be the anticipated procedural and clinical success rate. Clinical presentation, underlying etiology, and noninvasive imaging will help in this decision-making. If the decision to pursue with revascularization has been made, then noninvasive imaging will help delineate the arterial anatomy and best strategy to approach the problem (in terms of access and equipment). If the expertise is available, endovascular strategy should be considered as a

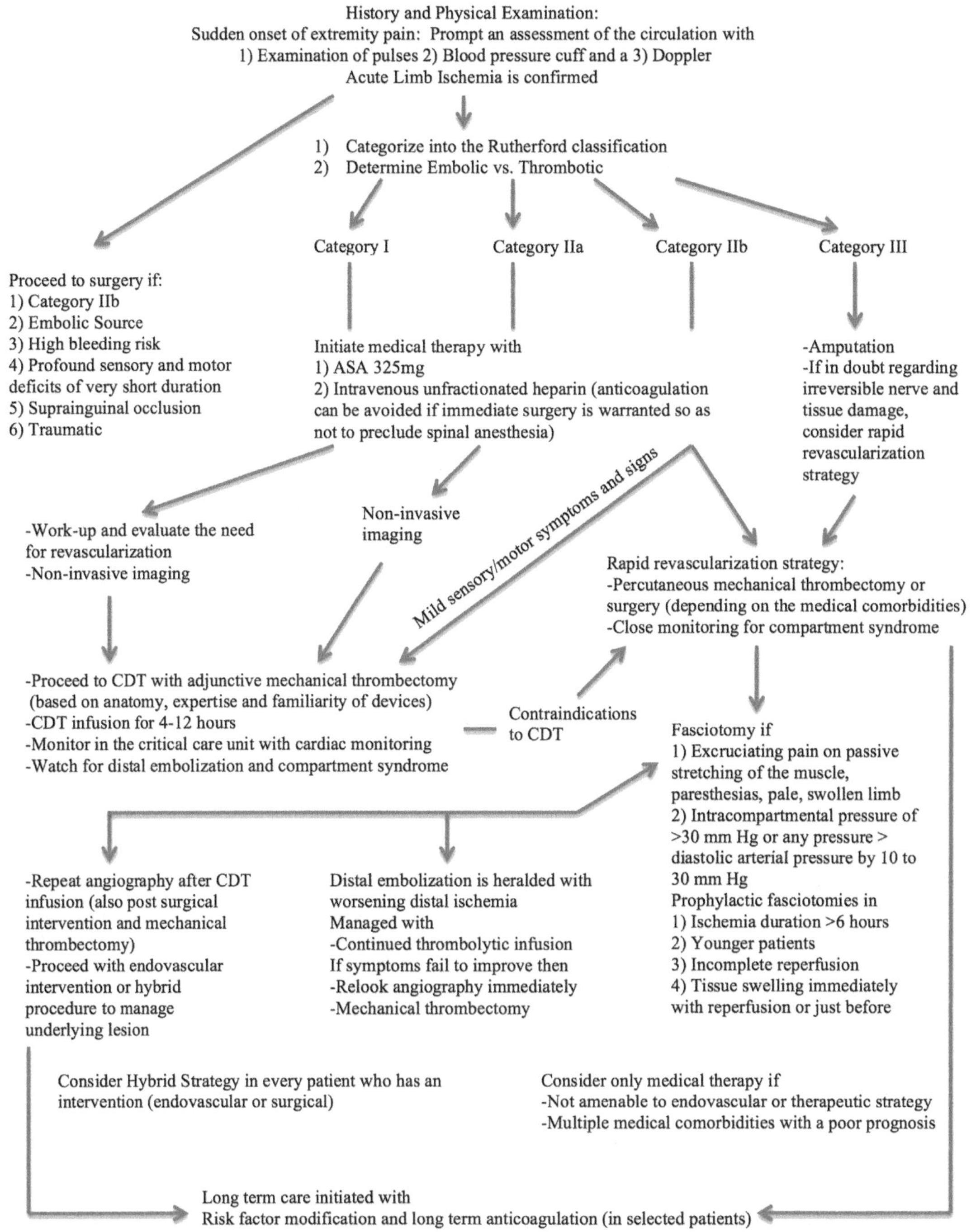

Fig. 1. Management algorithm for ALI.

first-line approach. However, the threshold to convert into a hybrid procedure should be low. PMT can be used if the anatomy permits and the expertise is available, especially if the patient has a high risk of bleeding. Patients falling under category IIa are treated in a similar fashion as delineated in category I, with the following exceptions. Firstly, the threshold to perform revascularization should be lower. Secondly, the decision to perform non-invasive imaging should be based on the extent, the limb is threatened. If it is marginally threatened, then noninvasive imaging can be considered. However, if it appears closer to category IIb, then there should be no delay in proceeding with revascularization. Once again, PMT should be considered, as it helps reduce the infusion dose, duration, and bleeding complications. Patients in category IIb are the most challenging to manage. It is of utmost importance to revascularize as soon as possible to maximize the chance of limb salvage. The standard CDT strategy, which requires prolonged infusion of the thrombolytic, may not be able to achieve this goal. Thus, PMT or surgical revascularization are the dominant strategies. Adjunctive thrombolysis (bolus dosing) with PMT can be considered. Finally, patients in category III are best managed with amputation. One exception to this rule would be an acute embolic presentation of 1 to 2 hours. Rapid revascularization strategy with percutaneous mechanical thrombectomy or surgery should be attempted. After such revascularization, the patients should be monitored closely, as they are at the highest risk for compartment syndrome and other systemic complications. Sometimes differentiation between a salvageable and unsalvageable extremity might be very difficult or near impossible. If in doubt, surgical or endovascular revascularization can be strongly considered.

The TASC I[81] consensus statement recommended surgery as the first-line strategy in patients with ALI. However, the TASC II consensus statement[2] concludes that "it seems reasonable to recommend CDT as initial therapy, to be potentially followed by surgical revascularization as needed." The 2005 American College of Cardiology/American Heart Association guidelines on PAD,[29] which were produced in collaboration with major vascular medicine, vascular surgery, and interventional radiology societies, concluded that there was general consensus that CDT is indicated in patients with ALI of less than 14 days' duration. The guidelines also state that the weight of evidence was in favor of PMT as an adjunctive therapy for ALI. The European Society of Cardiology (guidelines on the diagnosis and treatment of peripheral artery disease)[82] echoes with the other professional societies with regard to their recommendations on ALI management. Their class I recommendations were urgent revascularization in category II, urgent endovascular therapy in the combination form of CDT and PMT in category IIa, and surgical intervention in category IIb with motor or severe sensory deficit. Finally, the 2012 American College of Chest Physicians guideline[83] on antithrombotic therapy for peripheral arterial disease suggested CDT as a first-line treatment in patients with ALI.

REFERENCES

1. Dormandy J, Heeck L, Vig S. Acute limb ischemia. Semin Vasc Surg 1999;12:148–53.
2. Norgren L, Hiatt WR, Dormandy JA, et al. Inter-society Consensus for the Management of Peripheral Arterial Disease (TASC II). J Vasc Surg 2007;45(Suppl S):S5.
3. Brearley S. Acute leg ischemia. BMJ 2013;346:f2681.
4. National Patient Safety Agency. Early detection and treatment of acute limb ischemia. Signal. 2011. Available at: www.nrls.npsa.nhs.uk/resources/?EntryId45=130172. Accessed June 6, 2014.
5. Davies B, Braithwaite BD, Birch PA, et al. Acute leg ischemia in Gloucestershire. Br J Surg 1997;84:504–8.
6. Bergqvist D, Troeng T, Elfstrom J, et al. Auditing surgical outcome: ten years with the Swedish Vascular Registry—Swedvasc. The Steering Committee of Swedvasc. Eur J Surg 1998;(581):3–8.
7. Earnshaw JJ. Demography and etiology of acute leg ischemia. Semin Vasc Surg 2001;14:86–92.
8. Sobieszczyk PS. Acute arterial occlusion. In: Creager MA, Beckman JA, Loscalzo J, editors. Vascular medicine: a companion to Braunwald's heart disease. 2nd edition. Philadelphia: Elsevier Saunders; 2013. p. 557–71.
9. Eyers P, Earnshaw JJ. Acute non-traumatic arm ischemia. Br J Surg 1998;85:1340–6.
10. Klonaris C, Georgopoulus S, Katsargyris A, et al. Changing patterns in the etiology of acute lower limb ischemia. Int Angiol 2007;26:49–52.
11. Ouriel K, Veith FJ, Sasahara AA. A comparison of recombinant urokinase with vascular surgery as initial treatment for acute arterial occlusion of the legs. Thrombolysis or Peripheral Arterial Surgery (TOPAS) Investigators. N Engl J Med 1998;338:1105–11.
12. Abbott WM, Maloney RD, McCabe CC, et al. Arterial embolism: a 44-year perspective. Am J Surg 1982;143:460–4.
13. Elliott JP Jr, Hageman JH, Szilagyi E, et al. Arterial embolization: problems of source, multiplicity, recurrence, and delayed treatment. Surgery 1980; 88:833–45.
14. Sheiner NM, Zeltzer J, MacIntosh E. Arterial embolectomy in the modern era. Can J Surg 1982;25:373–5.

15. Burgess NA, Scriven MW, Lewis MH. An 11-year experience of arterial embolectomy in a district general hospital. J R Coll Surg Edinb 1994;39:93–6.
16. Greenfield LJ, Mulholland MW, Oldham KT, et al. Surgery, scientific principles and practice. 3rd edition. Philadelphia: Lippincott Williams & Wilkins; 2001.
17. Katz SG, Kohl RD. Direct revascularization for the treatment of forearm and hand ischemia. Am J Surg 1993;165:312–6.
18. Peeters P, Verbist J, Keirse K, et al. Endovascular management of acute limb ischemia. J Cardiovasc Surg 2010;51:329–36.
19. Brearley S, Shearman CP, Simms MH. Peripheral pulse palpation: an unreliable physical sign. Ann R Coll Surg Engl 1992;74:169–71.
20. Collins R, Burch J, Cranny G, et al. Duplex ultrasonography, magnetic resonance angiography, and computed tomography angiography for diagnosis and assessment of symptomatic, lower limb peripheral arterial disease: systematic review. BMJ 2007;334:1257.
21. Menke J, Larsen J. Meta-analysis: accuracy of contrast-enhanced magnetic resonance angiography for assessing steno-occlusions in peripheral arterial disease. Ann Intern Med 2010;153:325–34.
22. Met R, Bipat S, Legemate DA, et al. Diagnostic performance of computed tomography angiography in peripheral arterial disease: a systematic review and meta-analysis. JAMA 2009;301:415–24.
23. Eliason JL, Wainess RM, Proctor MC, et al. A national and single institutional experience in the contemporary treatment of acute lower extremity ischemia. Ann Surg 2003;238:382–9.
24. Earnshaw JJ, Whitman B, Foy C. National Audit of Thrombolysis for Acute Leg Ischemia (NATALI): clinical factors associated with early outcome. J Vasc Surg 2004;39:1018–25.
25. Henke PK. Contemporary management of acute limb ischemia: factors associated with amputation and in-hospital mortality. Semin Vasc Surg 2009;22:34–40.
26. Jivegard L, Holm J, Schersten T. Acute limb ischemia due to arterial embolism or thrombosis: influence of limb ischemia versus pre-existing cardiac disease on post operative mortality rate. J Cardiovasc Surg (Torino) 1988;29:32–6.
27. Braithwaite BD, Davies B, Birch PA, et al. Management of acute leg ischemia in the elderly. Br J Surg 1998;85:217–20.
28. Smith SC Jr, Allen J, Blair SN, et al. AHA/ACC guidelines for secondary prevention for patients with coronary and other atherosclerotic vascular disease: 2006 update: endorsed by the National Heart, Lung, and Blood Institute. Circulation 2006;113:2363–72.
29. Hirsch AT, Haskal ZJ, Hertzer NR, et al. ACC/AHA 2005 Practice Guidelines for the management of patients with peripheral arterial disease (lower extremity, renal, mesenteric, and abdominal aortic): a collaborative report from the American Association for Vascular Surgery/Society for Vascular Surgery, Society for Cardiovascular Angiography and Interventions, Society for Vascular Medicine and Biology, Society of Interventional Radiology, and the ACC/AHA Task Force on Practice Guidelines (Writing Committee to Develop Guidelines for the Management of Patients With Peripheral Arterial Disease): endorsed by the American Association of Cardiovascular and Pulmonary Rehabilitation; National Heart, Lung, and Blood Institute; Society for Vascular Nursing; TransAtlantic Inter-Society Consensus; and Vascular Disease Foundation. Circulation 2006;113:e463–654.
30. Dotter CT, Rosch J, Seaman AJ. Selective clot lysis with low-dose streptokinase. Radiology 1974;111:31–7.
31. Berridge DC, Gregson RH, Hopkinson BR, et al. Randomized trial of intra-arterial recombinant tissue plasminogen activator, intravenous recombinant tissue plasminogen activator and intra-arterial streptokinase in peripheral arterial thrombolysis. Br J Surg 1991;78:988–95.
32. Karnabatidis D, Spiliopoulos S, Tsetis D, et al. Quality improvement guidelines for percutaneous catheter-directed intra-arterial thrombolysis and mechanical thrombectomy for acute lower-limb ischemia. Cardiovasc Intervent Radiol 2011;34:1123–36.
33. Shortell CK, Ouriel K. Thrombolysis in acute peripheral arterial occlusion: predictors of immediate success. Ann Vasc Surg 1994;8:59–65.
34. Hynes BG, Margey RJ, Ruggiero N II, et al. Endovascular management of acute limb ischemia. Ann Vasc Surg 2012;26:110–24.
35. Razavi MK, Lee DS, Hofmann LV. Catheter-directed thrombolytic therapy for limb ischemia: current status and controversies. J Vasc Interv Radiol 2003;14:1491–501 [Erratum appears in J Vasc Interv Radiol 2004;15:13–23].
36. McNamara TO, Fischer JR. Thrombolysis of peripheral arterial and graft occlusions: improved results using high-dose urokinase. AJR Am J Roentgenol 1985;144:769–75.
37. Thomas SM, Gaines P. Avoiding the complications of thrombolysis. J Vasc Interv Radiol 1999;10(Suppl):246.
38. Riggs P, Ouriel K. Thrombolysis in the treatment of lower extremity occlusive disease. Surg Clin North Am 1995;75:633–45.
39. Working party on Thrombolysis in the management of Limb Ischemia. Thrombolysis in the management of lower limb peripheral arterial occlusion

consensus document. J Vasc Interv Radiol 2003; 14(9 Pt 2):S337–49.
40. Berride DC, Makin GS, Hopkinson BR. Local low dose intra-arterial thrombolytic therapy: the risk of stroke or major haemorrhage. Br J Surg 1989;76: 1230–3.
41. Tiwari A, Haq AI, Myint F, et al. Acute compartment syndromes. Br J Surg 2002;89:397–412.
42. Mubarak SJ, Hargens AR. Acute compartment syndromes. Surg Clin North Am 1983;63:539–65.
43. Wagner HJ, Starck EE. Acute embolic occlusions of the infrainguinal arteries: percutaneous aspiration embolectomy in 102 patients. Radiology 1992;182:403–7.
44. Zehnder T, Birrer M, Do DD, et al. Percutaneous catheter thrombus aspiration for acute or subacute arterial occlusion of the legs: how much thrombolysis is needed? Eur J Vasc Endovasc Surg 2000; 20:41–6.
45. Wagner HJ, Starck EE, Reuter P. Long term results of percutaneous aspiration embolectomy. Cardiovasc Intervent Radiol 1994;17:241–6.
46. Wagner HJ, Muller-Hulsbeck S, Pitton MB, et al. Rapid thrombectomy with a hydrodynamic catheter: results from a prospective, multicenter trial. Radiology 1997;205:675–81.
47. Muller-Hulsbeck S, Kalinowski M, Heller M, et al. Rheolytic hydrodynamic thrombectomy for percutaneous treatment of acutely occluded infra-aortic native arteries and bypass grafts: midterm follow-up results. Invest Radiol 2000;35:131–40.
48. Reekers JA, Kromhout JG, Spithoven HG, et al. Arterial thrombosis below the inguinal ligament: percutaneous treatment with a thrombosuction catheter. Radiology 1996;198:49–53.
49. Henry M, Amor M, Henry I, et al. The Hydrolyser thrombectomy catheter: a single-center experience. J Endovasc Surg 1998;5:24–31.
50. Kasirajan K, Gray B, Beavers FP, et al. Rheolytic thrombectomy in the management of acute and subacute limb-threatening ischemia. J Vasc Interv Radiol 2001;12:413–21.
51. Vesely TM, Hovsepian DM, Darcy MD, et al. Angioscopic observations after percutaneous thrombectomy of thrombosed hemodialysis grafts. J Vasc Interv Radiol 2000;11:971–7.
52. Sedghi Y, Collins TJ, White CJ. Endovascular management of acute limb ischemia. Vasc Med 2013;5: 307–13.
53. Rilinger N, Gorich J, Scharrer-Pamler R, et al. Mechanical thrombectomy of embolic occlusion in both the profunda femoris and superficial femoral arteries in critical limb ischemia. Br J Radiol 1997;70:80–4.
54. Lauer CG, Burge R, Tang CB, et al. Effect of ultrasound on tissue-type plasminogen activator-induced thrombolysis. Circulation 1992;86:1257–64.
55. Nyborg WL, Ziskin MC. Biological effects of ultrasound. New York: Churchill Livingstone; 1985. p. 1–33.
56. Rosenschein U, Rozenszajn LA, Kraus L, et al. Ultrasonic angioplasty in totally occluded peripheral arteries: initial clinical, histological, and angiographic result. Circulation 1991;83:1976–86.
57. Seigel RJ, Fishbein MC, Luo H, et al. Ultrasonic plaque ablation. A new method for recanalization of partially or totally occluded arteries. Ciruculation 1988;78:1443–8.
58. Steffen W, Fishbein MC, Luo H, et al. High intensity, low frequency catheter delivered ultrasound dissolution of occlusive coronary artery thrombi: an in vitro and in vivo study. J Am Coll Cardiol 1994; 24:1571–9.
59. Francis CW, Blinic A, Lee S, et al. Ultrasound accelerates transport of recombinant tissue plasminogen activator into clots. Ultrasound Med Biol 1995;21:419–24.
60. Braaten JV, Goss RA, Francis CW. Ultrasound reversible disaggregates fibrin fibres. Thromb Haemost 1997;78:1063–8.
61. Motarjeme A. Ultrasound-enhanced thrombolysis. J Endovasc Ther 2007;14:251–6.
62. Schrijver AM, Reijnen MM, van Oostayen JA, et al. Initial results of catheter-directed ultrasound-accelerated thrombolysis for thromboembolic obstructions of the aortofemoral arteries: a feasibility study. Cardiovasc Intervent Radiol 2012;35:279–85.
63. Wissgott C, Richter A, Kamusella P, et al. Treatment of critical limb ischemia using ultrasound-enhanced thrombolysis (PARES Trial): final results. J Endovasc Ther 2007;14:438–43.
64. Schrijver AM, Reijnen MM, Oostayen JA, et al. Dutch randomized trial comparing standard catheter-directed thrombolysis versus ultrasound-accelerated thrombolysis for thromboembolic infrainguinal disease (DUET): design and rationale. Trials 2011;12:20.
65. Available at: http://www.businesswire.com/news/home/20130415005520/en/Randomized-Controlled-Multi-Center-Trial-Demonstrates-Reduced-Treatment#.U0nrvV5v1g0. Accessed April 12, 2014.
66. Stone GW, Cox DA, Low R, et al. Safety and efficacy of a novel device for treatment of thrombotic and atherosclerotic lesions in native coronary arteries and saphenous vein grafts: results from the multicenter X-Sizer for treatment of thrombus and atherosclerosis in coronary applications trial (X-TRACT) study. Catheter Cardiovasc Interv 2003; 58:419–27.
67. Kornowski R, Ayzenberg O, Halon DA, et al. Preliminary experiences using X-sizer catheter for mechanical thrombectomy of thrombus-containing lesions during acute coronary syndromes. Catheter Cardiovasc Interv 2003;58:443–8.

68. Stanek F, Ouhrabkova R, Prochazka D. Mechanical thrombectomy using the Rotarex catheter—safe and effective method in the treatment of peripheral arterial thromboembolic occlusions. Vasa 2010;39: 334–40.
69. Fogarty TJ, Cranley JJ, Krause RJ, et al. A method for extraction of arterial emboli and thrombi. Surg Gynecol Obstet 1963;116:241–4.
70. Ouriel K, Shortell CK, DeWeese JA, et al. A comparison of thrombolytic therapy with operative revascularization in the initial treatment of acute peripheral arterial ischemia. J Vasc Surg 1994;19:1021–30.
71. Results of a prospective randomized trial evaluating surgery versus thrombolysis for ischemia of the lower extremity. The STILE trial. Ann Surg 1994; 220:251–66.
72. Berridge DC, Kessel DO, Robertson I. Surgery versus thrombolysis for initial management of acute limb ischaemia. Cochrane Database Syst Rev 2013;(6):CD002784.
73. Nilsson L, Albrechtsson U, Jonung T, et al. Surgical treatment versus thrombolysis in acute arterial occlusion: a randomised controlled study. Eur J Vasc Surg 1992;6(2):189–93.
74. Ouriel K, Veith FJ, Sasahara AA. Thrombolysis or peripheral arterial surgery: phase I results. J Vasc Surg 1996;23:64–73.
75. Plecha FR, Pories WJ. Intraoperative angiography in the immediate assessment of arterial reconstruction. Arch Surg 1972;105:902–7.
76. Setacci C, De Donato G, Setacci F, et al. Hybrid procedures for acute limb ischemia. J Cardiovasc Surg 2012;53(1 Suppl 1):133–43.
77. Davies MG, O'Malley K, Feeley M, et al. Upper limb embolus: a timely diagnosis. Ann Vasc Surg 1991; 5:85–7.
78. Pentti J, Salenius JP, Kuukasjarvi P. Outcome of surgical management in acute upper limb ischemia. Ann Chir Gynaecol 1995;84:25–8.
79. Hernandez-Richter T, Angele MK, Helmberger T, et al. Acute ischemia of the upper extremity: long term results following thromboembolectomy with the Fogarty catheter. Langenbecks Arch Surg 2001;386:261–6.
80. Turner EJ, Loh A, Howard A. Systematic review of the operative and non-operative management of acute upper limb ischemia. J Vasc Nurs 2012;30:71–6.
81. Dormandy JA, Rutherford RB. Management of peripheral arterial disease (PAD). TASC Working Group. TransAtlantic Inter-Society Consensus (TASC). J Vasc Surg 2000;31(1 Pt 2):S1–296.
82. Tendera M, Aboyans V, Bartelink ML, et al. ESC Guidelines on the diagnosis and treatment of peripheral artery diseases: document covering atherosclerotic disease of extracranial carotid and vertebral, mesenteric, renal, upper and lower extremity arteries: the Task Force on the Diagnosis and Treatment of Peripheral Artery Diseases of the European Society of Cardiology (ESC). Eur Heart J 2011;32:2851–906.
83. Alonso-Coello P, Bellmunt S, McGorrian C, et al. Antithrombotic therapy in peripheral artery disease: Antithrombotic Therapy and Prevention of Thrombosis, 9th ed: American College of Chest Physicians Evidence-Based Clinical Practice Guidelines. Chest 2012;141:e669S.
84. Hynes BG, Margey RJ, Rosebfield K, et al. Acute limb ischemia: overview, thrombolysis, and mechanical thrombectomy. In: Casserly IP, Sachar R, Yadav JS, editors. Practical peripheral vascular intervention. 2nd edition. Philadelphia: Lippincott Williams & Wilkins; 2011. p. 194–219.

Management of Infrapopliteal Arterial Disease: Critical Limb Ischemia

Jihad A. Mustapha, MD[a,b,*], Larry J. Diaz-Sandoval, MD[a,b]

KEYWORDS

- Chronic total occlusion (CTO) cap analysis • Infrapopliteal artery disease
- Critical limb ischemia (CLI)

KEY POINTS

- The TransAtlantic Inter-Society Consensus Document on Management of Peripheral Arterial Disease (TASC II) document states, "there is increasing evidence to support a recommendation for angioplasty in patients with critical limb ischemia (CLI) and infrapopliteal artery occlusion."
- Management of infrapopliteal (IP) artery disease starts with proper diagnosis using modern preprocedural noninvasive and invasive imaging.
- Interventionalists need to learn the role of chronic total occlusion (CTO) cap analysis and collateral zone recognition in angiosome-directed interventions for the management of patients with critical limb ischemia.
- Interventionalists should be familiar with proper equipment and device selection and a stepwise approach to set up for endovascular interventions for the treatment of complex IP disease.
- Interventionalists need to know which crossing tools to use to successfully cross complex CTO caps.

INTRODUCTION

CLI represents the terminal stage of peripheral arterial disease (PAD) and it occurs when arterial blood flow is restricted to the point that the capillary beds are inadequately perfused and unable to sustain tissue viability. It is defined by the presence of rest pain and/or tissue loss for at least 2 to 4 weeks that can be attributed to occlusive arterial disease. The European Consensus Conference has also included the need for analgesia for more than 2 weeks or ischemic tissue loss with an ankle pressure of less than 50 mm Hg as part of the definition.[1] Anatomically, CLI is characterized by multilevel and multivessel (ie, aortoiliac, femoropopliteal [FP], and IP), but fewer than 10% of CLI patients have hemodynamically significant disease in all 3 levels.[1–3] These arterial stenoses and occlusions create a severe imbalance between supply and demand of oxygen in the affected tissues, compromising its viability and threatening limb loss. In less severe circumstances, compensatory mechanisms, such as angiogenesis and arteriogenesis,[4] are sufficient to overcome the increased demand imposed by the lack of adequate tissue perfusion; however, in patients with CLI, these mechanisms have been exhausted and/or are defective. Inadequate perfusion of the skin and surrounding tissues leads to endothelial dysfunction, chronic inflammation,[5] and muscle damage.[6–8] CLI represents the "point of no return" or end stage in the clinical spectrum

The authors have nothing to disclose.

[a] Department of Clinical Research, College of Osteopathic Medicine, Michigan State University, 5900 Byron Center Ave SW, Wyoming, MI 49519, USA; [b] Department of Medicine, Metro Health Hospital, 5900 Byron Center Avenue, Southwest, Wyoming, MI 49519, USA
* Corresponding author. Department of Medicine, Metro Health Hospital, 5900 Byron Center Avenue, Southwest, Wyoming, MI 49519.
E-mail address: jihad.mustapha@metrogr.org

Intervent Cardiol Clin 3 (2014) 573–592
http://dx.doi.org/10.1016/j.iccl.2014.07.002

of patients with PAD. In patients with diabetes, the risk of PAD is 3- to 4-fold higher and it tends to be more aggressive than in patients without diabetes, with a major amputation rate 5 to 10 times higher, whereas typical below-the-knee (BTK) diabetic arterial disease is characterized by long, multilevel disease involving all 3 IP vessels.[9,10] Among patients with infrainguinal disease (FP and IP), approximately one-third have predominantly isolated IP disease and the remaining two-thirds a combination of FP and IP disease.[10–13] Isolated IP disease is mainly seen in elderly (>80 years old), diabetic, or dialysis-dependent patients.[11] These patients have higher risk for amputation and shorter amputation-free survival (AFS) compared with those with FP and IP disease (median AFS: 17 months vs 37 months; $P = .001$).[12]

It is presumed that this prognostic difference is at least in part secondary to an individual patient's ability to develop collateral systems that have been observed to mature in 4 major zones, which are of paramount importance for angiosome-directed therapy (ADT). The number and quality (diameter) of these collaterals is related to the degree of disease (high-grade stenosis vs CTOs [**Fig. 1**]) and patient comorbidities. Advanced age, history of coronary artery disease, hypertension, smoking, and elevated low-density lipoprotein cholesterol levels affect the number and migratory capacity of endothelial progenitor cells, which are known to be involved in the process of collateral formation.[14] The authors have recently described the PRIME collateral zones (**Fig. 2**), which group the collateral systems of the lower extremity in 4 distinct areas that have direct clinical implications in the management of CLI patients.

PRIME collateral zones

- Zone 1: collaterals originate primarily from the profunda and to a lesser extent from the proximal superficial femoral artery (SFA).
- Zone 2: collaterals originate in the distal SFA and the P1 and P2 segments of the popliteal artery (PA), depending on the occlusive state.
- Zone 3: collaterals originate from the P3 segment of the PA and the proximal tibial arteries, including the tibioperoneal trunk (TPT).
- Zone 4: collaterals originate from the distal tibial arteries, primarily from the peroneal artery (PrA) and, to a lesser extent, from the anterior tibial (AT) and posterior tibial (PT) arteries.

Continuous advances in the field of interventional endovascular medicine have facilitated the performance of IP interventions through the development of different technologies. These include low-profile sheaths, balloon and stent catheters, steerable and

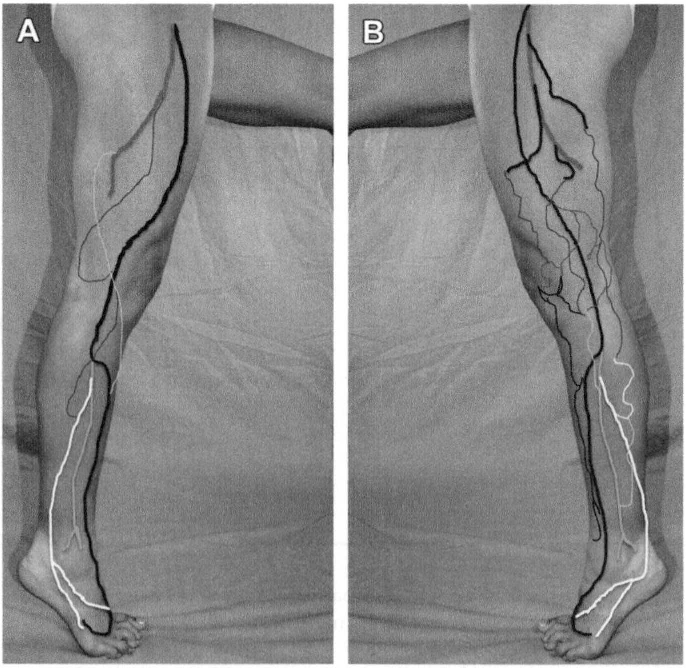

Fig. 1. Collateral systems of the lower extremity in patients with advanced PAD and critical limb ischemia. (*A*) Collaterals developed in patients with high-grade stenosis. (*B*) More robust collateral system, typically seen with CTOs. (*Adapted from* Mustapha JA, Diaz-Sandoval L, Saab F. Angiosome-directed therapy for the CLI patient. Endovasc Today 2014;13(5):65–70.)

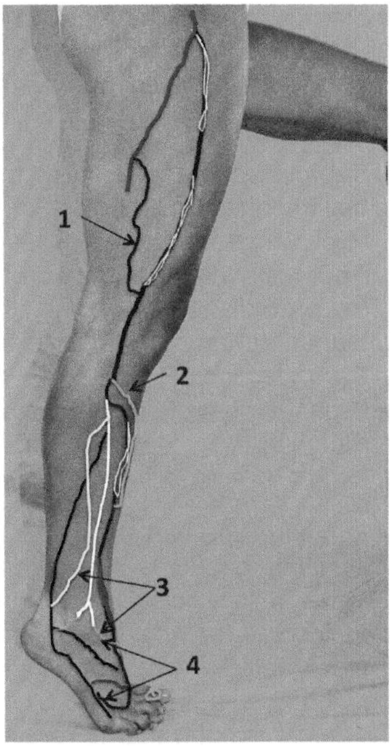

Fig. 2. Multiple level CTOs, typical in CLI patients. PRIME collateral zones keep limbs intact while metabolic supply and demand are balanced (stable state). PRIME zone 1: the collateral paths from the profunda to the popliteal and genicular branches. PRIME zone 2: the collateral paths from the popliteal and genicular branches to the tibial arteries. PRIME zone 3: the collateral path from the proximal to the distal tibials. PRIME zone 4: the pedal loops collateral paths. (*Adapted from* Mustapha JA, Diaz-Sandoval L, Saab F. Angiosome-directed therapy for the CLI patient. Endovasc Today 2014;13(5):65–70.)

hydrophilic guide wires, road mapping capabilities, atherectomy devices, CTO crossing devices, low-profile re-entry devices, use of extravascular ultrasound (EVUS) to aid in the diagnosis of IP disease[15] as well as to guide arterial access[16] and interventions, vasodilators, and antiplatelets, among other advances. IP endovascular interventions, such as angioplasty and stenting, have accrued a significant amount of clinical data and become the first-line treatment of BTK arterial occlusive disease.[17] Primary goals of CLI treatment are relief from ischemic pain, improvement of patient's functionality and quality of life, wound healing, limb salvage, and AFS.[5] Mechanical revascularization, via endovascular or surgical interventions, is necessary to achieve these goals. For some patients, primary amputation may be the only option. Treatment should also focus on diagnosis and management of a patient's cardiovascular risk factors (hypertension, hyperlipidemia, diabetes, obesity, and tobacco abuse) as well as concomitant coronary and cerebrovascular disease.[5,18] Ultimately, the comprehensive treatment of CLI patients requires the participation of a multidisciplinary team involved in their longitudinal follow-up even after revascularization and wound healing have been attained, because this peculiar cohort of patients is always at risk for new disarrays in their compromised metabolic balance.

DIAGNOSTIC IMAGING

Modern preprocedural imaging includes noninvasive modalities, such as multidetector CT angiography (MD-CTA), contrast-enhanced magnetic resonance angiography (CE-MRA), and high-frequency duplex ultrasound (DUS)[5,19–21] as well as the invasive digital subtraction angiography (DSA). The choice of the optimal preprocedural imaging modality should be individualized on a case-by-case basis and it largely depends on local expertise. Although all of these modalities are appropriate in evaluating the large-diameter supragenicular arterial tree, the small-caliber BTK outflow vessels are best depicted by either time-resolved CE-MRA or superselective DSA with the catheter positioned just above the IP trifurcation.[19,22,23] CE-MRA has been reported to detect significantly more distal pedal arteries than selective DSA, even in patients with diabetes, which could influence the pre- and intraprocedural BTK revascularization strategy.[24] The authors visualize the pedal arteries by DSA with placement of a 0.018-inch catheter as distal as possible in the tibial arteries and even into the below-the-ankle (BTA) vessels. MRA evaluation of in-stent stenosis is poor. MD-CTA of small-caliber calcified arteries is limited by artifacts, such as calcium blooming and beam hardening, which sometimes interfere with adequate assessment of severity of stenoses. DUS is operator dependent, and, although the IP arterial evaluation is compromised by inflow occlusions, obesity, and calcifications, it can be useful in assessing pedal artery morphology, patency, and physiology.[25] In patients with advanced chronic kidney disease (CKD) (stages 3 and 4 and predialysis), sole preoperative DUS is recommended because intravenous (IV) administration of contrast agents containing iodine can cause contrast-induced nephropathy, and IV use of gadolinium may cause nephrogenic systemic fibrosis.[26] The authors typically map the arterial tree with DUS in all patients with CLI and perform intraprocedural imaging with a combination of DUS and CO_2 angiography in patients with CKD. This allows minimizing radiation and contrast exposure. Pretreatment imaging in patients scheduled to undergo IP interventions should provide accurate information regarding the inflow and

IP vessels as well as the status of the pedal loops and arches. Evaluation of the iliacs, common femoral arteries (CFAs), superficial femoral arteries (SFA), and popliteal and tibial arteries is essential for the choice of treatment and procedural planning (access site, materials, and procedural time). Patency of the iliac and CFA is of practical importance, because it plays a role in determining whether an ipsilateral antegrade or contralateral retrograde common femoral approach is used. Most IP revascularization procedures should ideally be performed via antegrade CFA or SFA access because the ability to deliver coaxial force in a unilinear vector increases the likelihood of successful crossing of long, complex CTOs. This access strategy should be combined with retrograde tibial pedal access in cases where the CTO cap analysis indicates that the distal cap has retrograde congruous concavity (discussed later). Antegrade access also provides ability to perform distal injections to assess the status of the pedal vessels more accurately and ultimately provides the ability to potentially treat BTA vessels in the event of embolization, dissection, or other distal complications, which would be potentially impossible to perform with a contralateral approach (specially in tall patients). Optimal preprocedural imaging should identify the severity and length of the IP arterial lesions, provide detailed information about the distal foot vasculature and locate the distal point of reconstitution of the target vessels. To obtain procedural technical and clinical success, the IP vessel that feeds the ischemic angiosome should be (whenever possible) the target of the intervention.

An angiosome is a 3-D anatomic unit of tissue (consisting of skin, subcutaneous tissue, fascia, muscle, and bone) fed by a source artery and drained by specific veins. The foot and ankle angiosome is a topographic map conformed by 5 territories provided by 3 main arteries and their branches (**Fig. 3**):

- The PT provides 3 angiosomes: the medial calcaneal (medial plantar aspect of the heel), the medial plantar, and lateral plantar (supplying the corresponding plantar surfaces).
- The PrA provides 1 angiosome: the lateral calcaneal (lateral aspect of the heel and ankle)
- The AT provides the DP angiosome, supplying the dorsum of the foot and anterior aspect of the ankle.

ADT refers to the establishment of flow to the topographic area of the foot where the wound is located. This can be achieved via direct flow (DF), defined as in-line, pulsatile flow through the affected angiosome source artery, or indirect flow (IF), represented by the strategy whereby flow to the wound area is provided by collaterals fed by an arterial conduit that is revascularized, because no DF is considered feasible. When this approach is used, the recommendation is to open as many vessels as possible to increase the volume of blood to the foot (volume concept).

Based on recent studies of patients with CLI comparing limb salvage rates (LSRs), direct revascularization of the source artery with the DF strategy[27–30] seems more effective than revascularization of a nonspecific artery with reliance on collateral arteries (IF), despite the increased volume of blood provided to the foot by an increasing number of postprocedural patent IP arteries.[31]

In more recent studies of selected diabetic patients with CLI, the DF versus IF strategy did not influence outcomes nor did the number of revascularized tibial vessels,[32] as long as there was

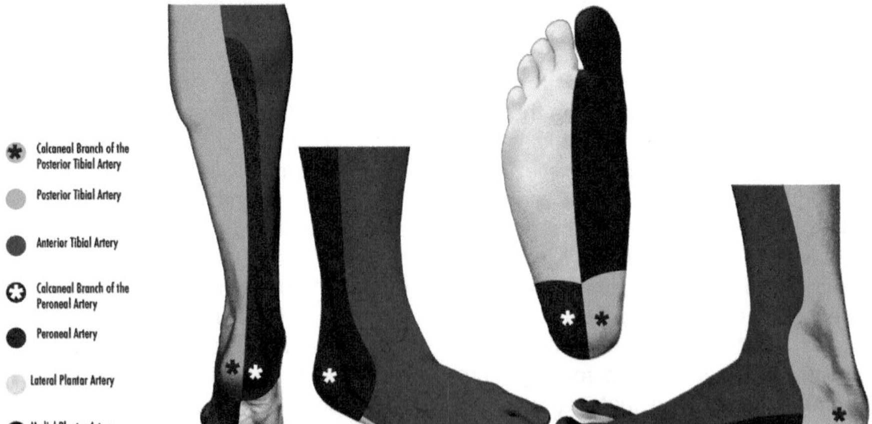

Fig. 3. Angiosomes and supplying arteries.

1 patent vessel runoff to the foot, in contraposition to the results obtained by Lejay and colleagues,[33] who found that in a similar population undergoing open revascularization, the LSR was superior when DF was achieved after ADT. One important observation to be made about all of these studies is that they share a retrospective design.

Until now, only 1 prospective study has been published comparing the strategies of DF and IF to the ischemic angiosome in 64 CLI patients with single-vessel runoff to the foot. Ulcer healing at 1, 3, and 6 months was superior among patients treated with the DF strategy. There was no statistically significant difference, however, in LSRs.[34]

One of the most significant hurdles in the real world is that DF to the ischemic angiosome may not be attainable in a large number of CLI patients. Berceli and colleagues[35] reported on the efficacy of DP bypass for ischemic forefoot and heel ulcerations. According to the angiosome concept and this strategy, the forefoot would receive DF, whereas the heel would be perfused via IF. They achieved an LSR of 86%, indicating that heel ulcerations can heel with IF, even in the absence of an intact pedal arch, presumably through inter-angiosome connections for perfusion.

As new techniques are developed and carried into practice, including US-guided tibial pedal access and interventions, transcollateral tibial interventions, digital and transmetatarsal artery access, and interventions, it seems that the future holds promise in regard to the ability to intervene in these complex patients.[36,37]

Box 1
TASC II classification of infrapopliteal lesions

TASC A

- Single stenosis shorter than 1 cm in the tibial or peroneal vessels

TASC B

- Multiple focal stenoses of the tibial or peroneal vessels (each <1 cm in length)
- One or 2 focal stenoses, each less than 1 cm in length at the tibial trifurcation
- Short tibial or peroneal stenosis in conjunction with an FP lesion

TASC C

- Stenoses 1–4 cm in length
- Occlusions 1–2 cm in length of the tibial or peroneal vessels
- Extensive stenoses of the tibial trifurcation

TASC D

- Tibial or peroneal occlusions greater than 2 cm
- Diffusely diseased tibial or peroneal vessels

From Norgren L, Hiatt WR, Dormandy JA, et al, on behalf of the TASC II Working Group. Inter-society consensus for the management of peripheral arterial disease (TASC II). Eur J Vasc Endovascular Surg 2007;33 Suppl 1:S1–75.

INDICATIONS AND CONTRAINDICATIONS

The primary goal of IP endovascular therapy is to obtain relief from the ischemic rest pain, facilitate healing of ulcer or gangrene, prevent limb loss or limit the extent of amputation, and permit wound healing after any type of amputation. Amputation above the ankle is generally defined as a major amputation; amputation at the ankle or BTA is a minor amputation. In critically ill patients, patients unable to cooperate, and patients with recent myocardial infarction, severe arrhythmia, or electrolyte imbalance, treatment should be discussed and undertaken in the presence of a cardiologist, anesthesiologist, or both. In patients with impaired renal function, alternative CO_2 use instead of standard contrast media can be considered. The TASC II classification is listed in **Box 1**.[5] Generally, in IP lesions classified as TASC A or B, endovascular treatment is preferred whereas in TASC D lesions, surgical vein bypass has been recommended until recently. The TASC II document states that "there is increasing evidence to support a recommendation for angioplasty in patients with CLI and IP artery occlusion."[5] In TASC C lesions, surgery is the preferred treatment in good-risk patients while considering the patient's comorbidities and preferences as well as the operator's success rates. In the absence of a suitable vein and/or adequate distal runoff vessels, however, and in high-risk surgical patients, endovascular treatment represents the only valid therapeutic option for CLI. It is, therefore, no surprise that in real-world practice with older and fragile patients, with poor surgical risk, numerous comorbidities, and poor inflow and/or outflow as well as without suitable conduits, endovascular treatment is often the first line of treatment and should be attempted even in difficult TASC C and D lesions. BTK interventions in patients with severe lifestyle-limiting intermittent claudication remain controversial.

EQUIPMENT FOR INFRAPOPLITEAL INTERVENTIONS

A complete array of dedicated BTK equipment is essential to perform tibial interventions in an effective and safe manner. The choice of wires used in treating tibioperoneal occlusions spans the spectrum from workhorse wires to dedicated, specialized CTO crossing wires. The operator alternates between the 2 groups, depending on the stage of CTO crossing.

The dedicated CTO wires are mainly used to actually cross the CTO caps, whereas the workhorse wires are used mainly to deliver catheters to their desired location. The idea is to minimize the use of the more-aggressive dedicated CTO wires, thereby decreasing complications.

DEVICE SELECTION

There are many wires, catheters, and crossing tools available for the treatment of tibioperoneal lesions, and operators must be familiar with the most important features of these devices. Pertaining to wires, the most important features include the platform, tip load, coating, and length.

The most commonly used platforms are 0.014-inch, 0.018-inch, and 0.035-inch. The tip load, core design, and wire length determine the transmission of force at the tip of the wire as well as the control in its maneuverability and the tactile feedback to the operator.

Below is a sample of some of the most used wires, catheters, and crossing devices that should be in the shelf of a CLI program as well as tools under development:

Workhorse 0.014-inch wires

- Runthrough NS (Terumo, Somerset, New Jersey). Hydrophilic wire with hydrophobic cap for tactile feedback and 1:1 torque. The Nitinol ribbon provides tip durability.
- Journey (Boston Scientific, Natick, Massachusetts). Steerable, hydrophilic wire, with uncoated tip, has 1:1 torque. Works well with the Crosser device (Bard, Tempe, Arizona).
- Regalia (Asahi, Burlington, Massachusetts)
- Mailman (Boston Scientific, Natick, Massachusetts). Stiff wire used for support.
- Command (Abbott Vascular, Santa Clara, California). A hybrid wire of Nitinol and stainless steel.

CTO crossing 0.014-inch wires

- Approach (Cook, Bloomington, Indiana). 12, 18, and 25 g.
- Astato XS (Asahi, Burlington, Massachusetts). 20 g.
- Porter (Bard, Tempe, Arizona). 3, 6, and 12 g; 195 and 300 cm length.

Workhorse 0.018-inch wires

- Glidewire Gold (Terumo, Somerset, New Jersey)
- SV5 (Cordis, Bridgewater, New Jersey). Provides excellent supportive rail.
- V-18 (Boston Scientific, Natick, Massachusetts). Has an atraumatic and shapeable tip that is designed for negotiation of tortuous anatomy, making it especially useful in pedal cases due to the support provided by its body. It is available in different lengths (cm): 60, 145, 180, 260, 300.

CTO crossing 0.018-inch wires

- Treasure (Asahi, Burlington, Massachusetts). 12 g. Has a 1-piece core and steerable tip.
- Astato (Asahi, Burlington, Massachusetts). 30 g.

Workhorse 0.035 inch

- Glidewire (Terumo, Somerset, New Jersey) (Soft and Stiff). Used mainly to traverse major vascular conduits.
- Glide wire Advantage (Terumo, Somerset, New Jersey). Useful in tortuous supragenicular anatomy due to its atraumatic tip and supportive body.
- Magic Torque (Boston Scientific, Natick, Massachusetts). Stiff wire that provides support that is used to advance sheaths from a contralateral approach as well as to advance catheters through tight stenoses/occlusions in the supragenicular vessels.

Crossing Catheters

0.035-Inch catheters

1. NaviCross (Terumo, Somerset, New Jersey) (angled and straight). It is available in 90, 135, and 150 cm. Double-braided catheter. Provides excellent support and its hydrophilic/atraumatic tip allows its advancement without necessarily having a wire in front of it.
2. Glide Catheter (Terumo, Somerset, New Jersey) (angled and straight).

Two platform catheters (0.035 inch and 0.014 inch):

1. Valet Micro catheter (Volcano, San Diego, California)

Multiple platform catheters (0.035 inch, 0.018 inch, and 0.014 inch):

1. CXI (Cook, Bloomington, Indiana)
2. TrailBlazer (Covidien, Plymouth, Minnesota)
3. Quick-Cross (Spectranetics, Colorado Springs, Colorado)
4. Seeker (Bard, Tempe, Arizona)

0.014-Inch catheters

1. FineCross MG (Terumo, Somerset, New Jersey)
2. Corsair microcatheter (Asahi, Burlington, Massachusetts). This is a specialty coronary catheter that the authors are applying in the tibial pedal vessels.

CTO crossing devices

1. Crosser (Bard, Tempe, Arizona). 14S, 14P, S6.
2. Frontrunner (Cordis, Bridgewater, New Jersey)
3. Viance (Covidien, Plymouth, Minnesota)
4. TruePath (Boston Scientific, Natick, Massachusetts)
5. Turbo Elite Laser 0.9, 1.4, and 1.7 (Spectranetics, Colorado Springs, Colorado)
6. Kitty-cat, Ocelot/PIXL (Avinger, Redwood City, California). Not currently available in the United States.

Re-entry devices

Enteer (Covidien, Plymouth, Minnesota)

INTERVENTIONAL SET-UP STEP BY STEP

Both groins should undergo sterile skin preparation. In CLI patients, the authors recommend painting the limb to be intervened on with betadine/chlorhexidine all the way from the groin to the toes. If there are any ulcerated wounds, these are covered with sterile materials. The entire limb is exposed on top of a sterile field to allow for EVUS imaging of the entire limb, which facilitates the retrograde US-guided access in the tibial pedal vessels and assists in guiding the intervention, maximizing the chance of staying inside of the true lumen. The site and direction of the arterial access (antegrade ipsilateral or retrograde contralateral) depend on the inflow status. Iliac disease can be treated during the same intervention via a contralateral retrograde CFA approach, provided there are no limitations in the use of contrast due to underlying renal disease. Traditionally, the inflow is revascularized before the BTK intervention. CLI patients, however, frequently have supragenicular lesions that cannot be treated with an antegrade CFA or SFA approach and need the assistance of a tibial pedal access with a retrograde wire and catheter support to actually cross the supragenicular CTO and allow for complete revascularization. Antegrade (CFA/SFA) and retrograde (Tibial/Pedal) combined arterial access should be pursued to achieve complete limb revascularization in the same setting, based on information obtained from the CTO cap analysis. When concomitant ipsilateral CFA occlusive disease is present, surgical patch atherectomy and BTK revascularization can be performed simultaneously if the institution counts with a hybrid suite and CLI team. If this is not available, a contralateral puncture can be performed immediately or soon after endarterectomy, or the endovascular treatment can be scheduled at least 2 weeks after surgery to facilitate the ipsilateral CFA or SFA puncture with safety. In nonobese patients without iliac, CFA, or very proximal SFA lesions, a direct antegrade puncture is preferable because it offers superior pushability, trackability, and torqueing of the crossing devices because the entire force applied to the device is transmitted to the lesion in a unidirectional vector, allowing crossing of hard, calcified distal occlusions as well as easier catheter and guide wire maneuvers. The retrograde crossover technique can be almost impossible in cases of extremely tortuous iliac arteries, hostile aortic bifurcations, Y prosthesis, or abdominal aortic stent grafts. In contralateral access, a long sheath or a guide catheter positioned into the ipsilateral external iliac artery or the SFA allows selective angiographic visualization of the BTK vessels. The contralateral up-and-over approach is only recommended in instances were an antegrade approach is not feasible, such as severely diseased CFA. When this approach is used, there is a deconstruction of the force vector into 4 (**Fig. 4**A) to 8 or more (see **Fig. 4**B) vectors depending on the tortuosity of the aortoiliac bifurcation, resulting in small transmission of the crossing force to the tip of the crossing device and, therefore, decreasing the likelihood of success.

INFRAPOPLITEAL INTERVENTION STEP BY STEP

US-guided puncture is used to facilitate fast and precise arterial access. With US guidance, the operator can choose to access either the CFA or the SFA selectively. Puncture of the SFA has the advantage of a more direct route but is associated with more bleeding complications. Popliteal and tibial pedal access should be performed under US guidance. Some investigators advocate the use of fluoroscopic guidance when there are vessel wall calcifications. US guidance is recommended because it allows precise visualization of the needle path, vessel depth, and surrounding veins and nerves as well as the ideal puncture site along the vessel path (depending on lumen size, calcification, occluded segments, and so forth).[16] A small real-time injection of contrast should be performed after sheath placement to adjust the position of the sheath in case it is

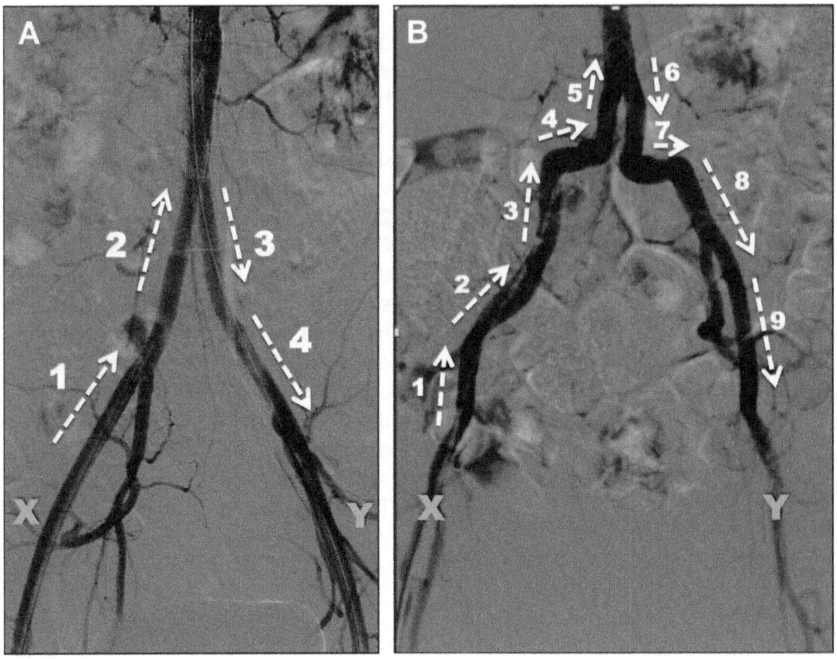

Fig. 4. The dashed arrows represent the vectors into which a force applied at point X would decompose before reaching point Y. (*A*) The force vector decomposes in at least 4 vectors with a narrow angle. (*B*) The force vector decomposes in 8 or more vectors with multiple changes in direction and narrow angles. (*Adapted from* Mustapha JA, Diaz-Sandoval L, Saab F. Tibioperoneal CTOs in patients with critical limb ischemia. Endovasc Today 2014;13(5):42–54.)

occluding the inflow.[38] Baseline selective and superselective arteriograms are obtained, preferably at a separate date preceding the intervention, in an attempt to minimize dye and radiation exposure as well as to aid in the planning of the interventional strategy, which includes the planning of the necessary ancillary staff (US technician, anesthesia support, assisting scrub nurse, and physician for dual-access complex cases) as well as the setup of the room for the intervention. For selective angiography, the catheter is positioned at the level of the SFA. Superselective angiography is performed with the catheter at the P3 segment of the popliteal artery or the tibial trifurcation. In cases where the pedal circulation is the target of the intervention, selective antegrade tibial angiography is performed if feasible with the aid of intra-arterial vasodilators. In general, optimal visualization of the upper and mid-third of the tibial arteries is gained in an ipsilateral oblique projection. Imaging of the distal tibial arteries and the foot is best achieved in a contralateral oblique projection with foot abduction that produces a lateral arteriogram of the foot. The optimal projection to visualize the common plantar artery bifurcation, the DP artery, and the pedal-plantar loop is the lateral oblique projection. To visualize the pedal-plantar loop and the tarsal and metatarsal arteries, an anteroposterior (AP) projection of the foot should be obtained.[24] The target tibial vessel is generally catheterized with a 0.018-inch support catheter. The tibial pedal lesions are crossed with a 0.014-inch or 0.018-inch guide wire. Retrograde tibial pedal access is gained with a 2.9-Fr sheath (sometimes only the dilator is used) and the authors typically use an atraumatic 0.014-inch wire, manipulated under US guidance. Once a point is reached where this is no longer useful, a 0.018-inch catheter is advanced and the wire exchanged for a CTO wire. In very distal lesions, a low-profile 2- or 2.5-mm balloon catheter may support the wire. In cases of subintimal crossing, a 0.018-inch guide wire is appropriate. Over-the-wire balloon platforms are used given their superior pushability, ability to inject through, and ability to exchange wires if needed. Heavily calcified vessels represent a challenge for both intraluminal (suboptimal inflation) and subintimal (difficulty in reentering into the true lumen and increased risk of rupture) angioplasties. Data regarding the duration of balloon inflation are scarce; to the authors' knowledge, there are no reliable studies on this topic in the literature covering peripheral endovascular interventions. Studies of coronary stenting have suggested a minimal inflation time of 25 seconds.[39] The authors traditionally use prolonged (2 minutes), low-pressure (2–4 ATMs) inflations, based on a theoretic decrease in the likelihood of barotrauma to the vessel wall. In case of suboptimal results due to inadequate dilation, elastic recoil, and/or dissection, a second inflation with a smaller diameter balloon for a longer period of time can be performed. If the dissection is flow limiting, the balloon should be kept inflated for a period of 3 to 5 minutes at a pressure not to exceed the nominal balloon pressure. If this does not work, the lesion can be stented (try to avoid this especially in the distal third of the tibial vessels). The stent types available for BTK include balloon and self-expandable bare metal stents as well as balloon expandable drug-eluting stents.[40,41]

Efforts should be made to improve the tibial runoff with additional BTA angioplasty of significant distal stenoses because the longevity of tibial artery patency may be jeopardized in the absence of adequate outflow. Stenting BTA is not recommended with currently available technology, because a potential future surgical bypass always is an option if an undamaged, unstented landing zone is preserved. Traditionally, in cases where the antegrade approach has failed, various retrograde techniques can be used in an effort to obtain limb salvage. The authors routinely use the antegrade-retrograde approach before even failing once through the antegrade-only approach (based on knowledge gained from CTO cap analysis).

In cases of occluded SFAs that cannot be recanalized, antegrade popliteal access may also be considered to address the tibioperoneal disease in CLI patients.[42]

CTO CAP ANALYSIS

The choice of crossing strategy is based on the type of tibial CTO to ensure a higher crossing success rate. There are many anatomic variations in CTOs of the IP arteries that are beyond the scope of this article. The authors have pursued a strategy based on the study of the different types of CTO caps, which have been classified according to their configuration and to the presence or absence of a hibernating lumen (HL). The HL is a segment of arterial lumen that is patent and located between 2 CTO caps (**Fig. 5**) that typically have a heterogeneous distribution of calcium (**Fig. 6**).

When an HL is present, each CTO cap is said to have 2 surfaces (depending on whether the lesion is approached in an antegrade or retrograde fashion [**Fig. 7**]).

The next step is to determine the configuration of each surface pertaining to the proximal and distal caps. These can be either concave or convex (**Fig. 8**). Based on this example, both the proximal and distal caps are classified as antegrade concave/retrograde convex.

Antegrade analysis is performed by comparing the antegrade surfaces of both proximal and distal caps (in the example in **Fig. 9**, antegrade

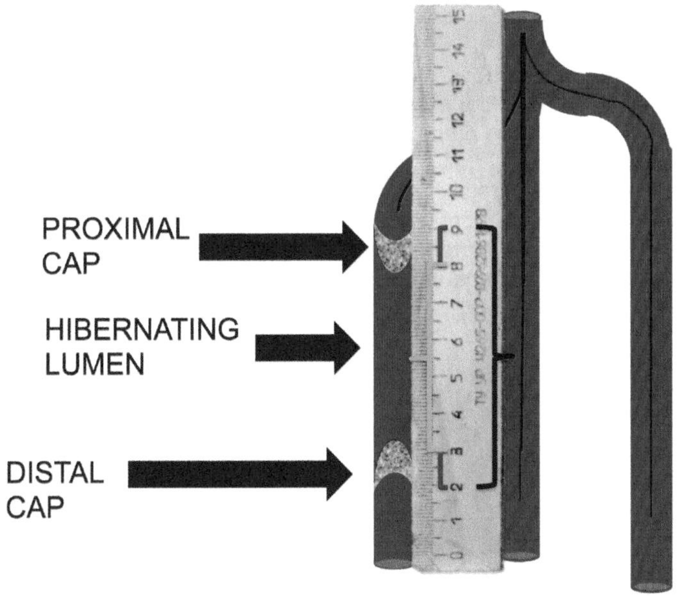

Fig. 5. The cartoon represents a total occlusion of the PT artery. With conventional angiography, it seems that this occlusion is 7 cm long (*black marker*). The true occlusion is limited, however, to the thickness of each cap, which is a total of 2 cm (*red markers*). The remaining 5 cm (*green marker*) represent the length of the HL. (*Adapted from* Mustapha JA, Diaz-Sandoval L, Saab F. Tibioperoneal CTOs in patients with critical limb ischemia. Endovasc Today 2014;13(5):42–54.)

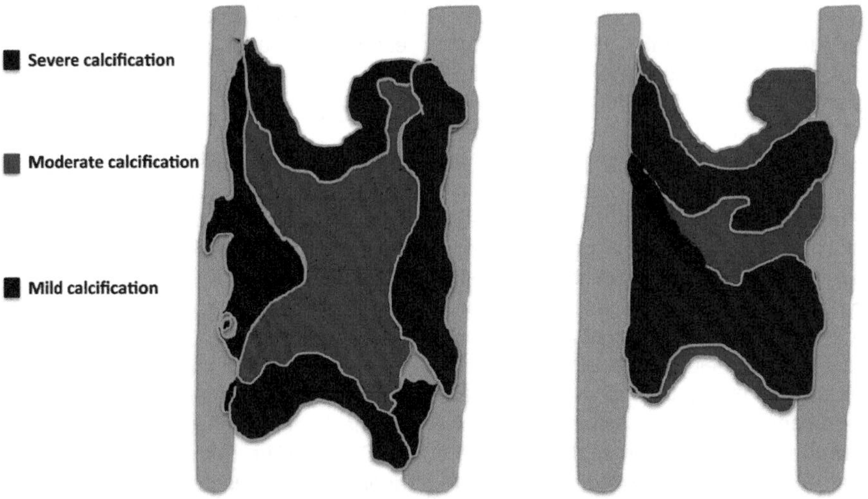

Fig. 6. Each CTO cap is composed of variable layers and isolated islands of different calcium densities, which can range from mild to severe and may be located in the lumen, intima, and media and even reach the adventitia. (*Adapted from* Mustapha JA, Diaz-Sandoval L, Saab F. Tibioperoneal CTOs in patients with critical limb ischemia. Endovasc Today 2014;13(5):42–54.)

concave/antegrade concave). When the same surface of each cap has the same configuration, the lesion is defined as having a congruous configuration in the surface described. In this example, the lesion has antegrade congruous concavity.

Retrograde analysis is performed by comparing the retrograde surfaces of both proximal and distal caps. The example shown in **Fig. 10** is retrograde convex/retrograde convex. This represents a lesion with retrograde congruous convexity.

In general, the intervention should be carried out following the direction of the concavity, because this configuration increases the likelihood of central intraluminal crossing (**Fig. 11**). In the example in **Fig. 11**, the intervention should be carried out using an antegrade approach.

In tibial CTOs, it is not uncommon to see a situation where the lesion has retrograde congruous concavity. In this situation, the best strategy is to intervene from a retrograde tibial pedal access approach (**Fig. 12**).

In more complex tibioperoneal CTOs, both antegrade and retrograde surfaces exhibit different configurations (mix of concave/convex). This is termed, *incongruous concavity*. In these cases, the best approach is a combined antegrade-retrograde access and intervention (**Fig. 13**).

In lesions of no identifiable HL, it is presumed that the entire length of the arterial segment not highlighted by contrast is occupied by fibrous/plaque material. In these cases, each cap only has 1 analyzable surface and configuration (**Figs. 14** and **15**).

Anterior Tibial Artery

The most common AT CTO is proximal, usually found 10 to 30 mm distal to the ostium of the tibial artery. The AT is frequently occluded at the site of the take-off of its large anterolateral branch, preserving the proximal 10 to 30 mm of its course. The most common distal reconstitution is located

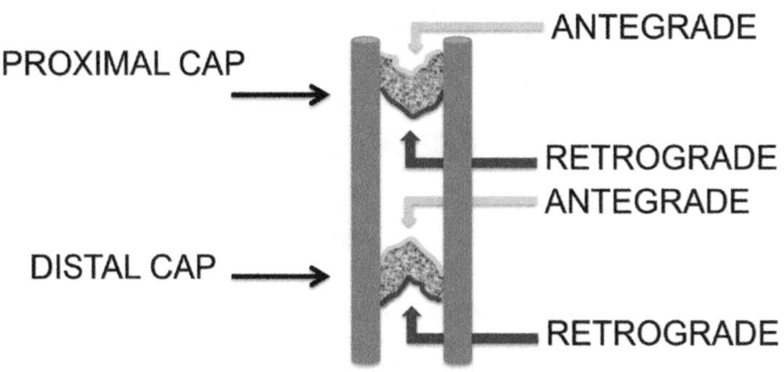

Fig. 7. Each CTO cap has an antegrade and a retrograde surface. (*Adapted from* Mustapha JA, Diaz-Sandoval L, Saab F. Tibioperoneal CTOs in patients with critical limb ischemia. Endovasc Today 2014;13(5):42–54.)

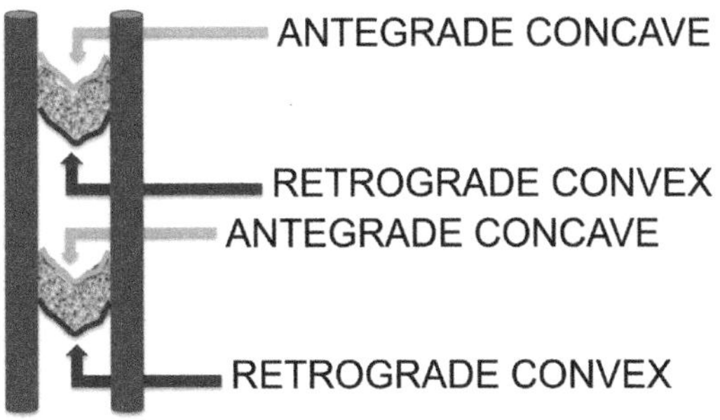

Fig. 8. The next step is to determine the configuration of each surface of both caps. Configuration can be either concave or convex. (*Adapted from* Mustapha JA, Diaz-Sandoval L, Saab F. Tibioperoneal CTOs in patients with critical limb ischemia. Endovasc Today 2014;13(5):42–54.)

around the anterior communicating artery (ACA), which usually fills the distal AT via the PrA (**Fig. 16**).

This example demonstrates the CTO approach of the AT and the PT by using retrograde tibial access and antegrade CFA access as well as selective tibial pedal angiography and simultaneous antegrade-retrograde selective angiography (**Fig. 17**).

These figures illustrate the value of combined antegrade/retrograde arterial access and selective angiography, which significantly enhance visualization of HLs, real length of occlusions, and morphology of CTO caps, which provide an unparalleled and unprecedented ability to plan and perform endovascular interventions for limb salvage cases.

TYPES OF TIBIAL CTOS AND CROSSING STRATEGIES

Posterior Tibial Artery

The most common site of a proximal PT CTO is localized either at the ostium or within the first 10 mm (see **Figs. 16**A and **17**A). The most common reconstitution site of the PT CTO is around the posterior communicating artery (PCA), in the distal third of the leg above the ankle. This vessel also feeds the distal run-off via the PrA (see **Figs. 16**B and **17**B, C; **Fig. 18**C, D).

Tibioperoneal Trunk and Peroneal Artery

The most common CTOs of the TPT and PrA occur at the ostium of the TPT and between the ostium and first 10 mm of the PrA (**Figs. 19**A and **20A**). The reconstitution of the PrA is usually in its distal one-third and mostly fills retrograde via the ACA, the PCA, or both. These branches communicate the PrA with the AT and PT, respectively (see **Figs. 19** and **20**).

CROSSING TECHNIQUES

The preferred access strategy for successful tibial CTO crossing is a combination of antegrade CFA or SFA with retrograde tibial single or double (AT, PT, or a combination), depending on the CTO cap analysis (discussed previously).

Tibial CTO Crossing Techniques

The best working view to cross the proximal AT, PT, and PA CTOs (if working with fluoroscopy guidance) is an ipsilateral oblique view at 30°. This opens the fibula and tibia and positions the AT, PT, and PA between the bones, making the arteries and crossing devices easier to visualize. This view also shows the bifurcation of the PT and PA, which helps identify these 2 vessels to more accurately. It is always best to start with a supporting device when crossing tibial CTOs, such as a catheter or sheath.

The most common antegrade approach is to place a long sheath, positioning the tip around the popliteal area, then engage the tibial artery with a variety of soft tip wires. When treating proximal PT and PA CTOs, make sure support catheter is within the proximal PT or PA prior to initiating the

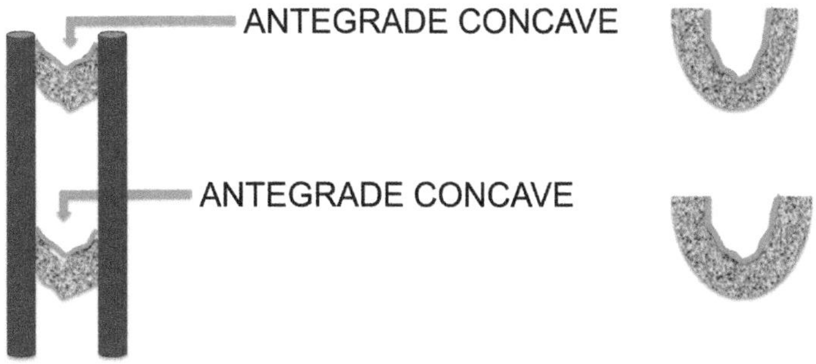

Fig. 9. If the antegrade surfaces of both the proximal and distal caps have the same configuration (concave), the lesion has antegrade congruous concavity. (*Adapted from* Mustapha JA, Diaz-Sandoval L, Saab F. Tibioperoneal CTOs in patients with critical limb ischemia. Endovasc Today 2014;13(5):42–54.)

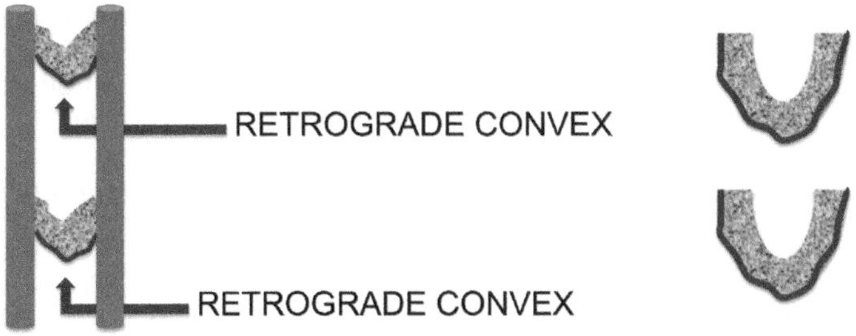

Fig. 10. If the retrograde surfaces of both the proximal and distal caps have the same configuration (convex), the lesion has retrograde congruous convexity. (*Adapted from* Mustapha JA, Diaz-Sandoval L, Saab F. Tibioperoneal CTOs in patients with critical limb ischemia. Endovasc Today 2014;13(5):42–54.)

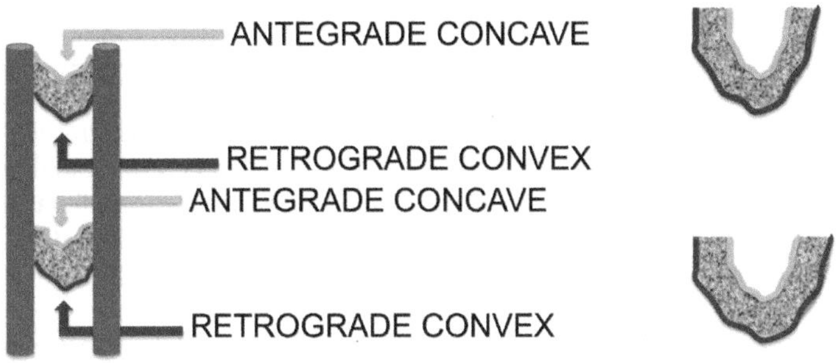

Fig. 11. When the caps are congruous from both approaches, the best strategy is to intervene following the direction of the concavity. (*Adapted from* Mustapha JA, Diaz-Sandoval L, Saab F. Tibioperoneal CTOs in patients with critical limb ischemia. Endovasc Today 2014;13(5):42–54.)

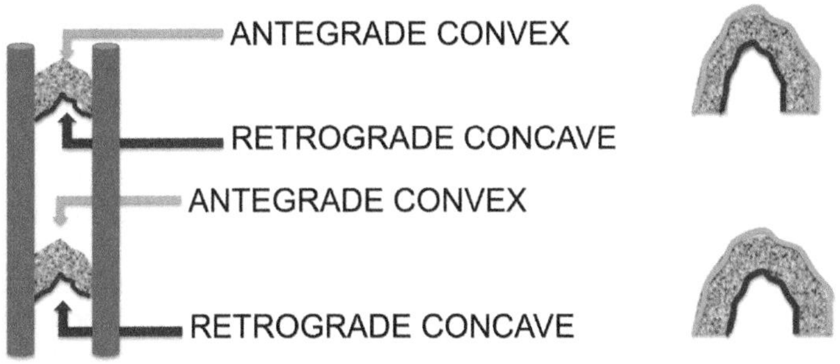

Fig. 12. A retrograde tibial pedal access and interventional approach is recommended in this example given the retrograde congruous concavity of the caps. (*Adapted from* Mustapha JA, Diaz-Sandoval L, Saab F. Tibioperoneal CTOs in patients with critical limb ischemia. Endovasc Today 2014;13(5):42–54.)

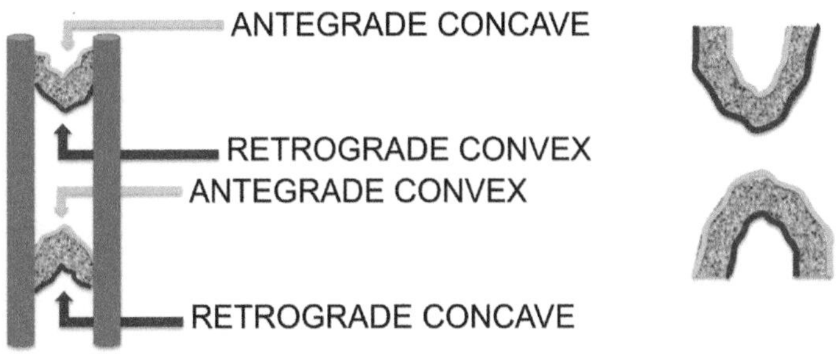

Fig. 13. If both surfaces reveal a different configuration, incongruous concavity is present. In cases of incongruous configurations, proceed with combined antegrade-retrograde access and intervention. (*Adapted from* Mustapha JA, Diaz-Sandoval L, Saab F. Tibioperoneal CTOs in patients with critical limb ischemia. Endovasc Today 2014;13(5):42–54.)

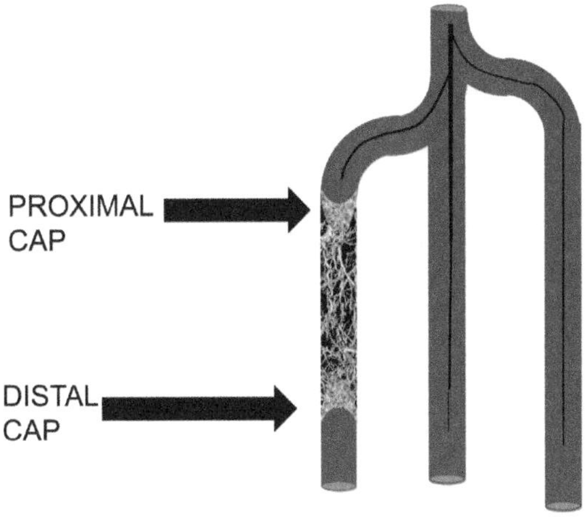

Fig. 14. There is no evidence of HL. The entire length of the segment not identified by angiography is occupied with plaque/fibrous material. (*Adapted from* Mustapha JA, Diaz-Sandoval L, Saab F. Tibioperoneal CTOs in patients with critical limb ischemia. Endovasc Today 2014;13(5):42–54.)

use of heavy gram tip wires. This technique allows you to protect the section of the distal TPT and the ostial PA (if crossing PT) or PT (if crossing PA) that are in close proximity. Keep in mind the majority of these patent proximal AT, PT, and PA segments do have plaque build-up in the range of 30% to 50% and, when crossing the ostium on the way to the CTO cap, it is necessary to avoid disruption of the nonocclusive plaque in the patent segment, which could lead to a devastating dissection or occlusion. To avoid this, start with a soft tip wire with an atraumatic tip-angled catheter, such as the 0.035-inch NaviCross 0.035-inch, 0.018-inch CXI, or angled 0.018-inch Quick Cross.

The Regalia, Journey, and Runthrough wires have an excellent 1:1 torque and atraumatic tip that is easily maneuvered to the proximal AT, PT, and PA CTO cap and provide enough support to advance the angled support catheter.

Once the support catheter is at the CTO cap, crossing can be initiated with the use of specialized CTO wires such as the Treasure 12 g or 20 g, Astato 30 g, Approach 12 g, 18 g or 25 g, PT2 or Victory (Boston Scientific, Natick, Massachusetts). Crossing devices, such as the Crosser 14S or 14P, Viance, and the 0.9 or 1.4 Turbo Elite Laser devices, are excellent choices and particularly helpful in long TPT, PT, and PA CTOs (given their straighter course). If an operator has need to limit choices to 2 workhorse wires for tibial CTO crossing, the authors recommend starting with a soft tip wire and exchanging to a heavy gram tip wire of the operator's choice.

REAL WORLD PRACTICE

The following case shows a complex CTO, which starts in the distal SFA/P1 segment of the popliteal. There is no obvious reconstitution, except for a very short segment of the proximal AT and what seems to be the bifurcation of the PT and PA. Also shown is the anterolateral branch of the AT, which is typically seen when the AT has a proximal CTO and tends to be confused for the AT itself (**Fig. 21**).

This case represents a typical example of a patient who is referred for above-the-knee amputation. The apparent lack of tibial pedal runoff, typically leads teams of surgeons and endovascular specialists to dismiss potential treatment options. Detailed US mapping of the tibial vessels was performed and segments of patent (hibernating) lumen were identified in all the distal vessels. Then, US-guided antegrade CFA access and retrograde AT access were obtained. A 2.9-Fr Cook tibial pedal sheath was placed in the AT and heparin (60 U/kg) and nitroglycerin (200 μg) administered. A 0.014-inch Journey wire was manipulated from the retrograde AT sheath into the PrA. This was followed by retrograde transtibial balloon angioplasty of the AT into TPT/proximal PrA (**Fig. 22**A). Retrograde angiogram revealed improved tibial runoff (see **Fig. 22**B). A 0.035-inch NaviCross catheter was advanced in antegrade fashion and the proximal CTO cap (distal SFA) was crossed with a 6-g 0.018-inch wire under US guidance. The catheter was

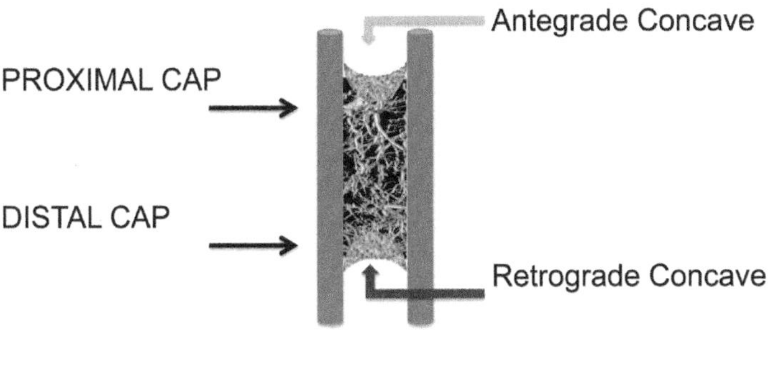

Fig. 15. Each cap only has 1 analyzable surface (proximal antegrade and distal retrograde) and configuration (proximal antegrade concave and retrograde distal concave). In this example, the lesion is considered incongruous; therefore, the recommendation is to proceed with antegrade-retrograde approach. (*Adapted from* Mustapha JA, Diaz-Sandoval L, Saab F. Tibioperoneal CTOs in patients with critical limb ischemia. Endovasc Today 2014;13(5): 42–54.)

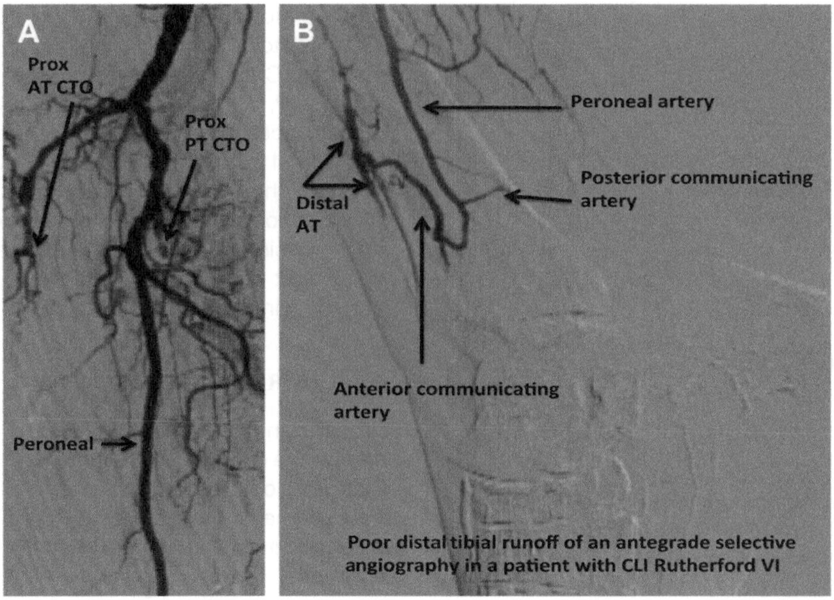

Fig. 16. (*A*) Proximal CTO cap in the proximal segment of both the AT and PT. (*B*) Distal reconstitution of the AT via the ACA. (*Adapted from* Mustapha JA, Diaz-Sandoval L, Saab F. Tibioperoneal CTOs in patients with critical limb ischemia. Endovasc Today 2014;13(5):42–54.)

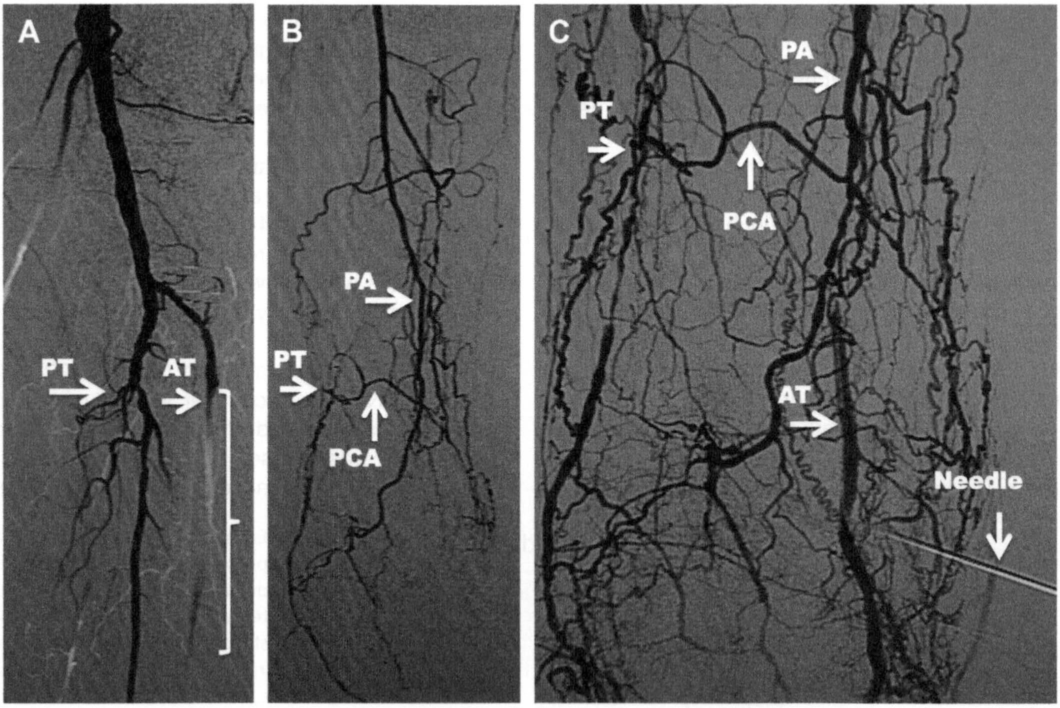

Fig. 17. (*A*) Selective antegrade popliteal angiogram with runoff. (*Arrows*) Ostial occlusion of the PT, without clear take off; proximal occlusion of the AT. (*Bracket*) Subtotal occlusion of the mid-AT. (*B*) Distal tibiopedal runoff from antegrade popliteal angiogram. (*C*) Simultaneous supraselective antegrade popliteal and retrograde AT angiogram (notice the wire inside the vessel from retrograde access). PA, peroneal artery. (*Adapted from* Mustapha JA, Diaz-Sandoval L, Saab F. Tibioperoneal CTOs in patients with critical limb ischemia. Endovasc Today 2014;13(5):42–54.)

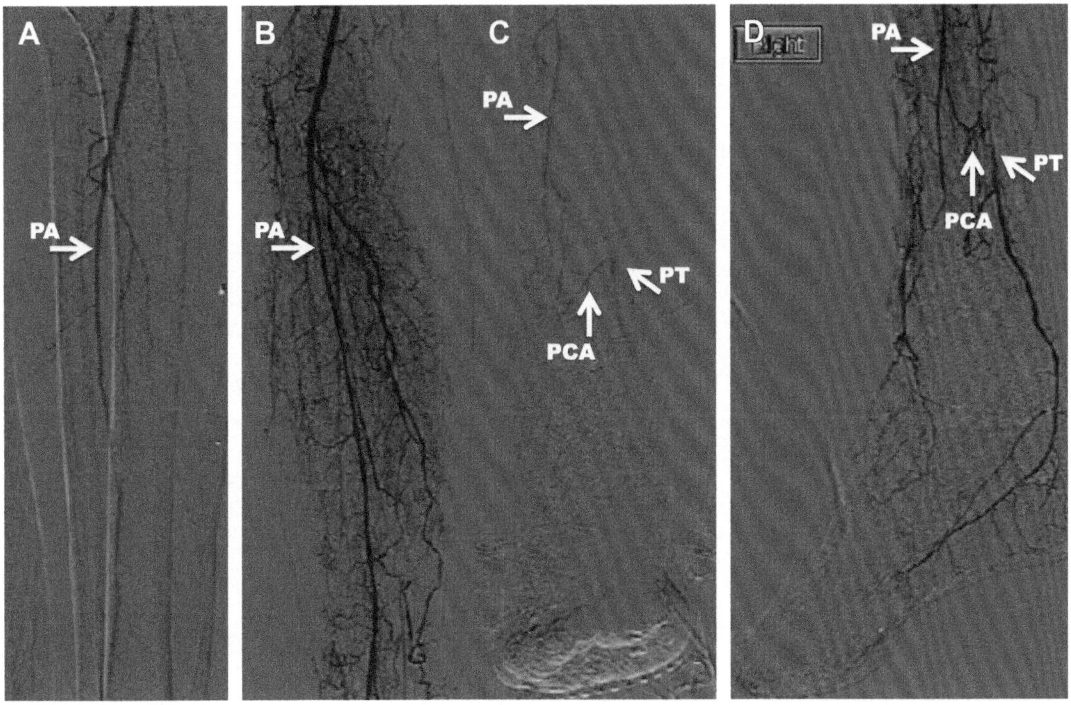

Fig. 18. (*A*) Distal popliteal, TPT, and peroneal artery (PA) visualized through nonselective abdominal angiogram with runoff. (*B*) Distal popliteal, TPT and peroneal visualized via selective popliteal angiogram with runoff. The PT is occluded at the ostium. A collateral is seen in the PT territory. (*C*) Distal PT reconstitution is seen via the PCA, visualized through nonselective abdominal angiogram with runoff. (*D*) Distal PT reconstitution is seen via the PCA, visualized through selective popliteal angiogram with runoff. (*Adapted from* Mustapha JA, Diaz-Sandoval L, Saab F. Tibioperoneal CTOs in patients with critical limb ischemia. Endovasc Today 2014;13(5):42–54.)

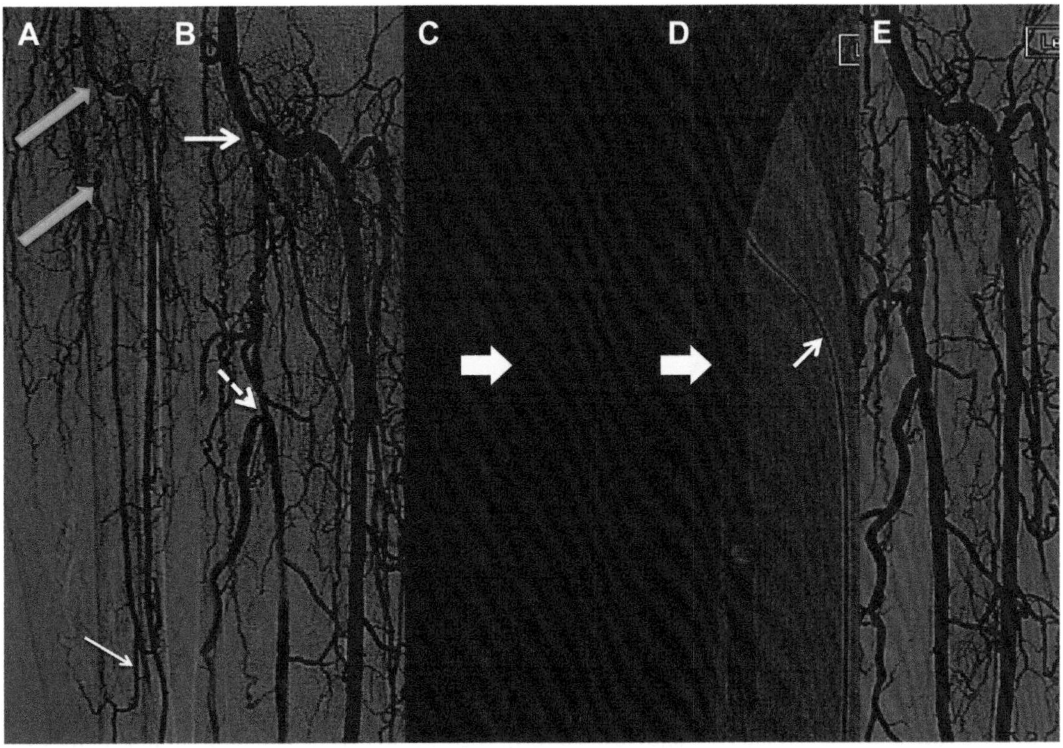

Fig. 19. (*A*) Totally occluded TPT/peroneal and PT. First blue arrow points to ostial TPT occlusion. Second blue arrow points to the origin of the peroneal. Thin white arrow points to the PCA, feeding the distal PT from the peroneal. (*B*) Reconstitution of the TPT (*solid arrow*) and the PT/peroneal bifurcation (*dashed arrow*). (*C*) Angioplasty of the TPT/peroneal (*thick arrow*). (*D*) Angioplasty of TPT/peroneal (*thick arrow*) with wire protecting the AT (*small arrow*). (*E*) Final angiogram after reconstruction of the TPT/peroneal. (*Adapted from* Mustapha JA, Diaz-Sandoval L, Saab F. Tibioperoneal CTOs in patients with critical limb ischemia. Endovasc Today 2014;13(5):42–54.)

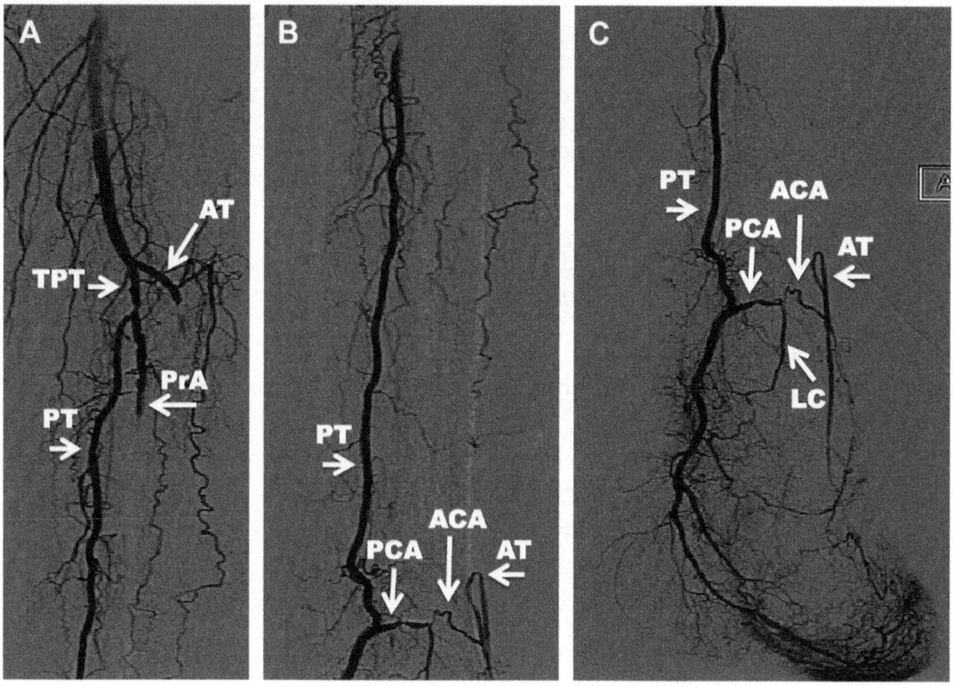

Fig. 20. CLI with 1 vessel runoff via the PT. (*A*) Proximal and mid-third of the IP vessels. Proximal occlusion AT. Total occlusion of the Peroneal (PrA). (*B*) Distal third of IP vessels at the ankle. The peroneal is not seen; however, the PCA to the PT and the ACA to the AT are seen. (*C*) Lateral calcanear branch of the peroneal. LC, Lateral Calcanear. (*Adapted from* Mustapha JA, Diaz-Sandoval L, Saab F. Tibioperoneal CTOs in patients with critical limb ischemia. Endovasc Today 2014;13(5):42–54.)

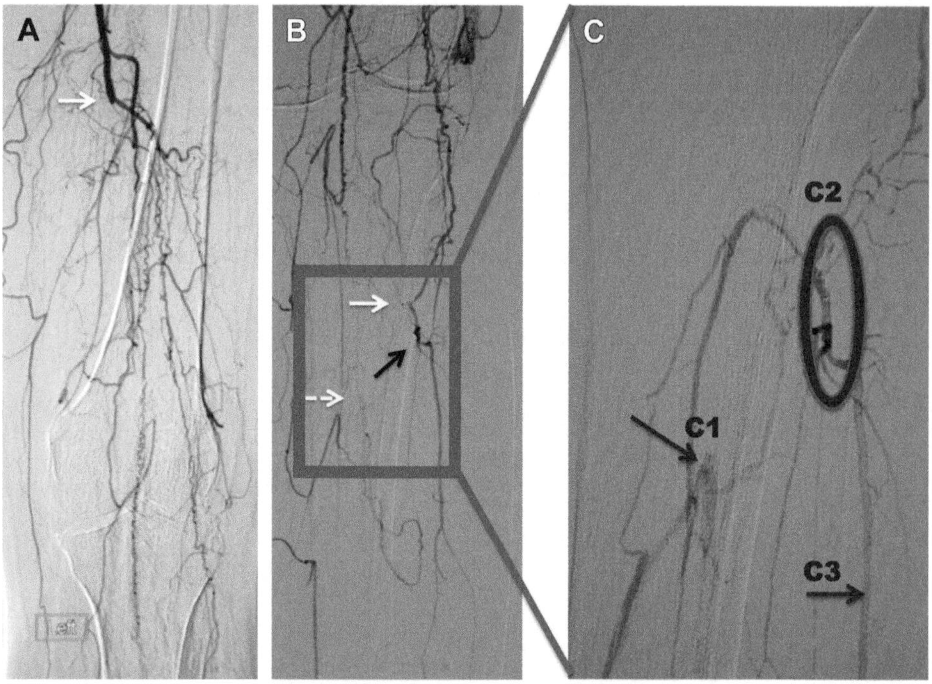

Fig. 21. (*A*) Totally occluded distal SFA (*arrow*) and popliteal in all 3 segments. (*B*) A hint of reconstitution of the AT (*white arrow*) and its anterolateral branch (*black arrow*). There seems to be a faint reconstitution of the PT/PA bifurcation (*dashed arrow*). (*C*) An amplified view of B. C1: reconstitution of the PT/PA bifurcation. C2: brief AT reconstitution and take off of the anterolateral branch (*inside oval*). C3: magnified view of the anterolateral branch of the AT. (*Adapted from* Mustapha JA, Diaz-Sandoval L, Saab F. Tibioperoneal CTOs in patients with critical limb ischemia. Endovasc Today 2014;13(5):42–54.)

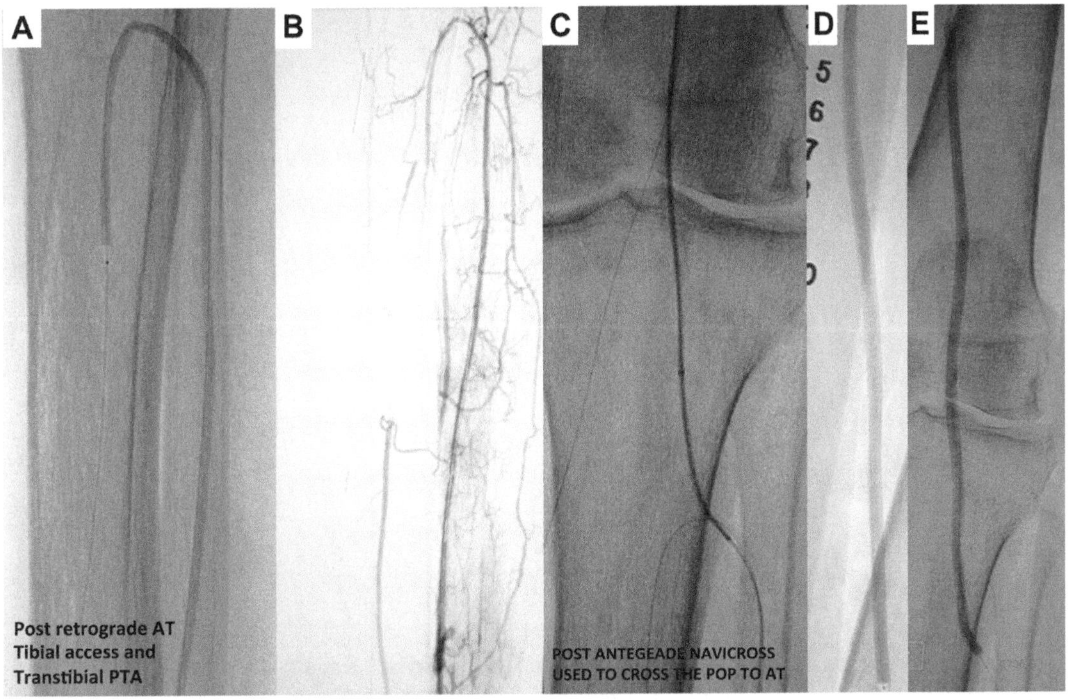

Fig. 22. (*A*) Transtibial retrograde angioplasty of the AT into the PrA. (*B*) Retrograde AT angiogram shows improved tibial flow. (*C*) Antegrade crossing of the CTO from distal SFA into the AT, followed by reversal of the retrograde access to finish the intervention in antegrade fashion. (*D, E*) Extensive angioplasty of the distal SFA, popliteal, and AT. (*Adapted from* Mustapha JA, Diaz-Sandoval L, Saab F. Tibioperoneal CTOs in patients with critical limb ischemia. Endovasc Today 2014;13(5):42–54.)

advanced under US guidance into the ostium of the AT and easily crossed with the wire (see **Fig. 22**C). The retrograde wire in the AT was introduced in the antegrade catheter using US guidance and the retrograde wire exteriorized at the groin. The NaviCross was removed and then a 0.018-inch CXI catheter was advanced in antegrade fashion into the distal AT. The retrograde wire was removed and introduced in antegrade fashion. The retrograde sheath was removed and the antegrade wire manipulated into the foot, past the point of retrograde access. Extensive antegrade balloon angioplasty was performed in the popliteal and AT using an Ultraverse balloon (Bard, Tempe, Arizona) (see **Fig. 22**D, E). Results of antegrade angioplasty were suboptimal and stenting of the distal SFA and entire popliteal (up to the AT/TPT bifurcation) was performed (**Fig. 23**A). Final angiogram revealed Thrombolysis in Myocardial Infarction grade 3 flow through the AT and PrA into the foot (see **Fig. 23**B).

Re-entry from the Tibial Subintimal Space to the True Lumen

The tibial arterial wall is thin and should be crossed primarily with a 0.014-inch wire system when possible. When crossed subintimally, re-entry is primarily accomplished with US guidance by use of an angled 0.018-inch catheter with a heavy tip wire featuring a short 90° bend at the tip, or by use of the Enteer catheter, which is a balloon-based device. It has 2 wire exit ports that can lead to the true lumen with a specialized angled wire that comes with the device.

In summary, IP intervention has already been shown to be safe and efficacious. As with any other interventional procedure, experience correlates with improved outcomes. As acknowledged by Liistro and colleagues,[43] in their study of drug-coated balloons, their impressive results may have been in part influenced by its single-center nature in a high-volume practice with a unique patient referral pattern, interventional technique, and integrated multidisciplinary approach. Ideally, operators and teams should strive to reproduce these features to make this kind of results more generalizable or real-world representative.

Further studies with longer follow-up are necessary to be able to answer some of the remaining queries about safety and efficacy, especially when referring to the potential use of these technologies into the next frontier for CLI therapies, currently represented by BTA interventions.

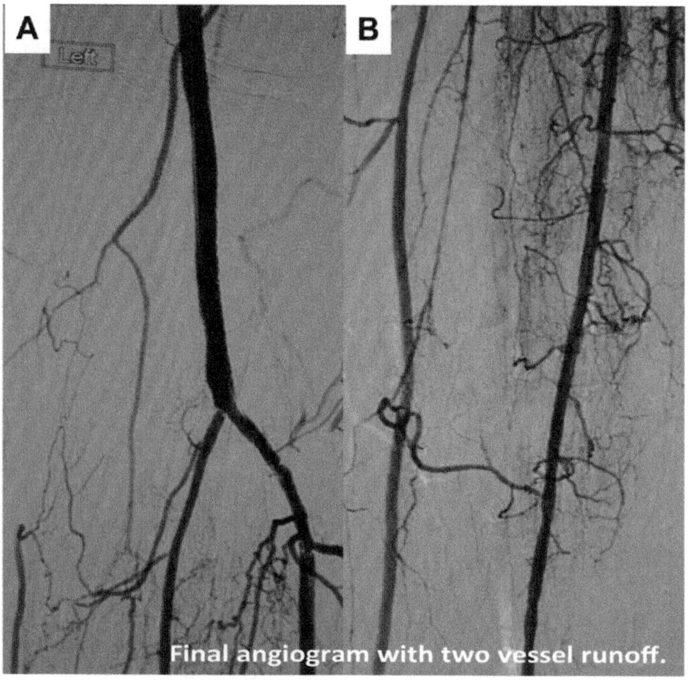

Fig. 23. (*A*) Status post stenting of the popliteal to the level of the AT/TPT bifurcation. (*B*) Two-vessel runoff to the foot via the AT and the peroneal. (*Adapted from* Mustapha JA, Diaz-Sandoval L, Saab F. Tibioperoneal CTOs in patients with critical limb ischemia. Endovasc Today 2014;13(5):42–54.)

REFERENCES

1. European Working Group on Critical Limb Ischemia. Second European consensus document on chronic critical leg ischaemia. Eur J Vasc Surg 1992; 6(Suppl A):1–32.
2. Wolfe JH, Wyatt MG. Critical and subcritical ischaemia. Eur J Vasc Endovasc Surg 1997;13: 578–82.
3. Aboyans V, Desormais I, Lacroix P, et al. The general prognosis of patients with peripheral arterial disease differs according to the disease localization. J Am Coll Cardiol 2010;55(9):898–903.
4. Varu V, Hogg M, Kibbe M. Critical limb ischemia. J Vasc Surg 2010;51:230–41.
5. Norgren L, Hiatt WR, Dormandy JA, et al, on behalf of the TASC II Working Group. Inter-Society Consensus for the Management of Peripheral Arterial Disease (TASC II). Eur J Vasc Endovasc Surg 2007; 33(Suppl 1):S1–75.
6. Pipinos I, Judge A, Selsby J, et al. The myopathy of peripheral arterial occlusive disease: part 1. Functional and histomorphological changes and evidence for mitochondrial dysfunction. Vasc Endovascular Surg 2008;41(6):481–9.
7. Pipinos I, Judge A, Selsby J, et al. The myopathy of peripheral arterial occlusive disease: part 2.Oxidative stress, neuropathy, and shift in muscle fiber type. Vasc Endovascular Surg 2008;42(2):101–12.
8. Lejay A, Georg Y, Tartaglia E, et al. Long-term outcomes of direct and indirect below-the-knee open revascularization based on the angiosome concept in diabetic patients with critical limb ischemia. Ann Vasc Surg 2014;28(4):983–9. http://dx.doi.org/10.1016/j.avsg.2013.08.026.
9. Spiliopoulos S, Katsanos K, Karnabatidis D, et al. Cryoplasty versus conventional balloon angioplasty of the femoropopliteal artery in diabetic patients: long-term results from a prospective randomized single-center controlled trial. Cardiovasc Intervent Radiol 2010;33:929–38.
10. Graziani L, Silvestro A, Bertone V, et al. Vascular involvement in diabetic subjects with ischemic foot ulcer: a new morphologic categorization of disease severity. Eur J Vasc Endovasc Surg 2007;33:453–60.
11. Gray BH, Grant AA, Kalbaugh CA, et al. The impact of isolated tibial disease on outcomes in the critical limb ischemic population. Ann Vasc Surg 2010; 24(3):349–59.
12. Sadek M, Ellozy SH, Turnbull IC, et al. Improved outcomes are associated with multilevel endovascular intervention involving the tibial vessels compared with isolated tibial intervention. J Vasc Surg 2009; 49:638–44.
13. Adam DJ, Beard JD, Cleveland T, et al. Bypass vs angioplasty in severe ischaemia of the leg (BASIL): multicentre, randomised controlled trial. Lancet 2005;366:1925–34.

14. Vasa M, Fichtlscherer S, Aicher A, et al. Number and migratory activity of circulating endothelial progenitor cells inversely correlates with risk factors for coronary artery disease. Circ Res 2001;89:e1–7.
15. Mustapha JA, Saab F, Diaz-Sandoval LJ, et al. Comparison between angiographic and arterial duplex ultrasound assessment of tibial arteries in patients with peripheral arterial disease: on behalf of the Joint Endovascular and Non-Invasive Assessment of LImb Perfusion (JENALI) Group. J Invasive Cardiol 2013;25(11):606–11.
16. Mustapha JA, Saab F, Diaz L, et al. Utility and feasibility of ultrasound-guided access in patients with critical limb ischemia. Catheter Cardiovasc Interv 2013;81(7):1204–11.
17. Van Overhagen H, Spiliopoulos S, Tsetis D. Below-the-knee interventions. Cardiovasc Intervent Radiol 2013;36:302–11.
18. Rooke TW, Hirsch AT, Misra S, et al. 2011 ACCF/AHA focused update of the guideline for the management of patients with peripheral artery disease (updating the 2005 guideline). Vasc Med 2011;16:452–76.
19. Haider CR, Riederer SJ, Borisch E, et al. High temporal and spatial resolution 3D time resolved contrast-enhanced magnetic resonance angiography of the hands and feet. J Magn Reson Imaging 2011;34:2–12.
20. Soulez G, Therasse E, Giroux MF, et al. Management of peripheral arterial disease: role of computed tomography angiography and magnetic resonance angiography. Presse Med 2011;40(9 Pt 2):e437–52.
21. Voth M, Haneder S, Huck K, et al. Peripheral magnetic resonance angiography with continuous table movement in combination with high spatial and temporal resolution time-resolved MRA with a total single dose (0.1 mmol/kg) of gadobutrol at 3.0 T. Invest Radiol 2009;44:627–33.
22. Collins R, Burch J, Cranny G, et al. Duplex ultrasonography, magnetic resonance angiography, and computed tomography angiography for diagnosis and assessment of symptomatic, lower limb peripheral arterial disease: systematic review. BMJ 2007; 334(7606):1257.
23. Manzi M, Cester G, Palena LM, et al. Vascular imaging of the foot: the first step toward endovascular recanalization. Radiographics 2011;31:1623–36.
24. Kreitner KF, Kunz RP, Herber S, et al. MR angiography of the pedal arteries with gadobenate dimeglumine, a contrast agent with increased relaxivity, and comparison with selective intra-arterial DSA. J Magn Reson Imaging 2008;27:78–85.
25. Hofmann WJ, Walter J, Ugurluoglu A, et al. Preoperative high-frequency duplex scanning of potential pedal target vessels. J Vasc Surg 2004;39: 169–75.
26. Stacul F, van der Molen AJ, Reimer P, et al. Contrast induced nephropathy: updated ESUR Contrast Media Committee guidelines. Eur Radiol 2011;21: 2527–41.
27. Iida O, Soga Y, Hirano K, et al. Long-term results of direct and indirect endovscular revascularization based on the angiosome concept in patients with critical limb ischemia presenting with isolated below-the-knee lesions. J Vasc Surg 2011;55: 363–70.
28. Attinger CE, Evans KK, Mesbahi A. Angiosomes of the foot and angiosome-dependent healing. In: Sidawy AN, editor. Diabetic foot, lower extremity disease and limb salvage. Philadelphia: Lipincott Williams & Wilkins; 2006. p. 341–50.
29. Iida O, Nanto S, Uematsu M, et al. Importance of the angiosome concept for endovascular therapy in patients with critical limb ischemia. Catheter Cardiovasc Interv 2010;75:830–6.
30. Varela C, Acin F, de Haro J, et al. The role of foot collateral vessels on ulcer healing and limb salvage after successful endovascular and surgical distal procedures according to an angiosome model. Vasc Endovascular Surg 2010;44:654–60.
31. Peregin J, Koznar B, Kovac J, et al. PTA of infrapopliteal arteries: long-term clinical follow-up and analysis of factors influencing clinical outcome. Cardiovasc Intervent Radiol 2010;33:720–5.
32. Acín F, Varela C, López deMaturana I, et al. Results of infrapopliteal endovascular procedures performed in diabetic patients with critical limb ischemia and tissue loss from the perspective of an angiosome-oriented revascularization strategy. Int J Vasc Med 2014;2014:270539, 1–13.
33. Lejay A, Georg Y, Tartaglia E, et al. Long-term outcomes of direct and indirect below-the-knee open revascularization based on the angiosome concept on diabetic patients with critical limb ischemia. Ann Vasc Surg 2013. http://dx.doi.org/10.1016/j.avsg. 2013.08.026.
34. Kabra A, Suresh KR, Vivekanand V, et al. Outcomes of angiosome and non-angiosome targeted revascularisation in critical lower limb ischemia. J Vasc Surg 2013;57:44–9.
35. Berceli SA, Chan AK, Pomposelli FB Jr, et al. Efficacy of dorsal pedal artery bypass in limb salvage for ischemic heel ulcers. J Vasc Surg 1999;30:499–508.
36. Mustapha J, Saab F, McGoff T, et al. Tibio-pedal arterial minimally invasive retrograde revascularization in patients with advanced peripheral vascular disease: the TAMI technique, original case series. Catheter Cardiovasc Interv 2013. http://dx.doi.org/ 10.1002/ccd.25227.
37. Palena LM, Brocco E, Manzi M. The clinical utility of below-the ankle using "transmetatarsal artery access" in complex cases of CLI. Catheter Cardiovasc Interv 2014;83(1):123–9.
38. Tsetis D, Belli AM. The role of infrapopliteal angioplasty. Br J Radiol 2004;77:1007–15.

39. Hovasse T, Mylotte D, Garot P, et al. Duration of balloon inflation for optimal stent deployment: five seconds is not enough. Catheter Cardiovasc Interv 2013;81(3):446–53.
40. Karnabatidis D, Spiliopoulos S, Katsanos K, et al. Below-the knee drug-eluting stents and drug-coated balloons. Expert Rev Med Devices 2012; 9:85–94.
41. Karnabatidis D, Spiliopoulos S, Diamantopoulos A, et al. Primary everolimus-eluting stenting versus balloon angioplasty with bailout bare metal stenting of long infrapopliteal lesions for treatment of critical limb ischemia. J Endovasc Ther 2011;18: 1–12.
42. Feiring AJ, Wesolowski AA. Antegrade popliteal artery approach for the treatment of critical limbs ischemia in patients with occluded superficial femoral arteries. Catheter Cardiovasc Interv 2007; 69(5):665–70.
43. Liistro F, Porto I, Angioli P, et al. Drug-eluting balloon in peripheral intervention for below the knee angioplasty evaluation (DEBATE-BTK): a randomized trial in diabetic patients with critical limb ischemia. Circulation 2013;128(6):615–21.

Chronic Venous Insufficiency

Karthik Gujja, MD, MPH, Jose Wiley, MD*, Prakash Krishnan, MD

KEYWORDS

- Chronic venous insufficiency (CVI) • Valvular incompetence • Plethysmography
- Superficial venous reflux • Radiofrequency ablation • Sclerotherapy • Phlebectomy
- Deep vein reflux

KEY POINTS

- Varicose veins are a common manifestation of chronic venous disease and affect approximately 25% of adults in the western hemisphere.
- The historical standard treatment has been surgery, with high ligation and stripping, combined with phlebectomies.
- In the past decade, alternative treatments such as endovenous ablation with laser, radiofrequency ablation, and ultrasonography-guided foam sclerotherapy have gained popularity.
- Performed as office-based procedures using tumescent local anesthesia, the new minimally invasive techniques have been shown in numerous studies to obliterate diseased veins, eliminate reflux, and improve symptoms safely and effectively.

INTRODUCTION

Chronic venous disease is a prevalent source of morbidity in western Europe and the United States. Varicose veins are a common manifestation of chronic venous insufficiency and affect approximately 25% of adults in the western hemisphere. The prevalence varies greatly by geographic area. The reported incidence of chronic venous insufficiency varies from less than 1% to 40% in women and from less than 1% to 17% in men. Estimates for varicose veins are higher; less than 1% to 73% in women and 2% to 56% in men.[1] These reported ranges reflect differences in the population distribution of risk factors, accuracy in the application of diagnostic criteria, and the quality and availability of medical diagnostic and treatment resources. Various risk factors are responsible for these incidences. These risk factors include older age, pregnancy (especially multiple), family history of venous disease, female gender, obesity, and occupations that involve long times standing resulting in significant orthostasis.[2] Venous insufficiency is most often associated with great saphenous vein (GSV) reflux, but can also be present in the small saphenous vein (SSV) or perforator veins.

The historical treatment has been surgery, with high ligation and stripping, combined with phlebectomies. Such treatment efficiently reduces symptoms, improves quality of life (QOL), and reduces the rate of reoperation compared with high ligation and phlebectomies only. However, the operation may occasionally be associated with significant postoperative morbidity, including bleeding, groin infection, thrombophlebitis, and saphenous nerve damage. Major complications are rare based on the current available data. Conventional surgery is often performed in hospital

The authors have nothing to disclose.
The Zena and Michael A. Weiner Cardiovascular Institute, The Mount Sinai School of Medicine, One Gustave L. Levy Place, Box 1030, New York, NY 10029, USA
* Corresponding author.
E-mail address: jose.wiley@mssm.edu

Intervent Cardiol Clin 3 (2014) 593–605
http://dx.doi.org/10.1016/j.iccl.2014.07.001
2211-7458/14/$ – see front matter

using general or regional anesthesia, which increases costs.

In the past decade, alternative treatments such as endovenous laser ablation (EVLA), radiofrequency ablation (RFA), and ultrasonography-guided foam sclerotherapy have gained popularity. Performed as office-based procedures using tumescent local anesthesia, the new minimally invasive techniques have been shown in numerous studies to obliterate the affected vein, eliminate reflux, and improve symptoms safely and effectively.[3]

PREDISPOSING FACTORS

Age and Gender

The prevalence of varicose veins in women is approximately twice that in men.[4] Advanced age has also been determined to be a risk factor in long-term studies.[5] Varicose veins have an estimated prevalence between 5% and 30% in the adult population, with a female to male predominance of 3 to 1, although a more recent study supports a higher male prevalence.[6] The Edinburgh Vein Study screened 1566 subjects for venous reflux and found chronic venous insufficiency (CVI) in 9.4% of men and 6.6% of women. After age adjustment, the prevalence increased with age (21.2% in men >50 years old, and 12.0% in women >50 years old).[7]

The Tampere study investigated a large cohort of 3284 men and 3590 women with varicose veins and showed a prevalence of 18% and 42%, respectively. The overall prevalence of varicose veins at ages 40, 50, and 60 years was 22%, 35%, and 41%, respectively.[8]

Pregnancy

Multiparity has been shown to be a major predisposing factor for development of varicose veins and part of its increase in prevalence has been attributed to female gender. In the Tampere study, the prevalence of varicose veins in women with 0, 1, 2, 3, and 4 or more pregnancies was 32%, 38%, 43%, 48%, and 59%, respectively.[8] The exact mechanism of pregnancy-induced venous insufficiency is not fully understood. It has been attributed to both hydrostatic and hormonal effects. Pressure of the gravid uterus on the pelvic vasculature is associated with lower extremity venous hypertension, venous distention, and valve rupture. High serum estradiol levels have been shown by Ciardullo and colleagues[9] to increase venous distensibility and varicose vein formation in menopausal women. The saphenous veins have been shown to contain estrogen and progesterone receptors that may enable the estradiol-rich hormonal state of pregnancy to exert a similar effect.[9]

Hereditary

A positive family history of varicose veins is associated with a significantly increased risk of development of varicose veins. One study conducted in Japan showed that 42% of women with varicose veins reported a positive family history compared with 14% without the disease.[10] Various genetic predispositions have been linked to development of varicose veins. Downregulation of the desmuslin gene affecting the smooth muscle cells in the saphenous vein wall, thrombomodulin mutation (−1208/−1209 TT deletion) caused by varicose vein formation via deep vein thrombosis, expression of structural genes regulating the extracellular matrix (ECM), cytoskeletal proteins, and myofibroblasts have all been shown to be associated with increased risk.

Certain mutations have been linked to a variety of syndromes, including Klippel-Trénaunay syndrome (translocation involving chromosome 8q22.3 and 14q13 [cutaneous capillary malformations, t tissues]), lymphedema distichiasis syndrome (FOXC2 mutation [extra eyelashes from meibomian glands, varicose veins, congenital heart defects, vertebral anomalies, extradural cysts, ptosis, and cleft palate]), cerebral autosomal dominant arteriopathy with subcortical infarcts and leukoencephalopathy (CADASIL; heterozygous mutation, -1279G > T), Chuvash polycythemia (autosomal recessive disorder caused by homozygous mutation of the von Hippel-Lindau gene [598 > T] on chromosome 3p25), and other genes have been associated with poor wound healing causing venous ulceration (F13A1 gene: factor XIII deficiency, HFE gene mutation, FGFR-2 [SNP 2451AG] mRNA instability, MMP-12 [SNP 82AA]; functional change predisposing to ulcer).[11]

Lifestyle

Sedentary work and prolonged standing at work are independent risk factors for development of venous insufficiency.[12] In the Tampere study, the prevalence of varicose veins in standing versus sitting workers was 36% and 27%, respectively. The Edinburg Vein Study has also shown predisposition of varicose veins in patients having prolonged standing time at their work places.

Body Habitus

Epidemiologic studies have shown that varicose veins are more common in female patients with increased body mass index (BMI) (especially >30 kg/m^2). It has been assumed that subcutaneous deposition of adipose and fibrous tissue disrupts the cutaneous venous network, impairs drainage, and promotes stasis. The Edinburgh Vein Study supported the findings that increased BMI in women is a risk factor. Callam,[2] in his epidemiologic review series, reached similar conclusions.

PATHOGENESIS OF CVI

Several theories have been proposed for the causal basis of CVI. There are 2 universally accepted theories: (1) primary valvular incompetence and (2) primary, congenital vein wall weakness.

Primary valvular incompetence is the oldest theory and was postulated by Sir William Harvey in 1628. It states that varicose veins develop as a sequela of central valvular incompetence related to paucity or atrophy of its valves. It causes venous hypertension in the vein segment below, which in turn damages adjacent peripheral valves and propagates varicose transformation in a central-to-peripheral direction. This theory conflicts with the fact that valves are strong structures capable of withstanding pressures of 200 mm Hg without leakage or degenerative changes in leaflets and that varicose veins can occur below or between competent valves.[13]

The primary vein wall weakness theory states that varicose veins develop from a defect in vein wall integrity rather than from a problem within the valves. The components of a normal vein wall include collagen matrix that provides strength, elastic fibers that provide compliance, and 3 smooth muscle layers (circular media surrounded by longitudinal intimal and adventitial layers) that control vascular tone. Histologic studies show that, compared with normal veins, varicose veins show proliferation of the collagen matrix with disruption and distortion of the muscle fiber layers. In the most diseased areas, the muscle layer is completely disrupted, leaving only elastic tissue and collagen as the sole components of the vein wall. This histologic alteration in turn causes loss of contractility, sagging of the muscular grid, and vessel dilatation in response to venous hypertension. The characteristic serpiginous appearance of varicose veins reflects segments of dilatation interspersed between segments of normal vein.[14]

Various factors influence the development of CVI:

Venous Stasis

This concept suggests that stagnant accumulation of blood in tortuous, nonfunctioning, dilated skin veins results in subsequent tissue anoxia and cell death leading to skin changes and ulceration. Arteriovenous fistulae in limbs with varicosities have also been attributed to low oxygen content and CVI skin changes.[15]

Venous Hypertension

This concept has been attributed to muscle pump dysfunction and venous ulceration. It has been hypothesized that venous hydrostatic pressure is equal in the deep and superficial venous systems both at rest and in the erect position. During calf muscle contraction, the pressure in the deep veins increases more than in the superficial veins. However, valve closure prevents the pressure from being transmitted to the superficial veins. In contrast, pump dysfunction or valvular incompetence causes venous pressure to be transmitted to the superficial veins leading to CVI symptoms and ulceration.[16–19]

Fibrin Cuff

Pericapillary fibrin cuff has been associated with restriction of oxygen diffusion across the vessel wall leading to edema and dermatosclerotic skin changes. Pericapillary fibrin cuffs may act as a barrier, a marker for endothelial cell damage, or as part of an overall mechanism of macromolecular leakage and trapping.[20]

Water Hammer Effect

This theory is the most widespread pathogenesis of CVI. It contends that reflux is mainly transmitted to the superficial veins through perforators. Studies by Raju and Fredericks have shown that this effect explains and correlates with most venous ulceration cases. At rest 20% to 25% of patients might have normal ambulatory venous pressure; nonetheless Valsalva-induced venous hypertension transmits pressure, resulting in skin changes and ulceration.[18,21]

Leukocyte Trapping

The concept of leukocyte trapping was described very early and explains most of the CVI symptoms. Because of stasis and venous pressure changes, margination of the white cells occurs resulting in capillary plugging with further tissue hypoxia and damage. These white cells also activate free radicals and cytokine (interleukin-1, tumor necrosis factor) release, resulting in tissue damage and apoptosis.[22] Unifying concepts of leukocyte trapping and venous hypertension have also been proposed.[16]

CLINICAL MANIFESTATIONS

CVI manifests at different stages. At first it may present as telangiectasia or reticular veins and advance to more complicated stages such as skin fibrosis and venous ulceration. The main clinical features of CVI are leg pain, leg edema, varicose veins, and cutaneous changes. Various pathogenic mechanisms produce different clinical manifestations (incompetent valves as varicose veins, venous obstruction as leg edema, and pump dysfunction as either symptom).

Varicose veins are dilated superficial veins that become progressively more tortuous and large. They are prone to develop bouts of superficial thrombophlebitis.

Edema begins in the perimalleolar region but ascends. Leg edema with dependent accumulation of fluid. The leg pain or discomfort is described as heaviness or aching after prolonged standing and is relieved by elevation of the leg. Edema produces pain by increasing intracompartmental and subcutaneous volume and pressure. Tenderness along varicose veins is in the result of venous distention. Obstruction of the deep venous system may lead to venous claudication, or intense leg cramping with ambulation.

Cutaneous changes include skin hyperpigmentation with hemosiderin deposition and eczematous dermatitis. Fibrosis also develops in the dermis and subcutaneous tissue (lipodermatosclerosis). There is an increased risk of cellulitis, leg ulceration, and delayed wound healing. Longstanding CVI may also lead to the development of lymphedema, representing a combined disease process.[23]

Several tools have been described to assess the severity of CVI and also monitor the effects of therapy. The CEAP (clinical, etiology, anatomic, pathophysiology) classification was the initial module developed by an international consensus conference to provide a basis for uniformity in reporting, diagnosing, and treating CVI. The CEAP classification takes into account all the diagnostic variables of CVI. In 2004, the CEAP revised consensus refined the class definitions and improved reproducibility of physician observations (**Box 1**, **Table 1**).[24–26] Because of limitations of the CEAP clinical classification in delineating categories, a venous severity score was developed to complement the CEAP classification. The venous clinical severity score consists of 10 attributes (pain, varicose veins, venous edema, skin pigmentation, inflammation, induration, number of ulcers, duration of ulcers, size of ulcers, and compressive therapy) with 4 grades (absent, mild, moderate, severe). The venous anatomic segmental score assigns a numerical value to segments of the venous system in the lower extremity that account for both reflux and obstruction (**Table 2**).[27,28] The venous disability score comes from the ability to perform normal activities of daily living with or without compressive stockings. The venous severity score has been mainly shown to be useful in evaluating the response to treatment.[29] The REVAS classification identifies patients with recurrent varices after surgery. In conjugation with the CEAP classification, it adds valuable information in evaluating patients with chronic venous disease after surgery.[30]

Box 1
Advanced CEAP classification

Superficial Veins

1. Telangiectasias/reticular veins
2. GSV above knee
3. GSV below knee
4. Lesser saphenous vein
5. Nonsaphenous veins

Deep veins

6. Inferior vena cava
7. Common iliac vein
8. Internal iliac vein
9. External iliac vein
10. Pelvic: gonadal, broad ligament veins, other
11. Common femoral vein
12. Deep femoral vein
13. Femoral vein
14. Popliteal vein
15. Crural: anterior tibial, posterior tibial, peroneal veins (all paired)
16. Muscular: gastrocnemial, soleal veins, other

Perforating veins

17. Thigh
18. Calf

This classification is the same as the basic classification with the addition that any of 18 named venous segments can be used as locators for venous disorders.

From Eklof B, Rutherford R, Bergan J, et al. Revision of the CEAP classification for chronic venous disorders: consensus statement. J Vasc Surg 2004;40:1248.

CVI: QOL AND ECONOMIC IMPACT

The impact of venous insufficiency on QOL was investigated by the Venous Insufficiency Epidemiologic and Economical Study (VEINES), an international survey. In VEINES, 65.2% of subjects with varicose veins had additional venous disease processes (edema, skin changes, ulceration),

Table 1
CEAP classification for chronic venous disorders

Clinical classification	
C0	No visible or palpable signs of venous disease
C1	Telangiectasias, reticular veins, malleolar flares
C2	Varicose veins
C3	Edema without skin changes
C4	Skin changes attribute to venous disease (eg, pigmentation, venous eczema, lipodermatosclerosis)
C4a	Pigmentation or eczema
C4b	Lipodermatosclerosis or atrophie blanche
C5	Skin changes as defined earlier with healed ulceration
C6	Skin changes as defined earlier with active ulceration
S	Symptomatic, including ache, pain, tightness, skin irritation, heaviness, and muscle cramps, and other complaints attributable to venous dysfunction
A	Asymptomatic
Causal classification	
Ec	Congenital
Ep	Primary
Es	Secondary (postthrombotic)
En	No venous cause identified
Anatomic classification	
As	Superficial veins
Ap	Perforator veins
Ad	Deep veins
An	No venous location identified
Pathophysiologic classification	
Pr	Reflux
Po	Obstruction
Pr,o	Reflux and obstruction
Pn	No venous pathophysiology identifiable

Therapy may alter the clinical category of chronic venous disease. Limbs should therefore be reclassified after any form of medical or surgical treatment.

Adapted from Eklof B, Rutherford R, Bergan J, et al. Revision of the CEAP classification for chronic venous disorders: consensus statement. J Vasc Surg 2004;40:1248.

and both physical and mental QOL scores concomitant with the severity of their venous disease.[31] In the most severe cases, those in which venous ulceration was present, the QOL rating was worse than with chronic lung disease, back pain, or arthritis.[32] The VEINES study has 2 components: a QOL assessment (VEINES-QOL), which estimates disease effect, and a symptoms questionnaire, which measures symptoms prevalence (VEINES-Sym). Other assessment programs used in clinical practice to assess the impact of CVI on QOL are the Aberdeen Varicose Vein Questionnaire (AVVQ), Charing Cross Venous Ulcer Questionnaire (CXVUQ), and Specific Quality of Life and Outcomes Response–Venous (SQOR-V) questionnaire.[33,34]

DIAGNOSIS OF CVI

Multiple modalities have shown benefit in diagnosing the cause of CVI. Physical examination is the most important one. A thorough physical examination is usually enough to diagnose CVI. It also provides guidance during therapy.

PHYSICAL EXAMINATION

Physical examination involves inspection of the skin for signs of CVI. Skin changes such as hyperpigmentation, stasis dermatitis, atrophic blanche (white scarring at the site of previous ulcerations with a paucity of capillaries), or lipodermatosclerosis are frequently seen. Varicose veins follow the path of superficial vein insufficiency.[23] Tenderness

Table 2
Revised venous clinical severity score

	Severity Score			
Attribute	**None: 0**	**Mild: 1**	**Moderate: 2**	**Severe: 3**
Pain or other discomfort (ie, aching, heaviness, fatigue, soreness, burning) Presumes venous origin	—	Occasional pain or other discomfort (not restricting regular daily activities)	Daily pain or other discomfort (interfering with but not preventing regular daily activities)	Daily pain or discomfort (limits most regular daily activities)
Varicose veins Varicose veins must be $\geq$3 mm in diameter to qualify in the standing position	—	Few: scattered (ie, isolated branch varicosities or clusters) Also includes corona phlebectatica (ankle flare)	Confined to calf or thigh	Involves calf and thigh
Venous edema Presumes venous origin	—	Limited to foot and ankle area	Extends above ankle but below knee	Extends to knee and above
Skin pigmentation Presumes venous origin Does not include focal pigmentation over varicose veins or pigmentation caused by other chronic diseases (ie, vasculitis purpura)	None or focal	Limited to perimalleolar area	Diffuse over lower third of calf	Wider distribution above lower third of calf
Inflammation More than just recent pigmentation (ie, erythema, cellulitis, venous eczema, dermatitis)	—	Limited to perimalleolar area	Diffuse over lower third of calf	Wider distribution above lower third of calf
Induration Presumes venous origin of secondary skin and subcutaneous changes (ie, chronic edema with fibrosis, hypodermitis). Includes white atrophy and lipodermatosclerosis	—	Limited to perimalleolar area	Diffuse over lower third of calf	Wider distribution above lower third of calf
Active ulcer number	0	1	2	3
Active ulcer duration (longest active)	N/A	<3 mo	>3 mo but <1 y	Not healed for >1 y
Active ulcer size (largest active)	N/A	Diameter<2 cm	Diameter 2–6 cm	Diameter>6 cm
Use of compression therapy	Not used	Intermittent use of stockings	Wears stockings most days	Full compliance: stockings

Abbreviation: N/A, not applicable.

From Vasquez MA, Rabe E, McLafferty RB, et al, American Venous Forum Ad Hoc Outcomes Working Group. Revision of the venous clinical severity score: venous outcomes consensus statement: special communication of the American Venous Forum Ad Hoc Outcomes Working Group. J Vasc Surg 2010;52(5):1387–96.

is almost always observed along the varicose veins. Skin edema is usually pitting, unless chronic edema makes the skin brawny and difficult to examine. Venous ulcerations are most common along the medial supramalleolar area at the site of a major perforator vein of high hydrostatic pressure. The classic tourniquet or Trendelenburg test may be performed at the bedside to help distinguish between deep and superficial reflux. The test is performed with the patient lying down to empty the lower extremity veins. The upright posture is then resumed after applying a tourniquet or using manual compression at various levels. In the presence of superficial disease the varicose veins remain collapsed if compression is distal to the point of reflux. With deep (or combined) venous insufficiency, the varicose veins appear despite the use of the tourniquet or manual compression. Although useful to help determine the distribution of venous insufficiency, this test does not help to determine the extent or severity of disease or to provide information about the cause.[35]

DUPLEX IMAGING

Doppler is an important tool in diagnosing CVI and monitoring therapy. The goal of Duplex imaging is to identify any obstruction or reflux in the deep veins, look for any presence of deep vein thrombosis, diagnose reflux in the superficial veins (great saphenous vein, perforator vein, and small saphenous vein), and localize branch varicose veins and perforator veins. Low-frequency transducers (2–3 MHz) are usually used to evaluate the iliac veins and inferior vena cava. High-frequency transducers (5–10 MHz) are used to evaluate lower extremity veins. Reflux thresholds for deep veins are greater than 1000 milliseconds, superficial veins greater than 500 milliseconds, and for perforators greater than 350 milliseconds.[36,37] The most common site for reflux is the confluence of the GSV and common femoral vein, contributing to 65% of all cases, in a review of 2036 patients.[38] However, duplex has a weak correlation with the severity of the disease. Physical examination and duplex scan can guide most therapy. Venous compressibility complimented with flow characteristics are key element in excluding thrombosis. The use of a cuff inflation-deflation method with rapid cuff deflation in the standing position is preferred to induce reflux.[39]

PLETHYSMOGRAPHY

Photoplethysmography (PPG) may be used to establish a diagnosis of CVI.[38] Relative changes in blood volume in the dermis of the limb can be determined by measuring the backscatter of light emitted from a diode with a photosensor. The venous refill time is the time required for the PPG tracing to return to 90% of the baseline after cessation of calf contraction. A venous refill time less than 18 to 20 seconds, depending on the patient's position during the study, indicates CVI. A venous refill time greater than 20 seconds suggests normal venous filling. The use of a tourniquet or low-pressure cuff allows superficial disease to be distinguished from deep venous disease. Refill time depends on several factors, including the volume of reflux and the vessel diameter. This technique has been used to assess emptying of the venous system during calf muscle contraction and venous outflow. PPG may provide an assessment of the overall physiologic function of the venous system, but it is most useful in determining the absence or presence of disease.[40,41]

Air plethysmography (APG) has the ability to measure each potential component of the pathophysiologic mechanisms of CVI: reflux, obstruction, and muscle pump dysfunction. Venous outflow is assessed during rapid cuff deflation on an elevated limb that has a proximal venous occlusion cuff applied. The outflow fraction at 1 second (or venous outflow at 1 second expressed as a percentage of the total venous volume) is the primary parameter used to evaluate the adequacy of outflow. A normal venous filling index is less than 2 mL/s, whereas higher levels (>4–7 mL/s) have been found to correlate with the severity of CVI. Complications of CVI, such as ulceration, have been shown to correlate with the severity of reflux assessed with the venous filling index and ejection capacity.[42,43]

COMPUTED TOMOGRAPHY AND MAGNETIC RESONANCE VENOGRAPHY

It is used in identifying more rare and complex causes of CVI. Computed tomography is an important tool in recognizing thromboembolic disease in the proximal veins, whereas magnetic resonance venography plays a major role in determining the age of thrombus. CVI syndromes such as May-Thurner syndrome, nutcracker syndrome, pelvic congestion syndrome, venous malformations, and atrioventricular malformations can be diagnosed effectively via these advanced imaging techniques.[44,45]

CVI TREATMENT

Initial Treatment: Behavioral Measures and Compression Garments

Conservative measures have been proposed to reduce symptoms caused by CVI and prevent secondary complications and progression of disease. Behavioral measures such as elevating the legs to minimize edema and reducing intra-abdominal pressure should be advocated. The use of compressive stockings is the mainstay of conservative management. The Bisgaard regimen has been proposed for the healing of venous ulcers. This regimen has 4 components: patient education, foot elevation, elastic compression garments, and evaluation subsequently with CEAP classification. Non-elastic ambulatory bellow-knee compression aggressively counters the impact of reflux from venous pump failure. Compression therapy is used for venous leg ulcers and can decrease blood vessel diameter and pressure, preventing blood from flowing backwards.[46,47] Compression is also used to decrease release of inflammatory cytokines, reduce capillary leak, prevent swelling, and delay clotting by decreasing activation of thrombin and increasing that of plasmin. Compression is applied using elastic bandages or boots specifically designed for the purpose. It is not clear whether non-elastic systems are better than multilayer elastic ones. Patients should wear as much compression as it is comfortable. The type of dressing applied beneath the compression does not seem to matter, and hydrocolloid has not been shown to be superior to simple low-adherent dressings. The use of graded elastic compressive stockings (with 20–50 mm Hg of tension) is well established in the treatment of CVI. Treatment with 30 to 40 mm Hg compression stockings results in significant improvement in pain, swelling, skin pigmentation, activity, and overall well-being as long as a compliance of 70% to 80% is achieved.[48] In patients with venous ulcers, graded compression stockings and other compressive bandage modalities are effective in both healing and preventing recurrences of ulcers. With a structured regimen of compression therapy, 93% of patients with venous ulcers can achieve complete healing at a mean of 5.3 months. Compression stockings have been shown to reduce residual volume fraction, an indicator of improvement in the calf muscle pump function, and to reduce reflux in vein segments.[49]

Failure of Conservative Therapy

Symptomatic patients who fail conservative therapy should be followed closely. These patients should have venous duplex studies and/or air plethysmography if conservative therapy fails or if there is any progression of symptoms in CEAP class. Further treatment is based on the results of noninvasive studies and specific treatment is based on severity of disease, with CEAP clinical classes 4 to 6 often requiring invasive treatment. Referral to a vascular specialist should be made for patients with CEAP classes 4 to 6 (and probably for CEAP class 3 with extensive edema). These patients with uncorrected advanced CVI are at risk for ulceration, recurrent ulceration, and nonhealing venous ulcers with progression to infection and lymphedema.

NONINVASIVE STUDY: VENOUS REFLUX DISEASE

Superficial Venous Reflux

Various therapies have been used for superficial venous reflux.

Cool-touch laser

The first procedure to replace ligation and stripping of the GSV was radiofrequency-mediated thermal ablation. Long-term experience with cool-touch endovenous laser ablation showed that tissue water within the vein wall has a specific target chromophore of 1320-nm laser and the presence or absence of red blood cells within the vessels is unimportant. Water is the main component in the walls of a vein. They are composed mainly of water and collagen. The chromophore for the 1.32-μm or 1320-nm wavelength laser is water. This wavelength penetrates as deep as 500 μm in tissue. This provides a safety margin by reducing the risks of penetration of laser energy beyond the vein wall. For even greater control of energy distribution, the 1320-nm CTEV is coupled with an automatic pullback device that can retract the fiber at a rate of 0.5, 1, or 2 mm/s.[50] Endovenous laser treatments at 810, 940, and 980 nm are designed to produce endothelial and vein wall shrinkage by nonspecific heating of the vessel.[51] This nonspecific heating is accomplished by creating a superheated coagulum at the fiber tip or by the heating of hemoglobin within red blood cells to create steam bubbles at extremely high temperatures. Without the presence of blood in the vein, such as an experimental situation in which the vein is filled with saline, laser-induced vessel wall injury is confined to the site of direct laser impact. By contrast, blood-filled veins show extensive thermal damage even in remote areas from the laser fiber, including the vein wall opposite to the laser impact. In the absence of blood, the situation is even worse; the areas of vein wall injury or burning result in intense postoperative pain and early recanalization of the treated vein. More importantly, superheating of hemoglobin leads to high temperatures (often higher than 1200°C), which results in vein perforations, hematoma, and postoperative pain.[52]

RFA therapy

Few studies have shown the superiority of RFA compared with EVLA in terms of pain, bruising, and postprocedure recovery, with GSV occlusion rates being comparable. The LARA study was a randomized control trial conducted to determine whether RFA of the GSV is associated with less pain and bruising than EVLA in 87 leg interventions.[53] In the bilateral group, RFA resulted in significantly less pain than EVLA on days 2 to 11 after surgery. RFA also resulted in significantly less bruising than EVLA on days 3 to 9. There were no significant differences in mean postoperative pain, bruising, and activity scores in the unilateral group. Both RFA and EVLA resulted in occlusion rates of 95% at 10 days after surgery.[54] The RECOVERY study randomized 87 veins in 69 patients to Closure FAST or 980-nm EVLA treatment of the GSV. It was a multicenter, prospective, randomized, single-blinded trial, performed at 5 American sites and 1 European site. All scores referable to pain, ecchymosis, and tenderness were statistically lower in the Closure FAST group at 48 hours, 1 week, and 2 weeks. Minor complications were more prevalent in the EVLA group ($P = .0210$); there were no major complications. Venous clinical severity scores and QOL measures were statistically lower in the Closure FAST group at 48 hours, 1 week, and 2 weeks. Radiofrequency thermal ablation was significantly superior to EVLA as measured by a comprehensive array of postprocedural recovery and QOL parameters.[55] The EVOLVeS trial studied the clinical outcomes of rates of recurrent varicosities, neovascularization, ultrasonography changes of the GSV, and QOL changes in patients undergoing RFA, ligation, or vein stripping. 2-year clinical results of radiofrequency obliteration are at least equal to those after high ligation and stripping of the GSV.[56]

Venous sclerotherapy

This treatment modality is used for obliterating telangiectasias, varicose veins, and venous segments with reflux. Sclerotherapy may be used as a primary treatment or in conjunction with surgical procedures in the correction of CVI. Sclerotherapy is indicated for a variety of conditions including spider veins (<1 mm), venous lakes, varicose veins of 1 to 4 mm in diameter, bleeding varicosities, and small cavernous hemangiomas (vascular malformation). The terminal interruption of reflux source technique involves blocking off the veins that drain the ulcer bed using Sotradecol or Polidocanol foam, administered under ultrasonography guidance.[57]

Patients with CVI need to be evaluated for surgical treatment if they have a nonhealing ulcer refractory to conservative and minimally invasive therapy resulting in delayed healing, recurrent varicose veins, CVI with disabling symptoms, persistent discomfort refractory to other therapy, noncompliant patients with conservative therapy, and to complement therapy with conservative measures.

Ligation and venous phlebectomy

Surgical ligation of the GSV has been shown to improve symptoms in patient with CEAP classes from 2 to 6. GSV removal with high ligation of the saphenofemoral junction has long been considered the standard treatment for patients with significant venous reflux, nonhealing ulcers, and symptomatic patients with concomitant deep venous reflux.[58] Transilluminated power phlebectomy (or TriVex) is a new surgical technique that uses tumescent dissection, transillumination, and powered phlebectomy. A prospective randomized controlled trial of 141 patients comparing conventional versus powered phlebectomy has shown a trend toward reduced operating time in extensive varicosities, and significantly fewer incisions. There was no difference in nerve injury, bruising, and cosmetic score during follow-up.[59] The ESCHAR study evaluated around 500 patients with venous ulcer and reflux of superficial and deep venous systems and randomized them to either conventional saphenous vein surgery with compression or to compression alone. The study showed a significant reduction in ulcer recurrence at 12 months in favor of surgery with compression compared with compression alone (12% vs 28%).[60] A follow-up study to observe the improvement in perforating vein incompetence included 261 patients from the ESCHAR trial. Surgical correction of superficial reflux was shown to abolish incompetence in some calf perforators but also helped wound healing and reflux symptoms by preventing development of new perforator incompetence.[61]

DEEP VENOUS REFLUX

Valve Reconstruction Surgery/Valvuloplasty

CVI has been shown to be partially attributable to venous valve injury and incompetence. Venous valve reconstruction of the deep vein valves has been performed in selected patients with advanced CVI who have recurrent ulceration with severe and disabling symptoms.[62] Open valve surgery was initially performed to repair the femoral vein valve but subsequently transcommissural valvuloplasty was developed for venous repair. Venous valvuloplasty has been shown to provide 59% competency and 63% ulcer-free recurrence at 30 months. Complications from valvuloplasty include bleeding (because patients need to remain anticoagulated), DVT, pulmonary embolism, ulcer recurrence, and wound infections.[63] This procedure is reserved for selected patients refractory to other therapies. Valve replacements and transposition procedures have been attempted successfully when native valves have postthrombotic valve destruction (not amenable to valvuloplasty). Valve transposition has been performed with the axillary vein valve, profunda femoris valve, or cryopreserved valve allografts. Cryopreserved vein valve allografts have also been shown to have early thrombosis, poor patency and competency, as well as high patient morbidity, precluding their use as a primary intervention.[64]

PERFORATOR REFLUX

Subfascial Endoscopic Perforator Surgery

Perforator vein incompetence has been proposed as a cause for CVI. Some surgical options have been proposed for the treatment of incompetent perforators, including subfascial endoscopic perforator surgery (SEPS). This procedure involves ligation of the incompetent perforator veins by gaining access from a remote site on the leg that is away from the area with lipodermatosclerosis or ulcers. The North American Study Group performed a study with 146 patients showing cumulative ulcer healing at 1 year of 88% (median time to healing was 54 days). Concomitant ablation of superficial reflux and lack of deep venous obstruction predicted ulcer healing ($P<.05$). Clinical score improved from 8.93 to 3.98 at the last follow-up ($P<.0001$). Cumulative ulcer recurrence at 1 year was 16% and at 2 years was 28% (standard error, <10%). Postthrombotic limbs had a higher 2-year cumulative recurrence rate (46%) than did those limbs with primary valvular incompetence (20%; $P<.05$).[65] The interruption of perforators with ablation of superficial reflux is effective in decreasing the symptoms of CVI and rapidly healing ulcers. SEPS in conjunction with vein ablation showed better ulcer healing and improvement in clinical severity score.[66]

NONINVASIVE STUDY: CHRONIC VENOUS FLOW OBSTRUCTION

Endovascular therapy in the treatment of CVI has become increasingly important to restore outflow of the venous system and provide relief of obstruction. Approximately 10% to 30% of patients with severe CVI can be diagnosed with a significant abnormality in venous outflow involving iliac vein segments that contributes to persistent symptoms. Before endovascular therapy, iliac vein stenosis and obstruction causing CVI was treated with surgical procedures such as cross-femoral venous bypass or iliac vein reconstructions with prosthetic materials. Because of the success of venous stenting, surgical venous bypass is infrequently performed. In a large single-center series of 429 patients with CVI and outflow obstruction, iliac vein stenting resulted in significant clinical improvement: 50% of patients were completely relieved of pain and 33% experienced complete resolution of edema. Furthermore, 55% of patients with venous ulcers experienced complete healing of their ulcers. Patency of iliac vein stents is good, with a primary patency of 75% at 3 years. Close follow-up is mandatory to ensure that stent patency is maintained. Also mandatory is to intervene early in patients with recurrent symptoms that may indicate in-stent restenosis, which occurs in approximately23% of patients.[67,68]

NONINVASIVE STUDY: MUSCLE PUMP DYSFUNCTION

Abnormalities in the calf and foot muscle pumps play a significant role in the pathophysiology of CVI. Graded exercise programs have been used in an effort to rehabilitate the muscle pump and improve CVI symptoms. In a small controlled study, 31 patients with CEAP class 4 to 6 CVI were randomized to structured calf muscle exercise or routine daily activities. Venous hemodynamics were assessed with duplex ultrasonography, air plethysmography, and muscle strength assessed with a dynamometer. After 6 months, patients receiving a calf muscle exercise regimen had normalized their calf muscle pump function parameters but experienced no change in the amount of reflux or severity scores. Padberg and colleagues[69] concluded that structured exercise to reestablish calf muscle pump function in CVI may prove beneficial as a supplemental therapy to medical and surgical treatment in advanced disease.

REFERENCES

1. Beebe-Dimmer JL, Pfeifer JR, Engle JS, et al. The epidemiology of chronic venous insufficiency and varicose veins. Ann Epidemiol 2005;15(3):175–84.
2. Callam MJ. Epidemiology of varicose veins. Br J Surg 1994;81:167–73.
3. Dwerryhouse S, Davies B, Harradine K, et al. Stripping the long saphenous vein reduces the rate of reoperation for recurrent varicose veins: five-year results of a randomized trial. J Vasc Surg 1999; 29:589–92.

4. Brand FN, Dannnenberg AL, Abbott RD, et al. The epidemiology of varicose veins: the Framingham study. Am J Prev Med 1988;4:96–101.
5. Sisto T, Reunanen A, Laurikka J, et al. Prevalence and risk factors of varicose veins in the lower extremities: Mini-Finland Health Survey. Eur J Surg 1995;161:405–14.
6. Evans CJ, Fowkes FG, Ruckley CV, et al. Prevalence of varicose veins and chronic venous insufficiency in men and women in the general population: Edinburgh Vein Study. J Epidemiol Community Health 1999;53:149–53.
7. Ruckley CV, Evans CJ, Allan PL, et al. Chronic venous insufficiency: clinical and duplex correlations. The Edinburgh Vein Study of venous disorders in the general population. J Vasc Surg 2002; 36(3):520–5.
8. Laurikka JO, Sisto T, Tarkka MR, et al. Risk indicators for varicose veins in forty- to sixty-year-olds in the Tampere varicose vein study. World J Surg 2002;26:648–51.
9. Ciardullo AV, Panico S, Bellati C, et al. High endogenous estradiol is associated with increased venous distensibility and clinical evidence of varicose veins in menopausal women. J Vasc Surg 2000;32:544–9.
10. Hirai M, Naiki K, Nakayama R. Prevalence and risk factors of varicose veins in Japanese women. Angiology 1990;41:228–32.
11. Anwa MA, Georgiadis KA, Shalhoub J, et al. A review of familial, genetic, and congenital aspects of primary varicose vein disease. Circ Cardiovasc Genet 2012;5:460–6. http://dx.doi.org/10.1161/CIRCGENETICS.112.963439.
12. Hobson J. Venous insufficiency at work. Angiology 1997;48:577–82.
13. Rose SS, Ahmed A. Some thoughts on the aetiology of varicose veins. J Cardiovasc Surg (Torino) 1986;27:534–43.
14. Lim CS, Davies AH. Pathogenesis of primary varicose veins. Br J Surg 2009;96:1231–42. http://dx.doi.org/10.1002/bjs.6798.
15. Gourdin FW, Smith JG Jr. Etiology of venous ulceration. South Med J 1993;86(10):1142–6.
16. Mustoe T. Understanding chronic wounds: a unifying hypothesis on their pathogenesis and implications for therapy. Am J Surg 2004;187(5A): 65S–70S.
17. Recek C. Calf pump activity influencing venous hemodynamics in the lower extremity. Int J Angiol 2013;22(1):23–30.
18. Recek C. Impact of the calf perforators on the venous hemodynamics in primary varicose veins. J Cardiovasc Surg (Torino) 2006;47(6):629–35.
19. Stanley AC, Lounsbury KM, Corrow K, et al. Pressure elevation slows the fibroblast response to wound healing. J Vasc Surg 2005;42(3):546–51.
20. Van de Scheur M, Falanga V. Pericapillary fibrin cuffs in venous disease. A reappraisal. Dermatol Surg 1997;23(10):955–9.
21. Raju S, Fredericks R. Evaluation of methods for detecting venous reflux. Perspectives in venous insufficiency. Arch Surg 1990;125(11):1463–7.
22. Hahn TL, Unthank JL, Lalka SG. Increased hind limb leukocyte concentration in a chronic rodent model of venous hypertension. J Surg Res 1999; 81(1):38–41.
23. Eberhardt RT, Raffetto JD. Chronic venous insufficiency. Circulation 2005;111:2398–409. http://dx.doi.org/10.1161/01.CIR.0000164199.72440.08.
24. Porter JM, Moneta GL. Reporting standards in venous disease: an update. International Consensus Committee on Chronic Venous Disease. J Vasc Surg 1995;21:635–45.
25. Eklof B, Rutherford R, Bergan J, et al. Revision of the CEAP classification for chronic venous disorders: consensus statement. J Vasc Surg 2004;40: 1248.
26. Carpentier PH, Cornu-Thenard A, Uhl JF, et al, Societe Francaise de Medecine Vasculaire, European Working Group on the Clinical Characterization of Venous Disorders. Appraisal of the information content of the C classes of CEAP clinical classification of chronic venous disorders: a multicenter evaluation of 872 patients. J Vasc Surg 2003;37:827–33.
27. Rutherford RB, Padberg FT, Comerota AJ, et al. Venous severity scoring: an adjunct to venous outcome assessment. J Vasc Surg 2000;31:1307–12.
28. Vasquez MA, Rabe E, McLafferty RB, et al, American Venous Forum Ad Hoc Outcomes Working Group. Revision of the venous clinical severity score: venous outcomes consensus statement: special communication of the American Venous Forum Ad Hoc Outcomes Working Group. J Vasc Surg 2010;52(5):1387–96.
29. Kakkos SK, Rivera MA, Matsagas MI, et al. Validation of the new venous severity scoring system in varicose vein surgery. J Vasc Surg 2003;38:224–8.
30. Perrin MR, Labropoulos N, Leon LR Jr. Presentation of the patient with recurrent varices after surgery (REVAS). J Vasc Surg 2006;43(2):327–34.
31. Abenhaim L, Kurz X. The VEINES study (VEnous INsufficiency Epidemiologic and economic Study): an international cohort study on chronic venous disorders of the leg. Angiology 1997;48:59–66.
32. Kurz X, Lamping DL, Kahn SR, et al. Do varicose veins affect quality of life? Results of an international population-based study. J Vasc Surg 2001; 34:641–8.
33. Lamping DL, Schroter S, Kurz X, et al. Evaluation of outcomes in chronic venous disorders of the leg: development of a scientifically rigorous, patient-reported measure of symptoms and quality of life. J Vasc Surg 2003;37(2):410–9.

34. Kahn SR, Lamping DL, Ducruet T, et al. VEINES-QOL/Sym questionnaire was a reliable and valid disease-specific quality of life measure for deep venous thrombosis. J Clin Epidemiol 2006;59(10):1049–56.
35. Bradbury A. Clinical assessment of patients with venous disease. In: Gloviczki P, Yao JS, editors. Handbook of venous disorders. 2nd edition. New York: Arnold; 2001. p. 71–83.
36. Van Bemmelen PS, Bedford G, Beach K, et al. Quantitative segmental evaluation of venous valvular reflux with duplex ultrasound scanning. J Vasc Surg 1989;10(4):425–31.
37. Malgor RD, Labropoulos N. Diagnosis of venous disease with duplex ultrasound. Phlebology 2013;28(Suppl 1):158–61.
38. García-Gimeno M, Rodríguez-Camarero S, Tagarro-Villalba S, et al. Duplex mapping of 2036 primary varicose veins. J Vasc Surg 2009;49(3):681–9.
39. Markel A, Meissner MH, Manzo RA, et al. A comparison of the cuff deflation method with Valsalva's maneuver and limb compression in detecting venous valvular reflux. Arch Surg 1994;129:701–5.
40. Nicolaides AN. Investigation of chronic venous insufficiency: a consensus statement. Circulation 2000;102:e126–63.
41. Abramowitz HB, Queral LA, Finn WR, et al. The use of photoplethsmography in the assessment of venous insufficiency: a comparison to venous pressure measurements. Surgery 1979;86:434–41.
42. Owens LV, Farber MA, Young ML. The value of air plethysmography in predicting clinical outcome after surgical treatment of chronic venous insufficiency. J Vasc Surg 2000;32:961–8.
43. Gillespie DL, Cordts PR, Hartono C, et al. The role of air plethysmography in monitoring results of venous surgery. J Vasc Surg 1992;16:674–8.
44. Meissner MH, Moneta G, Burnand K, et al. The hemodynamics and diagnosis of venous disease. J Vasc Surg 2007;46(Suppl S):4S–24S.
45. Davies MG, Lumsde AB, editors. Chronic venous insufficiency, vol. 1. 2011.
46. Van Gent WB, Wilschut ED, Wittens C. Management of venous ulcer disease. BMJ 2010;341:1092–6.
47. Motykie GD, Caprini JA, Arcelus JI, et al. Evaluation of therapeutic compression stockings in the treatment of chronic venous insufficiency. Dermatol Surg 1999;25:116–20.
48. Mayberry JC, Moneta GL, Taylor LM, et al. Fifteen-year results of ambulatory compression therapy for chronic venous ulcers. Surgery 1991;109:575–81.
49. Begbuna V, Delis KT, Nicolaides AN, et al. Effect of elastic compression stockings on venous hemodynamics during walking. J Vasc Surg 2003;37:420–5.
50. Goldman MP, Mauricio M, Rao J. Intravascular 1320-nm laser closure of the great saphenous vein: a 6- to 12-month follow-up study. Dermatol Surg 2004;30(11):1380–5.
51. Weiss RA. Comparison of endovenous radiofrequency versus 810 nm diode laser occlusion of large veins in an animal model. Dermatol Surg 2002;28(1):56–61.
52. Proebstle TM, Sandhofer M, Kargl A, et al. Thermal damage of the inner vein wall during endovenous laser treatment: key role of energy absorption by intravascular blood. Dermatol Surg 2002;28(7):596–600.
53. Goode SD, Chowdhury A, Crockett M, et al. Laser and radiofrequency ablation study (LARA study): a randomized study comparing radiofrequency ablation and endovenous laser ablation (810 nm). Eur J Vasc Endovasc Surg 2010;40(2):246–53.
54. Nordon IM, Hinchliffe RJ, Brar R, et al. A prospective double blind randomized controlled trial of radiofrequency versus laser treatment of the great saphenous vein in patients with varicose veins. Ann Surg 2011;254(6):876–81.
55. Lurie F, Creton D, Eklof B, et al. Prospective randomised study of endovenous radiofrequency obliteration (closure) versus ligation and vein stripping (EVOLVeS): two-year follow-up. Eur J Vasc Endovasc Surg 2005;29:67–73.
56. Almeida JI, Kaufman J, Göckeritz O, et al. Radiofrequency endovenous closure FAST versus laser ablation for the treatment of great saphenous reflux: a multicenter, single-blinded, randomized study (RECOVERY study). J Vasc Interv Radiol 2009;20(6):752–9.
57. Bush R. New technique to heal venous ulcers: terminal interruption of the reflux source (TIRS). Perspect Vasc Surg Endovasc Ther 2010;22(3):194–9.
58. Sarin S, Scurr JH, Coleridge Smith PD. Stripping of the long saphenous vein in the treatment of primary varicose veins. Br J Surg 1994;81:1455–8.
59. Aremu MA, Mahendran B, Butcher W, et al. Prospective randomized controlled trial: conventional versus powered phlebectomy. J Vasc Surg 2004;39(1):88–94.
60. Barwell JR, Davies CE, Deacon J, et al. Comparison of surgery and compression with compression alone in chronic venous ulceration (ESCHAR study): randomised controlled trial. Lancet 2004;363(9424):1854–9.
61. Gohel MS, Barwell JR, Wakely C, et al. The influence of superficial venous surgery and compression on incompetent calf perforators in chronic venous leg ulceration. Eur J Vasc Endovasc Surg 2005;29(1):78–82.
62. Kistner RL. Surgical repair of the incompetent femoral vein valve. Arch Surg 1975;110:1336–42.

63. Raju S, Berry MA, Neglen P. Transcommissural valvuloplasty: technique and results. J Vasc Surg 2000;32:969–76.
64. Neglen P, Raju S. Venous reflux repair with cryopreserved vein valves. J Vasc Surg 2003;38:1139–40.
65. Gloviczki P, Bergan JJ, Rhodes JM, et al. Mid-term results of endoscopic perforator vein interruption for chronic venous insufficiency: lessons learned from the North American subfascial endoscopic perforator surgery registry. The North American Study Group. J Vasc Surg 1999;29:489–502.
66. Bianchi C, Ballard JL, Abou-Zamzam AM, et al. Subfascial endoscopic perforator vein surgery combined with saphenous vein ablation: results and critical analysis. J Vasc Surg 2003; 38:67–71.
67. Danza R, Navarro T, Baldizan J. Reconstructive surgery in chronic venous obstruction of the lower limbs. J Cardiovasc Surg 1991;32:98–103.
68. Neglen P, Raju S. Intravascular ultrasound scan evaluation of the obstructed vein. J Vasc Surg 2002;35:694–700.
69. Padberg FT, Johnston MV, Sisto SA. Structured exercise improves calf muscle pump function in chronic venous insufficiency: a randomized trial. J Vasc Surg 2004;39:79–87.

Endovascular Treatment of Deep Vein Thrombosis

Julian J. Javier, MD

KEYWORDS

- Venous thromboembolism • Endovascular treatment of deep vein thrombosis
- Deep vein thrombosis • Catheter-directed thrombectomy

KEY POINTS

- Venous thromboembolism (VTE) is prevalent and undertreated, and it causes significant morbidity, mortality, and expense to the health care system.
- Recent guidelines from the ACCP and the American College of Cardiology/American Heart Association offer differing therapeutic options, creating clinical confusion. The ACCP has backpedaled and recommends mainly medical treatments, whereas the American Heart Association advocates more aggressive endovascular and surgical treatments.
- Despite the arrival of important new anticoagulation agents, medical treatment of VTE is associated with poor outcomes, particularly high rates of recurrence.
- Endovascular approaches include catheter-directed thrombolysis (CDT) and percutaneous mechanical thrombectomy or pharmacomechanical thrombolysis. Many innovative new devices are on the market to facilitate the endovascular treatment of VTE.
- Risks and benefits are associated with PMT and CDT, and treatment choices must be individualized for each patient.

INTRODUCTION

Venous thromboembolism (VTE), including deep vein thrombosis (DVT) and pulmonary embolism (PE), is prevalent, largely undertreated,[1] and responsible for significant morbidity and mortality.[2] An estimated 600,000 Americans are diagnosed each year with VTE.[3] About 60,000 to 100,000 Americans die of VTE each year, 10% to 30% within 1 month of diagnosis.[3] The first symptom in about 25% of people with PE is sudden death.[3] About half of patients experience long-term complications known as postthrombotic syndrome (PTS) and about one-third of patients with VTE experience recurrence within 10 years (**Fig. 1**).[3] The exact proportion of DVT versus PE is not known exactly, because PE is often clinically silent. Clinical studies of VTE without autopsy data often report DVT to be more prevalent than PE, whereas studies with autopsy data report a higher proportion of PE than DVT.[4] The prevalence of VTE may be as high as 80% among major trauma patients and patients in critical care.[5]

Known risk factors for VTE exist with synergistic interaction, such that the more risk factors, the greater likelihood an individual will develop VTE.[6] In broad strokes, these risk factors for DVT include overweight and obesity, cancer and its treatments, pregnancy and childbirth, hormone therapy for women (including contraceptives), smoking, advanced age, and ethnicity with whites and African-Americans more likely to develop DVT than Hispanics and other groups.[7] Other important risk factors are May-Thurner syndrome (compression of outflow tract) or iliac vein obstruction. Patients with specific multiple genetic mutations may be at elevated risk for DVT and/or PE.[8]

Despite innovative endovascular treatments and advanced pharmacologic therapy, including

The author has nothing to disclose.
Naples Vein Center, 1168 Goodlette Frank Road, Naples, FL 34102, USA
E-mail address: julianjjaviermd@aol.com

Intervent Cardiol Clin 3 (2014) 607–617
http://dx.doi.org/10.1016/j.iccl.2014.07.003

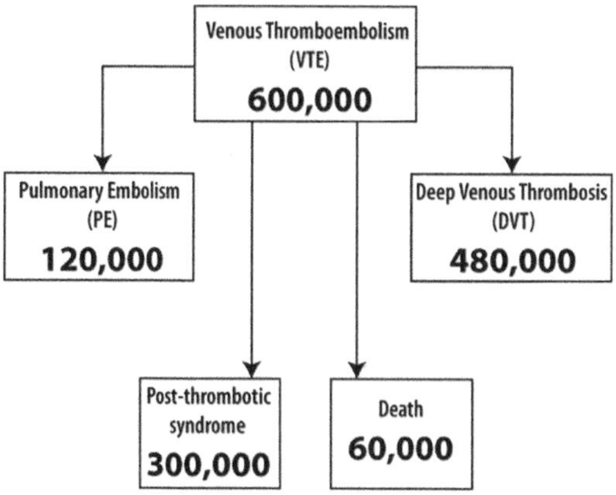

Fig. 1. Venous thromboembolism is associated with significant morbidity and mortality. (*Data from* Refs.[4,9,47–50])

anticoagulation, up to 75% of those treated with blood thinners develop PTS.[9] Anticoagulation therapy can be effective in reducing VTE recurrence, but the risk of associated bleeding complications makes it inappropriate for long-term use in some patients.[10] Novel therapeutic oral and parenteral agents have been added to the armamentarium of low-molecular-weight heparin (LMWH) for prevention and treatment of DVT.[11]

Despite promising new therapeutic approaches and technologies, VTE remains a substantial public health burden. The economic burden of VTE on the US health care system has been estimated to be more than $1.5 billion annually.[12] Although early treatment models exist and may be initially successful, they are associated with serious, long-term complications and decreased quality of life.[13] There is an urgent need for more and better treatment options for VTE.

ANTICOAGULATION THERAPY

Coagulation is an incompletely elucidated process that is currently thought to be mostly based at the cell surface, involving three stages: (1) initiation (when tissue-factor–expressing cells and microparticles are exposed to plasma), (2) amplification (thrombin incudes platelet activation and aggregation), and (3) propagation (forming Xase and prothombingase complexes and producing thrombin and cleaving fibrinogen to fibrin).[11]

Anticoagulants are available as oral and parenteral agents and can be grouped roughly as thrombin inhibitors, Factor Xa inhibitors, or indirect agents (eg, LMWH). New so-called direct oral anticoagulants have been found to be noninferior to LMWH plus vitamin K.[14] It remains unclear why many patients with DVT treated with anticoagulation therapy develop PTS. In a multicenter prospective study of 387 outpatients with DVT, 5.1% of patients with iliofemoral DVT treated with only anticoagulants alone experienced recurrence of DVT within 3 months.[15]

There are other problems associated with anticoagulation therapy. Warfarin and vitamin K antagonists (VKAs) have narrow therapeutic windows, necessitating close clinical monitoring for optimal results.[16] In a study of patients with atrial fibrillation, those who spent at least 70% of the time within the therapeutic range had a 79% reduced risk of stroke compared with patients who spent 30% or less time in the therapeutic range.[17]

VITAMIN K ANTAGONIST THERAPY

VKA therapy was evaluated in a meta-analysis (eight studies, a total of 2994 patients) and it was found that prolonged VKA therapy was associated with consistent reductions in the rates of VTE recurrence.[18] However, prolonged VKA therapy was also associated with an increased risk of bleeding complications.[18] This and other drawbacks, such as slow onset and offset of action, potential for drug-drug and drug-food interactions, a narrow therapeutic window, and large interpatient dose-response variability, have limited the use of VKAs in clinical practice.

COMPARISONS OF ANTICOAGULATION AGENTS

General recommendations about anticoagulation therapy appear in **Table 1**. Newer anticoagulation agents include rivaroxaban, apixaban, and edoxaban (Factor Xa inhibitors), and dabigatran (thrombin inhibitor). Dabigatran had a reduced rate of major bleeding compared with warfarin (1.6% vs 1.9%, respectively) but a higher rate of recurrent VTE (2.4% vs 2.1%, respectively).[19] In another study, recurrent VTE was 0.4% with dabigatran versus 5.6% with the comparator with low rates of major bleeding (0.3% for dabigatran vs 0 for the comparator).[20] Rivaroxaban had a 2.1% rate of recurrent VTE and a 0.8% rate of major bleeding compared with 3.0% VTE rate and 1.2% major bleeding rate of conventional therapy.[21]

In summary, novel oral anticoagulation agents are important additions to the therapeutic armamentarium and offer similar efficacy to warfarin but with greater safety. It remains unclear as to which patients with VTE are the ideal candidates for new anticoagulant therapy; clearly, patients who have poor international normalized ratio control with warfarin are suitable candidates for these new agents. It remains a matter of clinical

Table 1
Synopsis of anticoagulation strategies

Drug Class	Mechanism of Action	Interactions with Food, Drugs, Alcohol	Monitoring	Considerations
VKA	Acts on clotting factors that depend on vitamin K	Yes	Yes	INR 2–3
Direct thrombin inhibitors	Inhibits thrombin	Few	No	No reversal agents
Oral Factor XA inhibitors	Inhibits Factor XA	Few	No	No reversal agent

Abbreviation: INR, international normalized ratio.

judgment as to which other patients should take new anticoagulants. Those who have severe PE, extensive DVT, or hepatic or renal insufficiency likely should avoid these newer agents. An important consideration that often is not discussed is that there are no specific antidotes for some of these agents.

STANDARD OF CARE

Before 2008, the standard of care for DVT included anticoagulation therapy (heparin, LMWH, or Coumadin) and compression stockings. Clinical outcomes have been suboptimal with such treatments. Cumulative rates of recurrence increase with time and approach 30% at 8 years.[22] VTE recurrence rate after cessation of anticoagulation therapy depends on the cause of the original VTE. For example, in patients with continuing risk factors, such as cancer, or idiopathic VTE, the annual rate of recurrences is 10% or greater.[23] Mortality is also high. The RIETE registry found mortality was 17% and 6% in patients with VTE treated medically and surgically, respectively (**Table 2**).[24] The RIETE registry was also used to study patients with chronic obstructive pulmonary disease (COPD) with VTE (either PE or DVT) and found 3-month all-cause mortality to be 11.0%, significantly higher in patients with COPD/PE (12.5%) than patients with COPD/DVT (8.7%; *P* = .0001).[25] Moreover, patients with COPD who present with PE have an increased risk for PE recurrence.

In 2008, the US Surgeon General published a call to action to prevent DVT and PE and set forth the development of a coordinated strategy to raise awareness about these conditions, to more conscientiously apply evidence-based treatments, and to advance research.[26] The Surgeon General sounded the alarm because many cases of DVT and PE are clinically silent and about 10% of all in-hospital mortality may be related to PE. But the standard of care may have led to poor outcomes. For example, the greatest risk factor for PE is current or previous DVT, because PE often initiates as a clot in the deep veins of the leg. Although there are known risk factors for PE (major surgery, neurosurgery, cancer surgery, and cancer), about half of all PE cases occur in patients without known risk factors. PE is the most common preventable cause of death among hospital in-patients.[27]

More than a century ago, German pathologist Rudolf Virchow correctly identified the three main causes of blood clots: (1) vessel wall injury, (2) hypercoagulation, and (3) stasis.[7] The pre-2008

Table 2
Clinical outcomes after VTE treatment based on the RIETE registry (671 surgical and 1286 medical patients treated for VTE)

	Surgical (%)	Medical Treatment (%)	Odds Ratio, *P* Value
Mortality	6	17	0.36 (0.25–0.51); *P* = .0001
Fatal PE	0.8	3.3	0.22 (0.08–0.58); *P* = .0004
Fatal bleeding	0.2	1.3	0.11 (0.01–0.79); *P* = .0099
Major bleeding	1.5	4.0	0.36 (0.17–0.74); *P* = .002

Data from Monreal M, Kakkar AK, Caprini JA, et al. The outcome after treatment of venous thromboembolism is different in surgical and acutely ill medical patients. Findings from the RIETE registry. J Thromb Haemost 2004;2(11):1892–8.

standard of care may have contributed to PTS in patients with DVT. First of all, damage to the veins and valves is irreversible. Enlarged or distended veins may lead to improper valve closure and regurgitation. These conditions can reduce quality of life, cause pain and edema, and lead to disability. Thus, patients with DVT often developed PTS, a persistent or chronic condition that reduced their physical function.[28]

The American College of Chest Physicians (ACCP) issued its ninth edition of clinical practice guidelines for the prevention and treatment of VTE in 2012.[29] Compared with its 2008 guidelines, the ACCP no longer recognized iliofemoral DVT as a high-risk subset and no longer recommends venous thrombectomy or catheter-directed thrombolysis (CDT) to reduce the incidence of PTS. Overall, the 2012 ACCP guidelines offer little guidance for more aggressive treatment of VTE. In contrast, the American Heart Association issued guidelines calling for CDT in many instances (**Table 3**).[30]

POSTTHROMBOTIC SYNDROME

The most unfortunate long-term sequelae of DVT is PTS, which presents with chronic venous insufficiency and edema, ulceration, claudication, pain, discoloration, and varicose veins. These symptoms can be severe, sometimes necessitating amputation. PTS occurs in more than 10% of all patients with DVT at 1 year with the incidence increasing over time.[22] Patients with VTE are at particularly high risk of venous ulcers, with that risk likewise increasing over time.[31]

Table 3
Comparison of ACCP and AHA guidelines/guidance with respect to treatment of VTE and DVT

	ACCP 2012	AHA 2011
Acute DVT or PE	Initial parenteral anticoagulation (1B) or anticoagulation with rivaroxaban LMWH is preferred over IV UFH (2C) or subcutaneous UFH (2B)	Therapeutic anticoagulation with subcutaneous LMWH, IV or subcutaneous UFH with monitoring (IA); fibrinolysis is reasonable for patients with massive acute PE and acceptable risk for bleeding (IIaB); catheter embolectomy and fragmentation or surgical embolectomy is reasonable for patients with massive PE and contraindications to fibrinolysis (IIaC) or who are unstable after fibrinolysis (IIaC)
Active malignancy	3 mo of anticoagulation therapy (1B) with LMWH preferred over VKA (2B)	Anticoagulation therapy with LMWH for 3–6 mo or as long as cancer is under active treatment
Postthrombotic syndrome prevention	Compression stockings (2B)	Not specifically addressed
Acute iliofemoral DVT	No CDT recommended (in 2008, CDT was recommended)	Therapeutic anticoagulation with IV UFH (IA), UFH subcutaneously (IB), or LMWH (IA) or fondaprinux (IA); compression stockings recommended for at least 2 y (IB); patients with acute proximal DVT or acute PE who are contraindicated for anticoagulation should receive an inferior vena cava filter; CDT or PCDT is appropriate for such patients with limb-threatening circulatory compromise (IC)
Chronic thromboembolic pulmonary hypertension		Pulmonary endartectomy even if symptoms are mild (IC)

ACCP: Grade 1, strong recommendation; Grade 2, weak recommendation; A, high-quality evidence; B, moderate-quality evidence; C, low-quality evidence.

AHA: Class I, benefit >>>> risk; Class IIa, benefit >> risk; Class IIb, benefit $\geq$ risk; Class III, no benefit and/or harm; A, multiple populations evaluated; B, limited populations evaluated; C, very limited populations evaluated.

Abbreviations: ACCP, American College of Chest Physicians; AHA, American Heart Association; DVT, deep vein thrombosis; IV, intravenous; UFH, unfractionated heparin; VTE, venous thromboembolism.

The ACCP recommends in its guidelines the use of compression stockings to prevent PTS. This recommendation is not particularly helpful because of patient compliance issues and clinical outcomes. In a randomized, multicenter, placebo-controlled study of active versus placebo elastic compression stocking for the prevention of PTS in patients with DVT (N = 806), the cumulative incidence of PTS was similar in both groups (14.2% in the active and 12.7% in the placebo groups; $P = .58$).[32]

CHRONIC THROMBOEMBOLIC PULMONARY HYPERTENSION

Chronic thromboembolic pulmonary hypertension was once thought to be a relatively rare complication of PE, but it seems that 3% to 4% of patients with PE develop chronic thromboembolic pulmonary hypertension in 2 years (N = 223).[33] Chronic thromboembolic pulmonary hypertension is associated with substantial morbidity and mortality.

CATHETER-DIRECTED THROMBOLYSIS AND BEYOND

In 2008, CDT was recommended in the ACCP guidelines for management of iliofemoral DVT, but this recommendation was rescinded with the 2012 guidelines.[29] The main benefit of CDT is clot dissolution without valvular damage. The disadvantages associated with CDT are long treatment times and relatively high incidences of bleeding complications. It was likely based on these drawbacks that ACCP chose to withdraw its recommendation of CDT.

Several innovative endovascular treatment options and technologies are now available to help manage VTE. Percutaneous treatment options, such as percutaneous mechanical thrombectomy or pharmacomechanical thrombolysis, offer shorter treatment times and lower bleeding rates, and may be considered a viable alternative to CDT (Trellis; Bachuss Vascular, Santa Clara, CA, USA). The procedure uses mechanical wire maceration thrombolytics with proximal and distal balloon protection; aspiration then

Table 4
Selected new products for CDT and PMT

Product Name	Manufacturer	Technology	Mechanism of Action	Attributes
UniFuse	AngioDynamics	CDT	Drug infusion	Catheter 4–5F 5-, 10-, 20-, 30-, 40-, 50-cm treatment zone 45-, 90-, 135-cm length 0.035 wire
AngioJet	Possis Medical	PMT	Drug infusion with high-pressure fragmentation and aspiration	Catheter 6F Sheath 8F 90- to 1209-cm length 0.035 wire
Trellis	Bacchus Vascular	PMT	Dispersion wire, distal protection, drug infusion, aspiration	Catheter/device 6F 10-, 15-, 30-cm treatment zone Sheath 7F 60 min maximum time 80- to 120-cm length 0.035 wire
Omniwave	Omnisonics	PMT	Dispersion wire and drug infusion	Catheter 7F 8.4-cm treatment zone 10-min delivery time 100-cm length 0.018 wire
EkoSonic Mach 4	EKOS	PMT	Ultrasound and drug infusion	Catheter 5.2F 6-, 12-, 18-, 24-, 30-, 40-, 50-cm treatment zone Sheath 6F 106- to 135-cm length 0.035 guidewire

Note: Product names and manufacturer names may be trademarks or registered trademarks of their owners.
Abbreviations: CDT, catheter-directed thrombolysis; PMT, pharmacomechanical thrombolysis.

Table 5
Selected key studies on DVT therapy

Description	Population	End Points	Results	Comments
Meng et al,[38] 2013	155 patients with lower-extremity DVT	CDT performed; patients with residual stenosis >50% (N = 74) were randomized for stenting	Patency at last follow-up (87.5% vs 29.6%) and at 1 y (86.0% vs 54.8%) were higher in stented than control patients	Stenting of iliac vein after CDT may increase patency of the deep vein
Enden et al,[39] 2012 (CaVenT Study)	209 patients with first-time iliofemoral DVT	Randomized to CDT or no-CDT; all patients got standard medical treatment	At 24 mo, 41.1% of CDT vs 55.5% of control patients had PTS ($P = .047$)	Iliofemoral patency at 6 mo was 65.9% in CDT and 47.4% in control patients ($P = .012$)
Comerota et al,[40] 2012	71 iliofemoral DVT patients treated with CDT	CDT with and without mechanical techniques	Residual thrombus was significantly associated with PTS	It seems that when thrombus clearance is complete, PTS can be prevented
Elsharawy & Elzayat,[41] 2002	35 consecutive iliofemoral DVT patients	Randomized to CDT with anticoagulation or anticoagulation alone	At 6 mo, CDT patients had better patency rates (72% vs 12%; $P<.001$) and less venous reflux (11% vs 41%; $P = .04$) than anticoagulation-only patients	In the short term, CDT patients had significantly better patency than anticoagulation-only patients
Comerota et al,[42] 2000	Survey of ilifemoral DVT patients	Patients had been treated with CDT vs those treated with anticoagulation alone	CDT patients reported significantly better functioning ($P = .046$), less health distress ($P = .022$), and fewer postthrombotic symptoms ($P = .006$)	Successful lysis correlated significantly with health-related quality of life

ATTRACT[43]	Approximately 700 patients with acute proximal DVT	Pharmacomechanical CDT plus standard therapy vs standard therapy alone; primary end point is development of PTS at 2 y	Study is ongoing	Other endpoints include safety, quality of life, pain, and cost effectiveness
Trellis-8 Registry[44]	Retrospective analysis of 19 consecutive above-knee DVT patients	Patients treated with Trellis device (isolated thrombolysis catheter in single session of PMT combined with low-dose thrombolysis with tissue-plasminogen activator	Rapid inline venous flow restored in all cases and thrombus removal was 50%–95% in 82% of cases; mean treatment time was 91 min per limb, primary patency in treated venous segments at 2 d was 86%, and primary assisted patency at 30 d was 100%	No major complications reported, two patients in this study died of advanced malignancy
PEARL I Registry[45]	Prospective observational study of 452 patients with thrombosed hemodialysis ateriovenous grafts and fistulae of whom 72 had thrombosed access sites	Patients were treated with AngoJet for various thrombotic conditions	92% procedural access with significant improvement in vessel occlusion from baseline to final angiography (P<.0001) with 88% of access sites patent by end of procedure	5% mortality rate at 3 mo, no deaths deemed related to the procedure or device
PEARL II Registry[46]	371 DVT patients who had thrombi removed in the periphery using AngioJet rheolytic thrombectomy	Treatment times, effectiveness, stenting rates	Results presented at scientific sessions but not yet published	Could help establish this technology and procedure as outpatient treatment option for DVT

removes fragments. The disadvantages associated with pharmacomechanical thrombolysis are increased catheter laboratory time, a high likelihood of residual thrombus, hemolysis, risk of distal embolism, and risk of valve or vessel wall damage.

Microsonic ultrasound-accelerated CDT lowers the risk of bleeding, shortens lysis time, and may lower drug dosage (AngioJet; Possis Medical, Minneapolis, MN, USA). Microsonic ultrasound-accelerated CDT works with a pulse spray (Bernoulli effect) and is followed by aspiration; it is less likely to damage valves and because it does not break or disrupt the thrombus, it reduces the risk of emboli. Ultrasound-accelerated CDT is also a relatively fast procedure that may require less than a half-hour in the catheter laboratory. The use of ultrasound energy causes fibrin strands to thin and loosen, exposing plasminogen receptor sites. Thrombus permeability and thrombolytic penetration increase, while the ultrasonic waves force the drug deep into the clot.

NEW PRODUCT MATRIX

Several novel technologies have recently come to market for the treatment of DVT (**Table 4**).

PROCEDURE PEARLS

The most important goal of endovascular treatment of DVT is restoration of flow. A case-by-case evaluation is necessary and the weight value of conservative therapy must be considered. Following a complete patient history and physical examination, the physician must determine the severity venous score, review all imaging, and then follow a treatment plan. Once it is decided to perform an endovascular procedure, the anatomic location for endovascular access must be determined.

- Initial site of access should be the ipsilateral popliteal vein, if open. If the ipsilateral popliteal vein is occluded, try the ipsilateral posterotibial, and if occluded, then try the contralateral femoral vein.
- Enoxaparin preprocedure at 1 mg per kg.
- Do ultrasound-guided access with initial 5F catheter sheath and try to cross with a 4F Berenstein catheter and stiff guidewire. If unsuccessful, try to cross with 4F Berenstein catheter; if that does not work, try a Navicross support catheter (Terumo Medical, Somerset, NJ). Another option is a Triforce (Cook Medical Technology, Bloomington, IN) with a 6F catheter support system.
- Once across, do balloon angioplasty of the segment to the appropriate size. An iliac segment usually requires a 12- to 14-mm balloon, femoral an 8- to 10-mm balloon, and popliteal a 6- to 8-mm balloon.
- Once across and dilated with balloon, place the mechanical device for infusion of lytics overnight.
- Once lytics are infused, the next day return to catheter laboratory and consider repeat balloon angioplasty to segment.
- It is recommended that patients be discharged home with enoxaparin, subcutaneous 1 mg/kg twice a day for 1 month, and then changed to oral anticoagulants.

CLINICAL OUTCOMES

CDT can help to remove clots in proximal DVT and may reduce the incidence of PTS.[34] In a study of 92 patients with acute iliofemoral or proximal femoral DVT treated with CDT, successful lysis could be achieved in 90% with a mean clot resolution of 88%; patency at 24 months was 75.3%.[34] Pulse-spray CDT forcefully injects the thrombolytic agent into the thrombus to fragment it and increase its surface area for more extensive enzymatic action. In a study of 44 patients with lower-extremity ischemia, clinically successfully lysis occurred in 81.8% with an amputation rate of 9.1% and no mortality at 12 months.[35] Ultrasound-accelerated CDT was shown to be safe and effective in a study of 12 patients with DVT; 85% had successful thrombolysis and no cases of PE.[36] The DUET study is ongoing in the Netherlands to compare CDT with ultrasound-accelerated CDT for thromboembolic infrainguinal disease.[37] A summary of selected clinical trials for DVT appears in **Table 5**. Note that further study is warranted, in particular comparative studies.

Of great interest to this subject is the ongoing ATTRACT study, evaluating pharmacomechanical CDT in proximal DVT.[43] The role of endovascular therapy remains to be defined; the controversies that exist related to endovascular approaches mainly involve defining the appropriate candidates and timing for such interventions. For instance, most clinicians would agree that endovascular therapy should be considered for any patient with DVT at high risk for a fatal PE. Recurrent DVT, extension of the clot burden, compression by a pelvic tumor, and other conditions also warrant consideration of endovascular intervention. However, clinicians and even specialties are divided as to whether more routine patients with DVT should be treated with endovascular or surgical approaches.

In summary, the goals of endovascular intervention for DVT include the following:

- More rapid lysis via local administration of the drug
- Pain relief
- Decreased edema
- Prevention of PE, recurrent thrombosis, and PTS
- Restoration of vessel patency
- Preservation of proper valve function
- Correction of underlying anatomic lesions

These goals can often be attained with endovascular procedures, even when they are not achieved with conventional anticoagulation therapy alone.

SUMMARY

VTE is a prevalent condition associated with substantial morbidity and mortality that places an enormous clinical, financial, and public health burden on society. Treatment options for VTE exist and novel pharmacologic agents and new technologies are currently being developed. What remains is for the clinical community to better assess these treatment options and define appropriate patient populations and indications. Many endovascular approaches to VTE have been shown to be safe and effective, but their appropriate use is currently the subject of some controversy, even across specialties.

REFERENCES

1. Cohen AT, Tapson VF, Bergmann JF, et al. Venous thromboembolism risk and prophylaxis in the acute hospital care setting (ENDORSE study): a multinational cross-sectional study. Lancet 2008; 371(9610):387–94.
2. Goldhaber SZ, Visani L, De Rosa M. Acute pulmonary embolism: clinical outcomes in the International Cooperative Pulmonary Embolism Registry (ICOPER). Lancet 1999;353(9162):1386–9.
3. Centers for Disease Control and Prevention. Deep vein thrombosis (DVT)/pulmonary embolism (PE) – blood clot forming in a vein. Data and statistics. 2012. Available at: http://www.cdc.gov/ncbddd/dvt/data.html. Accessed May 2, 2014.
4. White RH. The epidemiology of venous thromboembolism. Circulation 2003;107(23 Suppl 1):I4–8.
5. Geerts WH, Pineo GF, Heit JA, et al. Prevention of venous thromboembolism: the Seventh ACCP Conference on Antithrombotic and Thrombolytic Therapy. Chest 2004;126(Suppl 3):338S–400S.
6. Bulger C, Jacobs C, Patel N. Epidemiology of acute deep vein thrombosis. Tech Vasc Interv Radiol 2004;7(2):50–4.
7. Makin A, Silverman SH, Lip GY. Peripheral vascular disease and Virchow's triad for thrombogenesis. QJM 2002;95(4):199–210.
8. Simsek E, Yesilyurt A, Pinarli F, et al. Combined genetic mutations have remarkable effect on deep venous thrombosis and/or pulmonary embolism occurrence. Gene 2014;536(1):171–6.
9. Parikh S, Motarjeme A, McNamara T, et al. Ultrasound-accelerated thrombolysis for the treatment of deep vein thrombosis: initial clinical experience. J Vasc Interv Radiol 2008;19(4):521–8.
10. Agnelli G, Becattini C. Treatment of DVT: how long is enough and how do you predict recurrence. J Thromb Thrombolysis 2008;25(1):37–44.
11. De Caterina R, Husted S, Wallentin L, et al. General mechanisms of coagulation and targets of anticoagulants (Section I). Position paper of the ESC working group on thrombosis–task force on anticoagulants in heart disease. Thromb Haemost 2013; 109(4):569–79.
12. Dobesh PP. Economic burden of venous thromboembolism in hospitalized patients. Pharmacotherapy 2009;29(8):943–53.
13. Lozano Sanchez FS, Sanchez Nevarez I, Gonzalez-Porras JR, et al. Quality of life in patients with chronic venous disease: influence of the sociodemographical and clinical factors. Int Angiol 2013;32(4):433–41.
14. Darius H. New direct oral anticoagulants (DOACs): indications of DOACs. Anasthesiol Intensivmed Notfallmed Schmerzther 2014;49(3):182–91.
15. Kahn SR, Shrier I, Julian JA, et al. Determinants and time course of the postthrombotic syndrome after acute deep venous thrombosis. Ann Intern Med 2008;149(10):698–707.
16. Oden A, Fahlen M, Hart RG. Optimal INR for prevention of stroke and death in atrial fibrillation: a critical appraisal. Thromb Res 2006; 117(5):493–9.
17. Gallagher AM, Setakis E, Plumb JM, et al. Risks of stroke and mortality associated with suboptimal anticoagulation in atrial fibrillation patients. Thromb Haemost 2011;106(5):968–77.
18. Hutten BA, Prins MH. Duration of treatment with vitamin K antagonists in symptomatic venous thromboembolism. Cochrane Database Syst Rev 2006;(1):CD001367.
19. Schulman S, Kearon C, Kakkar AK, et al. Dabigatran versus warfarin in the treatment of acute venous thromboembolism. N Engl J Med 2009; 361(24):2342–52.
20. Schulman S, Kearon C, Kakkar AK, et al. Extended use of dabigatran, warfarin, or placebo in venous thromboembolism. N Engl J Med 2013;368(8): 709–18.
21. EINSTEIN Investigators, Bauersachs R, Berkowitz SD, et al. Oral rivaroxaban for symptomatic venous

thromboembolism. N Engl J Med 2010;363(26):2499–510.
22. Prandoni P, Lensing AW, Cogo A, et al. The long-term clinical course of acute deep venous thrombosis. Ann Intern Med 1996;125(1):1–7.
23. Kearon C. Natural history of venous thromboembolism. Circulation 2003;107(23 Suppl 1):I22–30.
24. Monreal M, Kakkar AK, Caprini JA, et al. The outcome after treatment of venous thromboembolism is different in surgical and acutely ill medical patients. Findings from the RIETE registry. J Thromb Haemost 2004;2(11):1892–8.
25. Bertoletti L, Quenet S, Laporte S, et al. Pulmonary embolism and 3-month outcomes in 4036 patients with venous thromboembolism and chronic obstructive pulmonary disease: data from the RIETE registry. Respir Res 2013;14:75.
26. Office of the Surgeon General (US), National Heart, Lung, and Blood Institute (US). The Surgeon General's call to action to prevent deep vein thrombosis and pulmonary embolism. Rockville (MD): Office of the Surgeon General (US); 2008. Available at: http://www.ncbi.nlm.nih.gov/books/NBK44178/.
27. Dentali F, Douketis JD, Gianni M, et al. Meta-analysis: anticoagulant prophylaxis to prevent symptomatic venous thromboembolism in hospitalized medical patients. Ann Intern Med 2007;146(4):278–88.
28. Kahn SR, Ginsberg JS. Relationship between deep venous thrombosis and the postthrombotic syndrome. Arch Intern Med 2004;164(1):17–26.
29. Kearon C, Akl EA, Comerota AJ, et al. Antithrombotic therapy for VTE disease: antithrombotic therapy and prevention of thrombosis, 9th ed: American College of Chest Physicians evidence-based clinical practice guidelines. Chest 2012;141(Suppl 2):e419S–94S.
30. Jaff MR, McMurtry MS, Archer SL, et al. Management of massive and submassive pulmonary embolism, iliofemoral deep vein thrombosis, and chronic thromboembolic pulmonary hypertension: a scientific statement from the American Heart Association. Circulation 2011;123(16):1788–830.
31. Schulman S, Lindmarker P, Holmstrom M, et al. Post-thrombotic syndrome, recurrence, and death 10 years after the first episode of venous thromboembolism treated with warfarin for 6 weeks or 6 months. J Thromb Haemost 2006;4(4):734–42.
32. Kahn SR, Shapiro S, Wells PS, et al. Compression stockings to prevent post-thrombotic syndrome: a randomised placebo-controlled trial. Lancet 2014;383(9920):880–8.
33. Pengo V, Lensing AW, Prins MH, et al. Incidence of chronic thromboembolic pulmonary hypertension after pulmonary embolism. N Engl J Med 2004;350(22):2257–64.
34. Haig Y, Enden T, Slagsvold CE, et al. Determinants of early and long-term efficacy of catheter-directed thrombolysis in proximal deep vein thrombosis. J Vasc Interv Radiol 2013;24(1):17–24 [quiz: 26].
35. Chen YX, Liu CW, Zeng R, et al. Pulse-spray catheter directed thrombolysis in patients with recent onset or deterioration of lower extremity ischemia. Chin Med J 2012;125(2):188–92.
36. Grommes J, Strijkers R, Greiner A, et al. Safety and feasibility of ultrasound-accelerated catheter-directed thrombolysis in deep vein thrombosis. Eur J Vasc Endovasc Surg 2011;41(4):526–32.
37. Schrijver AM, Reijnen MM, van Oostayen JA, et al. Dutch randomized trial comparing standard catheter-directed thrombolysis versus ultrasound-accelerated thrombolysis for thromboembolic infrainguinal disease (DUET): design and rationale. Trials 2011;12:20.
38. Meng QY, Li XQ, Jiang K, et al. Stenting of iliac vein obstruction following catheter-directed thrombolysis in lower extremity deep vein thrombosis. Chin Med J 2013;126(18):3519–22.
39. Enden T, Haig Y, Klow NE, et al. Long-term outcome after additional catheter-directed thrombolysis versus standard treatment for acute iliofemoral deep vein thrombosis (the CaVenT study): a randomised controlled trial. Lancet 2012;379(9810):31–8.
40. Comerota AJ, Grewal N, Martinez JT, et al. Post-thrombotic morbidity correlates with residual thrombus following catheter-directed thrombolysis for iliofemoral deep vein thrombosis. J Vasc Surg 2012;55(3):768–73.
41. Elsharawy M, Elzayat E. Early results of thrombolysis vs anticoagulation in iliofemoral venous thrombosis. A randomised clinical trial. Eur J Vasc Endovasc Surg 2002;24(3):209–14.
42. Comerota AJ, Throm RC, Mathias SD, et al. Catheter-directed thrombolysis for iliofemoral deep venous thrombosis improves health-related quality of life. J Vasc Surg 2000;32(1):130–7.
43. Vedantham S, Goldhaber SZ, Kahn SR, et al. Rationale and design of the ATTRACT Study: a multicenter randomized trial to evaluate pharmacomechanical catheter-directed thrombolysis for the prevention of postthrombotic syndrome in patients with proximal deep vein thrombosis. Am Heart J 2013;165(4):523–30.e3.
44. O'Sullivan GJ, Lohan DG, Gough N, et al. Pharmacomechanical thrombectomy of acute deep vein thrombosis with the Trellis-8 isolated thrombolysis catheter. J Vasc Interv Radiol 2007;18(6):715–24.
45. Simoni E, Blitz L, Lookstein R. Outcomes of AngioJet(R) thrombectomy in hemodialysis vascular access grafts and fistulas: PEARL I Registry. J Vasc Access 2013;14(1):72–6.
46. Endovascular Today. PEARL registry's phase II results presented at ISET. 2013. Available at:

http://evtoday.com/2013/01/pearl-registrys-phase-ii-results-presented-at-iset. Accessed May 4, 2014.
47. Rosamond W, Flegal K, Friday G, et al. Heart disease and stroke statistics–2007 update: a report from the American Heart Association Statistics Committee and Stroke Statistics Subcommittee. Circulation 2007;115(5):e69–171.
48. Arcasoy SM, Kreit JW. Thrombolytic therapy of pulmonary embolism: a comprehensive review of current evidence. Chest 1999;115(6):1695–707.
49. Society of Interventional Radiology. Fact sheet. Fairfax (VA): Society of Interventional Radiology. Available at: http://www.sirweb.org/news/factSheet.shtml. Accessed July 2, 2014.
50. Recombinant plasmin from lemna minor - purification, characterization and in vitro comparison to human-plasma derived plasmin. Presented at 51st Annual Congress of the German Society of Thrombosis and Haemostasis Research. Dresden (Germany), February 21–24, 2007.

Index

Note: Page numbers of article titles are in **boldface** type.

Intervent Cardiol Clin 3 (2014) 619–625
http://dx.doi.org/10.1016/S2211-7458(14)00080-7
2211-7458/14/$ – see front matter

Q

R

S

W

X

Z

Printed and bound by CPI Group (UK) Ltd, Croydon, CR0 4YY
03/10/2024
01040379-0013